AF567037

ORTHOPAEDIC ANAESTHESIA

ORTHOPAEDIC ANAESTHESIA

Second Edition

Edited by
Alan Loach
MA, MB, BChir FRCA DA
Consultant, Nuffield Department of Anaesthetics
Consultant Anaesthetist, Nuffield Orthopaedic Centre
Honorary Clinical lecturer, University of Oxford, Oxford, UK

Edward Arnold
A member of the Hodder Headline Group
LONDON BOSTON MELBOURNE AUCKLAND

First published in Great Britain 1983 as
Anaesthesia for Orthopaedic Patients
Second Edition 1994

Distributed in the Americas by Little, Brown and Company
34 Beacon Street, Boston, MA 02108

British Library Cataloguing in Publication Data

Loach, Alan
Orthopaedic Anaesthesia. – 2Rev.ed
I. Title
617.9673

ISBN 0-340-56438-5

Whilst the advice and information in this book is believed to be true and accurate at the date of going to press, neither the author nor the publisher can accept any legal responsibility or liability for any errors or omissions that may be made. In particular (but without limiting the generality of the preceding disclaimer) every effort has been made to check drug dosages; however, it is still possible that errors have been missed. Furthermore, dosage schedules are constantly being revised and new side effects recognised. For these reasons the reader is strongly urged to consult the manufacturer's printed instructions before administering any of the drugs recommended in this book.

Typeset in 10/11pt Century Old Style by Rowland Phototypesetting Limited, Bury St Edmunds, Suffolk.
Printed and bound in Great Britain for Edward Arnold, a division of Hodder Headline PLC, Mill Road, Dunton Green, Sevenoaks, Kent TN13 2YA by Butler and Tanner Limited, Frome and London.

Contents

List of contributors

Neil Schofield, MA MB BChir FRCA
Consultant, Nuffield Department of Anaesthetics
Honorary Clinical Lecturer, University of Oxford

Peter J McKenzie, MD FRCA
Consultant Anaesthetist, Nuffield Department of Anaesthetics, Oxford

John Stevens, MB BS FRCA
Director, Paediatric Intensive Care Unit, John Radcliffe Hospital
Honorary Clinical Lecturer, University of Oxford

Jennifer Goy, MB BS FRCA
Consultant Anaesthetist, Stoke Mandeville Hospital

Part I

Elective Surgery

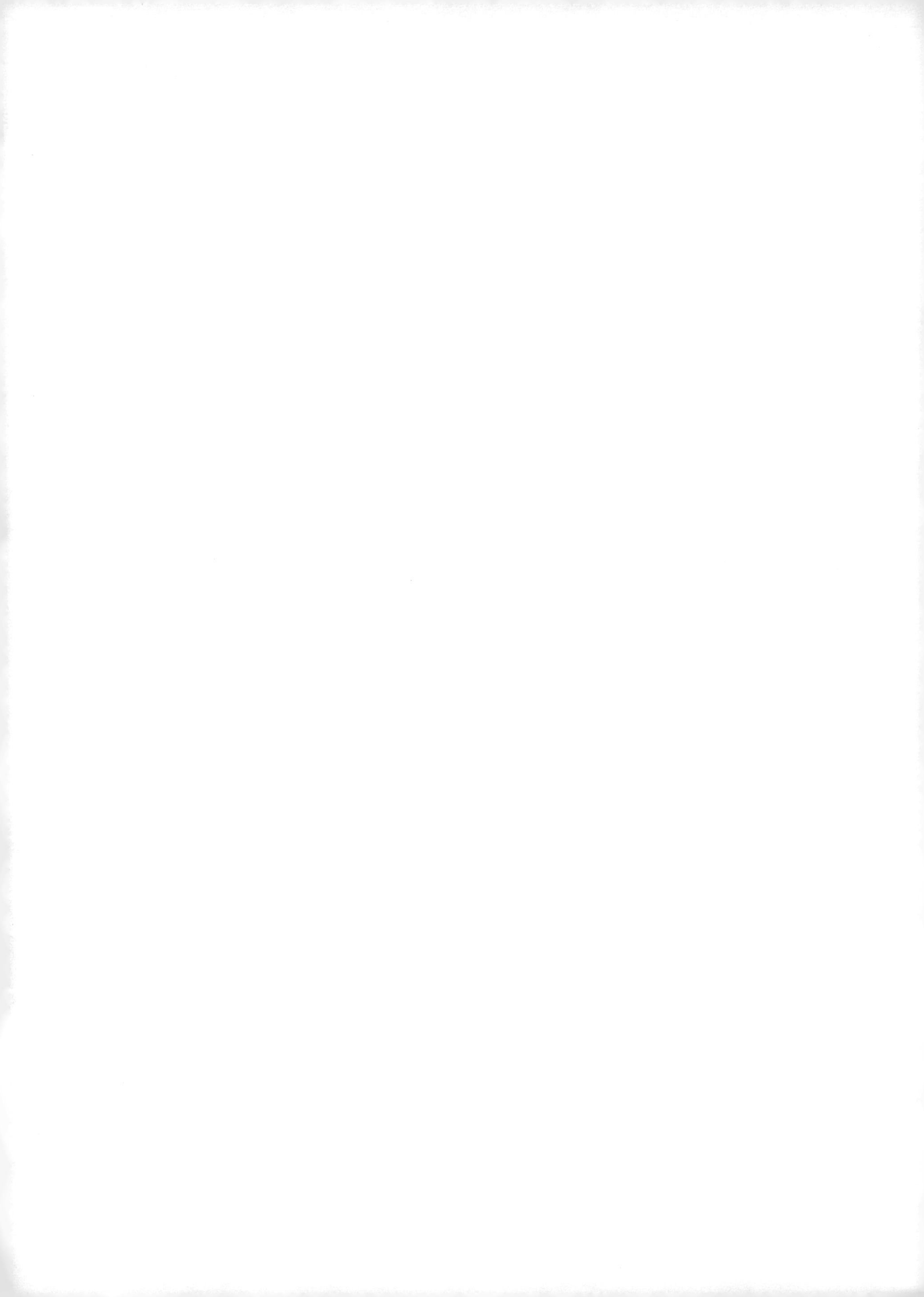

Chapter 1

Introduction

For I am so plagued in on[e] of my hippes that I am neither able to indevor to ride nor sitt on[e] hour.

Lord Sheffield to the Earl of Salisbury, explaining his failure to appear in Parliament, 1610

The development of orthopaedic surgery

Lord Sheffield was only 45 when he made the statement above complaining of pain in his hip joints. For elderly people the commonest reason for consulting a general practitioner is osteoarthritis and the proportion of onward referrals rises with age. Total hip replacement is now the commonest joint operation in the United Kingdom with over 50 000 procedures being performed each year. The surgical treatment of arthritis has stimulated the development of modern orthopaedic surgery and has been so successful that failure to provide adequate resources for this surgery has provoked political crises.

Before 1960 the work of an orthopaedic unit consisted chiefly of the management of infections of bone and joints, the treatment of fractures and trauma, the rehabilitation of patients disabled by paralytic poliomyelitis and the surgery of neoplasms of bone. Although by then in decline, tuberculosis of bone was still common. Thus most patients were adolescent to middle-aged and the duration of hospital admission was measured in weeks or months. Hospital schools were established to maintain the education of children who were admitted. However, whilst many patients were still treated with wedged plasters and braces, operative orthopaedic surgery was increasing, encouraged by the experience gained during the Second World War and the growing availability of effective antibacterial agents. The pattern of work now is quite different. Since 1985 an average of only 3 cases of paralytic poliomyelitis has been reported each year in England and Wales, and the number is falling: poliomyelitis should be eradicated by the end of the century. The surgery of tuberculosis and infections of bone has dwindled as systemic infection is treated more effectively at the outset, and the emphasis in orthopaedic surgery has thus shifted to reconstructive surgery in patients of all ages. The mean duration of hospital admission is now 11 days.

In the very young, operative procedures are increasingly being used to correct congenital malformations and to minimize the duration of hospital admission: direct repair is favoured over splinting. In adults, orthopaedic surgery is directed towards the repair of injuries sustained on the road, on the sports field, or at work. However, the most dramatic change in orthopaedic practice has been the development of reliable, efficient, joint prostheses which offer the prospect of pain-free mobility to all those crippled with osteoarthritis. As experience of the implanted prostheses accumulates, so, progressively, joint replacement is being offered to younger patients whose joints have been destroyed by a variety of pathological processes – inflammatory arthritis, renal disease, haemophilia and injury. However, although the age range of patients has widened, it is among the elderly that the greatest increase in numbers has occurred. Many of these patients have their own burden of chronic disease and have sometimes already undergone other reconstructive procedures in the past; heart valve replacement, renal transplantation and coronary artery grafts. Increasingly, the trend is to regard the elderly as an extension of the middle-aged when treatment is planned rather than a separate group of patients. Many who were previously considered unsuitable for surgery are now scheduled for major procedures. Although the provision of operations has risen steadily – by 30 per cent in the decade from 1976 (Seagroatt *et al.*, 1991) – there remains a very large unfilled need. One-fifth of the population is now aged 65 or over – the age group which consumes two-thirds of all joint replacements and this proportion is increasing.

In 1981 there were 500 000 people aged 85 or more in Britain and this figure will have doubled by 2006. The incidence of most diseases increases with age whilst that of fractured neck of femur increases exponentially with age.

Orthopaedic work in the future will have to cope with the explosion in demand for joint replacement whilst also managing the complications. Much operating time is likely to be spent revising previous operations as the large population of patients who have already received a prosthetic joint return when it eventually fails or works loose. In addition to hip and knee joints further prostheses for all the other limb joints are already in use or under development.

Introduction to anaesthesia for orthopaedic surgery

Before considering the general management of anaesthesia for orthopaedic surgery, it is worth discussing two major background problems which concern surgeon and anaesthetist alike. Venous thromboembolism and deep-seated infection are the major factors, respectively, in operative mortality and morbidity in orthopaedic surgery.

Deep vein thrombosis and pulmonary embolism

Deep venous thrombosis and its sequel, pulmonary embolism are major problems in orthopaedic surgery. Many orthopaedic patients are immobilized postoperatively; surgery is often extensive provoking maximal hormonal changes in response; and many patients are elderly with concurrent disease such as cardiovascular disease, treated malignancy or lung infections. Some patients smoke and others are obese from enforced inactivity. All these factors increase the risk. Preceding trauma is a further hazard, possibly because surgery then takes place with the hormonal response to stress already well established. Thus, deep vein thrombosis and pulmonary embolism are both more likely after surgery for a fractured hip than after elective hip surgery.

There are further risks in a population of elderly patients: they take longer to recover from an operation and more readily develop complications. Thus in a survey of 11 607 total hip replacements Seagroatt *et al.* (1991) found that postoperative case fatality rates and emergency re-admission rates increased with age. Deaths were due principally to cardiovascular causes and thromboembolism whilst the major cause of emergency readmission was thromboembolism. This survey differs from most surgical reports by including all deaths up to 90 days postoperatively and not restricting the report to the period of hospital admission.

After orthopaedic surgery immobility may be forced by extensive plasters or traction. After 3 week's immobility, the incidence of deep venous thrombosis has reached 90 per cent (Morris and Mitchell, 1977).

Without anticoagulant prophylaxis, deep vein thrombosis and fatal pulmonary embolism occur in 40–70 per cent and 1–5 per cent of patients respectively (Salzman and Hirsch, 1987). In particular, proximal thrombosis of the femoral vein occurs frequently with surgery of the hip although seldom seen elsewhere (Stamatakis, 1978). The thrombosis may be caused by stasis in the femoral vein during surgery, heat generated by the orthopaedic cement or by kinking of the femoral vessels as demonstrated by Planes *et al.* (1990) (Fig. 1.1, 1.2). A slightly smaller incidence of venous thrombosis (60–70 per cent) is found after major knee surgery or tibial osteotomy, and the deep veins of the calf are then more commonly involved.

Prevention of deep vein thrombosis

Venous thrombosis occurring with previous surgery is associated with an increased risk of further thrombosis and Johnson *et al.* (1977) advised that as long an interval as possible should be left between successive operations.

Oestrogen containing oral contraceptives induce a mildly hypercoagulable state; they should be stopped before elective surgery. Bonnar (1987) found an in-

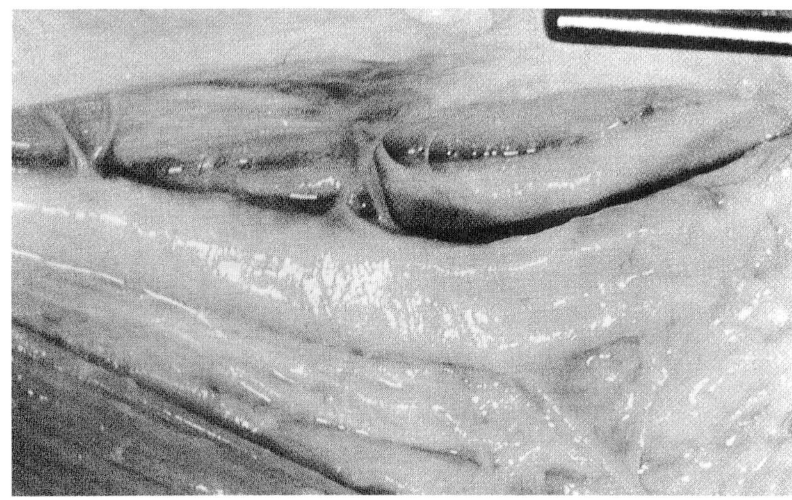

Fig 1.1 The femoral vessels at dissection, with the leg straight. Reproduced from Planes *et al.* (1990), with permission.

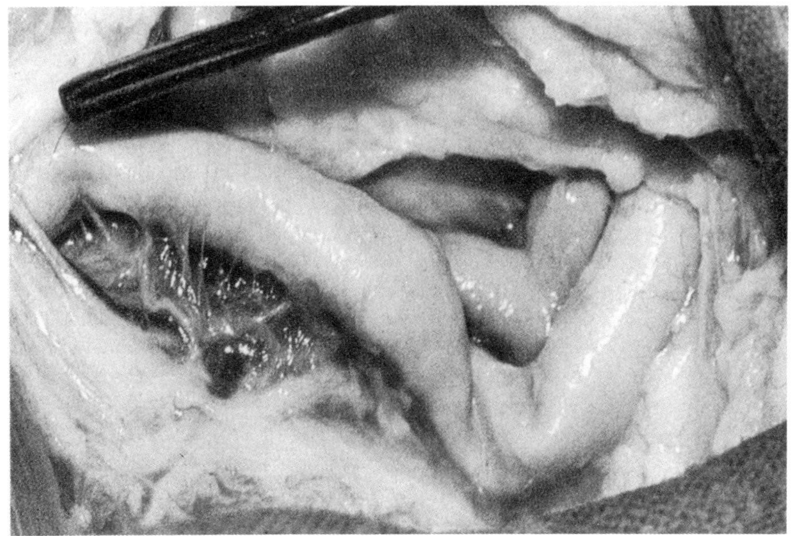

Fig 1.2 The femoral vessels at dissection, with the hip flexed and adducted as during hip replacement. Reproduced from Planes *et al.* (1990), with permission.

crease in plasma fibrinogen and factors II, VII, IX and XII together with an associated decrease in antithrombin III concentration in patients taking oral contraceptives. After stopping the pill there is a rebound phenomenon with antithrombin III increasing and fibrinogen decreasing before normal levels are restored by 8 weeks (Robinson *et al.*, 1991). Patients who are taking an oestrogen containing oral contraceptive should be advised to discontinue at least 4 weeks before surgery and to use an alternative form of contraception unless they will be ambulant within 24 hours and are not having surgery to the legs. For hormone replacement therapy the position is less clear but unless the drugs are essential to control disturbing climacteric symptoms there is little reason not to discontinue them prior to surgery as for oral contraceptives.

Active measures should be taken to avoid venous thromboembolism; a suitable regimen of pharmacological prophylaxis should be followed; a choice of anaesthetic technique made with regard to maintenance of leg blood flow (Chapter 3) and care should be taken when positioning patients to ensure that calf veins have free drainage: graduated compression should be applied to the calves using correctly fitting graduated compression stockings (TED stockings the Kendal company Ltd). In addition, specific prophylaxis should be considered for any patient who is to be immobilized after surgery and it is mandatory for all who have hip surgery.

Pharmacological prophylaxis

Oral anticoagulants

Oral anticoagulants in a variety of dosage regimens have been the mainstay of thromboembolism prophylaxis. To avoid increased surgical bleeding, oral anticoagulants are usually begun 24–48 hours after surgery when the risk of thrombosis is already diminishing: some surgeons are prepared to accept a two-step scheme of dosage which uses a low dosage preoperatively as a compromise before increasing dosage postoperatively to the full therapeutic range (Parker-Williams and Vickers, 1991). Whatever regimen is chosen however, these drugs require regular laboratory monitoring of effect and careful adjustment of dosage if potentially dangerous pathological bleeding is to be avoided. This close control is especially difficult to maintain over weekends and public holidays but even with perfect control, sudden severe bleeding from intestinal erosions of analgesic gastropathy may still occur.

Many agents which reduce platelet aggregation: aspirin, sulphinpyrazone, vitamin E, pyridoxine have been used for thromboprophylaxis but studies of their efficacy have produced conflicting results and no clear benefit for orthopaedic patients.

Heparin regimens

Unfractionated heparin is ineffective for thromboprophylaxis after total hip replacement although results can be improved if a venoconstrictor, dihydroergotamine, is added (Kakkar *et al.*, 1979). However, frequent administration is necessary due to its short half-life and many patients complain of pain at the injection site: heparin also interferes with platelet function increasing the haemorrhagic risk. Low molecular weight heparin is free of many of these disadvantages. It is a fractionated compound with higher bio-availability and a longer half-life so that only a single daily injection is needed. It has less effect on platelet function and a specific antifactor Xa activity. However, the study by Leyvraz *et al.* (1991) found no decisive advantage for low molecular weight heparin when compared with unfractionated heparin during hip replacement. More studies are needed to assess the place, if any, of low molecular weight heparin and of newer compounds such as Hirudin.

Dextran

Dextran as the 70 000 molecular weight form given in a volume of at least 500 ml during surgery and then daily for 2–5 days, offers effective prophylaxis at the period of high risk but its use is associated with increased bleeding during surgery and a greater likelihood of wound haematoma formation. In the elderly there is the additional possibility of circulatory overload. Dextran must therefore be given with care, monitoring the central venous pressure if there is any cause for concern. However, dextran infusion is an alternative to oral anticoagulants and may be used to give additional early prophylaxis in patients who are particularly at risk.

Physical methods of prophylaxis

Simple physical methods such as raising the legs and exercising the legs have given disappointing results except in patients over 60 years of age (Flanc *et al.*, 1969). Elastic compression stockings are similarly unrewarding unless they fit accurately and apply graduated compression (Lawrence and Kakkar, 1980). External pneumatic compression applied by devices which intermittently compress the calves is highly effective in most forms of surgery provided that it is continued for 24 hours or more. It has also been shown to prevent venous thrombosis after total knee replacement (McKenna *et al.*, 1980) but appears to be ineffective when used in patients undergoing hip surgery (Hirsch, 1981). This is puzzling since, although little direct effect upon femoral vein blood flow would be expected, external pneumatic compression has been shown to stimulate fibrinolysis (Allenby *et al.*, 1973) and to be effective in preventing deep vein thrombosis in the legs even when applied to the arms during and after operation (Knight and Dawson, 1976). The original compressive devices were cumbersome but the newer devices are more compact and more comfortable for patients to wear.

Despite the wide choice of treatments which diminish the risk of postoperative thromboembolism, a poll by Morris (1980) investigating the use of prophylaxis by general and orthopaedic surgeons gave surprising results: their use was inversely related to risk! Thus, 38 per cent of surgeons used prophylaxis routinely for hip fractures, 52 per cent for hip replacement and 62 per cent for major abdominal and thoracic operations. A similar percentage of use of prophylaxis was found by Brenkel and Clancy (1989) but the survey by Laverick *et al.* (1991) found that 83 per cent of surgeons used thromboprophylaxis after hip surgery.

Infection

The consequences of infection of bone or implanted prosthesis are little short of disastrous for the patient – years of pain, multiple surgical procedures and ultimately an inferior functional result – so every effort must be made to minimize the possibility of wound contamination. It is no exaggeration to say that the principal history of orthopaedic surgery has been the eradication of infection of bone – initially endogenous and latterly exogenous, due to surgery. The growing emphasis on joint replacement has intensified the drive towards lower operative infection rates: critical examination of operating theatre design led to the development of the clean-air enclosure (Charnley, 1972) (Fig. 1.3).

Details of design of enclosure vary, but in essence it consists of a working area within the operating theatre enclosed by glass panels on three sides and at the entrance by hangings which are draped and clipped around the patients (Fig. 1.4).

Within the enclosure a powerful vertical laminar downdraught from an air conditioning and filtration plant mounted in the roof delivers air at 30 m per minute, filtered to 3 μm with 400 air changes per hour. Those within the enclosure wear helmets and coverall gowns and their expired air is ducted away by body exhaust systems (Fig. 1.5).

Space within the enclosure is strictly limited and when bulky equipment is in use (e.g. *X*-ray screening equipment) or extra surgical assistants are required the area becomes congested. Enclosures have therefore been modified by reducing the side walls to permit greater ground level access and later enclosures are larger (Fig. 1.6).

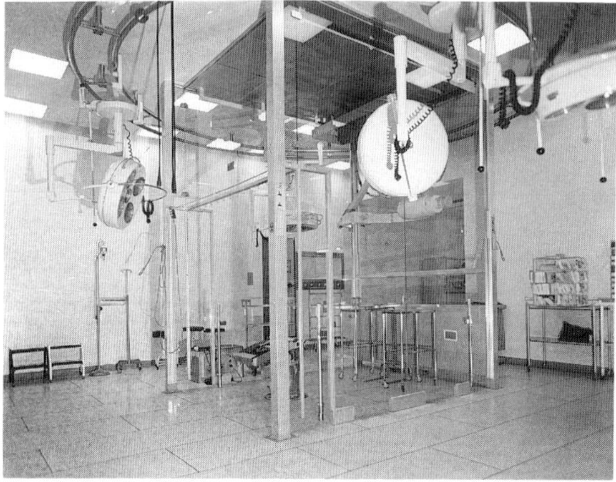

Fig 1.3 The clean air enclosure; the entrance is on the left.

Preliminary skin preparation and draping of the operation site are carried out in the anaesthetic room before the patient is wheeled into the enclosure where further skin preparation takes place. Use of the enclosure thus adds up to 30 minutes to operating time per case.

Preliminary reports suggesting that wound sepsis may be diminished by the clean-air enclosure were reinforced by a Medical Research Council multicentre trial (Lidwell *et al.*, 1982); this reported an

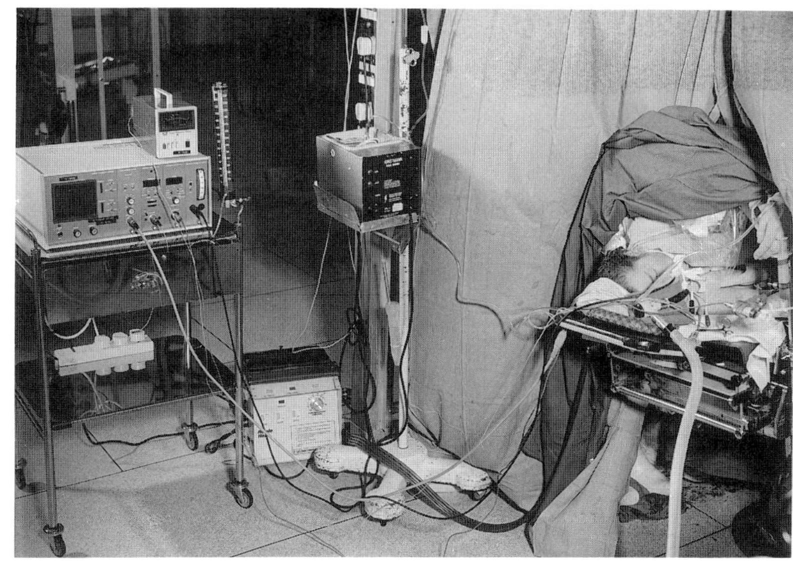

Fig 1.4 The clean air enclosure; the patient is now inside the enclosure, which is closed to the anaesthetist by hangings draped around the patient's neck.

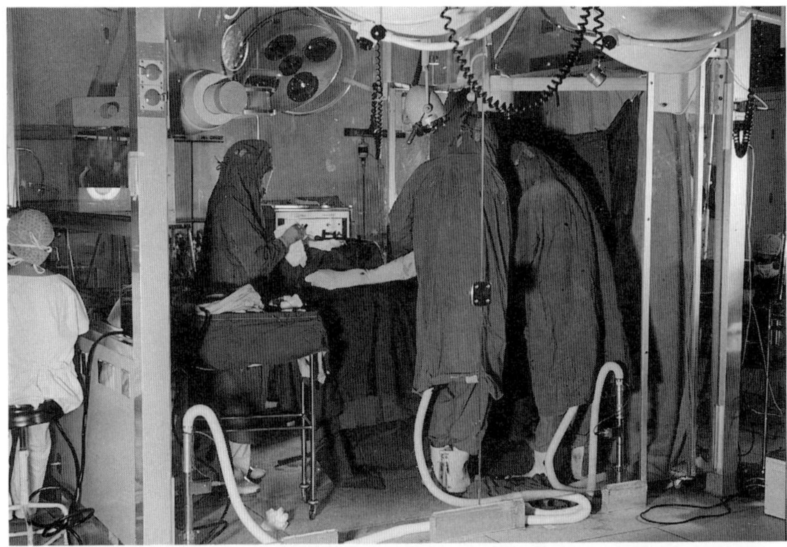

Fig 1.5 The clean air enclosure; only the patient and surgical team enter the enclosure. Instruments are passed in by the nurses (left) and the anaesthetist is excluded by drapes (right).

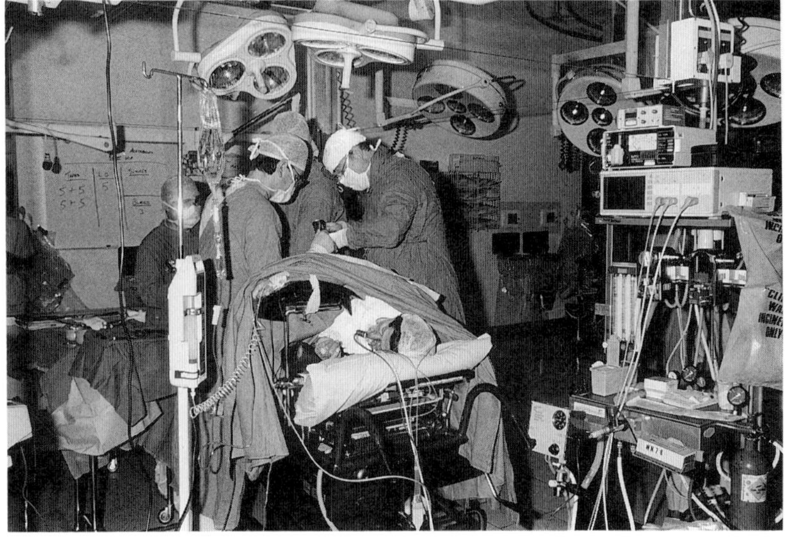

Fig 1.6 Modified clean air enclosure; the glass side walls now only extend part way down from the roof and serve to direct the down draught of clean air. Access is much improved.

overall incidence of sepsis for cases operated on in the clean-air enclosure with surgeons wearing exhaust ventilated suits, reduced to about a quarter of that found after operations performed in conventional theatres.

Sanderson and Bentley (1976) compared wound contamination in a conventional theatre with that in a Charnley enclosure – with both theatres situated in the same building and built contemporaneously – and found significant reduction both in bacterial sedimentation rate and in wound contamination in the Charnley enclosure. No actual wound infection occurred in any of the 42 patients studied. Since these studies were published, antibacterial prophylaxis has become widespread, so that the once clear, advantages of the clean-air enclosure have become eroded: few new ones are being built. However, four new Charnley type enclosures of advanced design enclosed in a 'high-tech barn' were commissioned in 1992 at the Robert-Jones and Agnes Hunt Orthopaedic Hospital at Oswestry and features of the design are likely to be incorporated in future operating theatres.

The clean-air enclosure is particularly suitable for surgery to patients who are hepatitis B or HIV positive, since all contaminated material is enclosed within a restricted space and may be disposed of with minimal risk.

There are two major difficulties for anaesthetists in this environment; little of the patient is immediately visible or accessible to the anaesthetist; and the cooling effect of the air flow upon the exposed patient is appreciable. Because little of the patient is visible and the surgeons are all screened off, surgical progress and blood loss are difficult to assess and great care must be taken to arrange adequate patient monitoring. Equally, little of the patient is accessible once in the enclosure, so all necessary infusions and monitoring must be installed before the patient is wheeled into the enclosure: it is best to devise a routine of preparation in the anaesthetic room so that no essential item (e.g. the indifferent plate of the diathermy!) is forgotten.

The dangers to patients of hypothermia in the operating theatre brought on by bodily exposure, suppressed shivering and the need to humidify dry gases breathed are already appreciated, particularly with regard to the very young and the very old. In the clean-air enclosure these problems are magnified by the chill factor of the air flow which is 10 times that of a conventional theatre. Every means available should therefore be used to maintain the patient's body temperature; heat conserving drapes of polythene or better, aluminized plastic, should be used and all fluids for infusion should be warmed, whilst the anaesthetic room should be kept as warm as is tolerable to minimize falls in temperature during induction.

After surgery, the recovery room beds should be warmed before the patients are transferred into them and aluminized space blankets should be used on the beds until body temperature is normal. All patients should receive oxygen by face mask for the first few hours postoperatively so that hypoxaemia during shivering is minimized and the recovery room staff should continue to record body temperature hourly until it is normal.

General management of orthopaedic anaesthesia

The importance of preoperative assessment

Whilst many orthopaedic patients are young and fit, a very large proportion are elderly or debilitated by chronic disease. Most orthopaedic procedures in these patients are elective in the sense that the operation is not intended to treat systemic illness, but rather to improve the quality of life. They are further elective in the sense that alternative lesser treatments may exist if the health of the patient precludes a major operation. Orthopaedic surgery contributes the majority of elective procedures carried out in the elderly and adequate preoperative assessment and careful selection of patients are of the greatest importance in achieving good results.

In many units preoperative assessment clinics have been established in order that patients recognized at surgical outpatients to pose difficulties for anaesthesia may be seen and assessed well before the pressure of an impending operation, and any necessary treatment carried out. For most patients, however, immediate preoperative assessment by an anaesthetist is all that is necessary. This is made easier when all patients are admitted to an admissions ward where a medical history is taken and they undergo a general examination before being prepared for theatre; preoperative ward rounds are simplified because the patients are grouped together. An experienced ward sister is often able to pick up details of a patient's medical history which have escaped the medical staff simply because she is with the patient longer: any particular worries or fears which patients are reluctant to explain to a doctor may be confided to her. It is also easier in these circumstances to establish a routine of preoperative work-up so that patients are fully investigated in advance of the anaesthetist's visit and less time is wasted waiting for results. Preoperative assessment is considered in detail in Chapter 2.

Repeat anaesthetics

Many orthopaedic patients undergo a series of anaesthetics, first for the initial procedure and then for subsequent manipulations or changes of plaster. It is essential that details of each anaesthetic are recorded in the patient's case notes so that repeated exposure to any inhalation agent may be avoided.

Positioning of patients on the operating table

Patients must be positioned carefully and securely on the operating table because considerable forces of traction and leverage are often deployed by the operating team. Patients must be fixed so that movement is minimal and they should be padded at every contact point in order that, particularly in the elderly, skin damage and contre-coup injuries will not be caused by table restraints. A plentiful supply of foam rubber pieces, Gamgee and elasticated bandages is essential as the restraints and supports supplied with proprietary operating tables seem crude and always require additional padding. For longer procedures the patient's feet should each be wrapped in a piece of foam rubber (Fig. 1.7) and bandaged to prevent skin damage at points of contact with the table, particularly the heels; further padding should be placed between the legs to prevent compression of the calves if a full or semilateral position is required.

The patient's head should rest upon a foam rubber ring and the neck should be supported by a piece of foam rubber (Fig. 1.8).

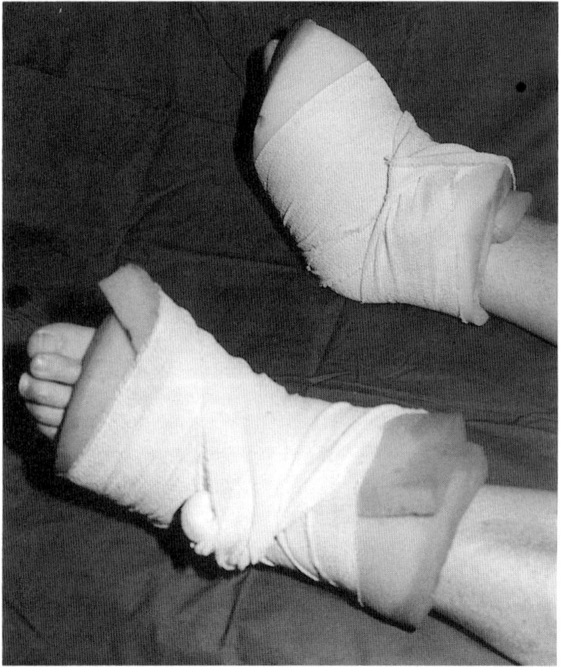

Fig 1.7 The patient's feet should be wrapped in foam rubber before lengthy surgery or if the patient is unusually frail.

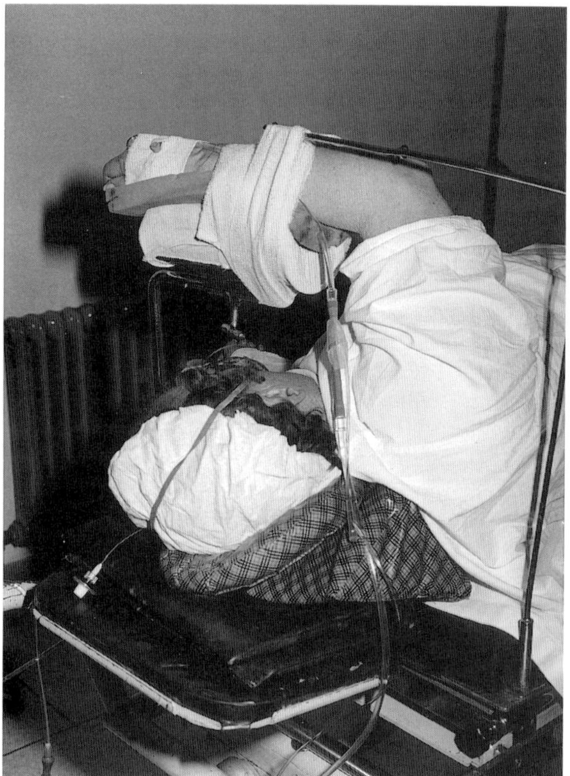

Fig 1.8 The patient's head and neck may be comfortably supported with a foam rubber ring and a triangular foam rubber wedge.

Limb tourniquets

Where possible, orthopaedic surgery is carried out in a bloodless field created by a proximal tourniquet inflated above arterial pressure. This makes identification of small structures easier, allows more precise dissection and is indispensable for finer work on the hand. Microsurgical repair of nerves and vessels becomes extremely difficult if a tourniquet cannot be used, but for surgery of the proximal part of the limb there may not be room to accommodate a tourniquet while remaining outside the surgical field. Careful haemostasis during surgery is necessary and should be maintained postoperatively by the application of a compression dressing to the wound before the tourniquet is released. The tightness of the compression dressing can be a source of considerable pain postoperatively and adequate analgesia must be provided (see Chapter 5). The preferred type of tourniquet is the pneumatic cuff, which has improved markedly over the last few years (Fig. 1.9). Pressure is maintained constant in the cuff by an automatic pressure-maintaining device powered from a cylinder of compressed gas. The pressure is displayed on a manometer and the apparatus also incorporates a simple timing device which sounds an alarm after a preset time interval. The accuracy of the tourniquet manometer should be checked regularly.

An alternative pneumatic tourniquet is operated by a bicycle pump but this apparatus lacks a timer and is small enough to be hidden by bedclothes at the end of surgery and thus accidentally left in position. (The Esmarch rubber bandage should not be used as a tourniquet since there is no indication of the pressure beneath it and it is therefore obsolete for all but exsanguination.)

The cuff should be applied snugly over either the upper thigh close to the groin or a little above the midpoint of the upper arm. In each situation there is ample muscle bulk to cushion arteries and nerves, although for thin subjects the limb should be bound with Gamgee to add further padding. Care should be taken over the application of the tourniquet; if it is applied loosely, it may not expand enough to occlude the artery and there is a risk that it may spring open when inflated; severe bruising of superficial tissues will result if the cuff is pulled tight and the skin puckered beneath it. For surgery of the foot, the cuff is better positioned over the thigh than the calf to prevent direct trauma to deep veins of the calf.

Any antibiotics prescribed prophylactically must be given before the tourniquet is inflated if adequate

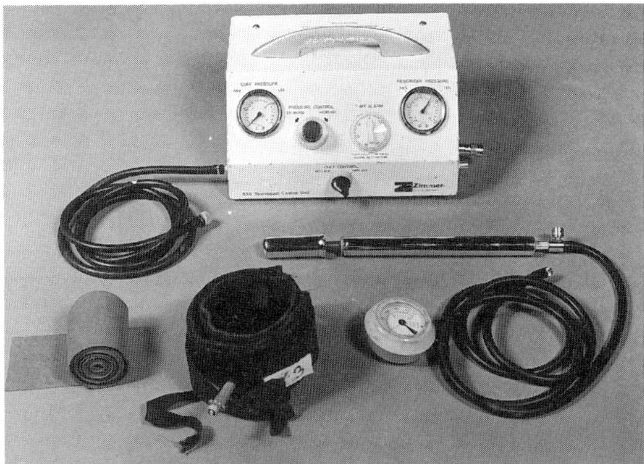

Fig 1.9 Types of tourniquet. At rear, an automatic tourniquet powered by compressed gas and equipped with a manometer and a timer; front, bicycle pump tourniquet with a manometer. Centre, cuff for both types. Left, rubber Esmarch bandage used for exsanguination.

concentrations are to be achieved in the wound during surgery.

When the cuff is in position and before inflation, the limb is exsanguinated by winding on a spiral Esmarch bandage from the periphery to the margin of the cuff, using moderate tension. Limbs should not be exsanguinated in this way when glass or other foreign bodies are embedded or when a neoplasm is present. Exsanguination of the lower limb is also best avoided if a deep vein thrombosis might be present, since pulmonary embolism has been provoked by this manoeuvre (Hoffman and Wyatt, 1985; Wilke, 1992). If the limb contains a cystic swelling, that area should not be exsanguinated because of the likelihood of rupturing the cyst. Simple elevation of the limb with a finger compressing the artery of supply will in most cases provide effective exsanguination.

After exsanguination of the limb the tourniquet cuff is inflated to a pressure 30–50 mmHg higher than systolic arterial pressure for the arm, and 50–70 mmHg higher for the leg where the greater bulk of tissue requires more compression. In children, for whom appropriately smaller cuffs are available, a lower pressure should be used. In the elderly with compensated cardiac failure, the simultaneous increase in circulating blood volume and the increase in peripheral resistance imposed by the tourniquet could precipitate congestive cardiac failure, and the procedure should therefore be carried out slowly: only one tourniquet at a time should be permitted.

The length of time that a tourniquet may be left inflated will vary from patient to patient. An accepted guide is 1 hour for the arm and 1½ hours for the leg. In the early stages of tourniquet compression, direct pressure damage to nerves and vessels may occur, and thin patients are particularly prone to nerve injury in this way. Ischaemic tissue damage becomes more likely with increasing duration of arterial occlusion. If required, the tourniquet may be re-inflated after 15 minutes of free perfusion for a further period of ischaemia lasting half the initial period. Although Spira, *et al.* (1965) have shown that some perfusion of the limb occurs through the nutrient vessels of bone beneath a tourniquet, the degree of perfusion is very variable and cannot be predicted, so this finding cannot be used to justify increased tourniquet times.

Tourniquets should not be used on patients with marked peripheral vascular disease or if the limb shows evidence of ischaemia. For patients with sickle cell disease, if a tourniquet must be used, it should be for the minimum time necessary; in a series reported by Homi *et al.* (1979), 4 patients with sickle cell disease undergoing orthopaedic surgery had tourniquets applied uneventfully.

The need for a tourniquet must be considered when planning local anaesthetic techniques, since adequate proximal analgesia must be provided for the ischaemic pain caused by the tourniquet itself. If it is intended that any drugs enter the limb – antibiotics or muscle relaxants – these must be given before the tourniquet is in place.

When the tourniquet is released, there follows a marked reactive hyperaemia in the limb, which may increase limb blood flow up to 4-fold. This is caused by massive vasodilatation in response to local tissue hypoxia, anaerobic metabolism and lactic acid production. Hyperaemia is minimized by compression dressings and elevation of the limb. After removal of the tourniquet, the development of reactive hyperaemia confirms restoration of normal circulation in the limb; its absence, with the limb remaining blanched, is suggestive of vascular damage and merits further close observation.

Monitoring

Since the previous edition of this book the need for comprehensive monitoring at all times has become widely accepted. Despite the heavy initial capital cost of monitoring equipment, the expenditure can be justified by the likelihood of avoiding heavy litigation costs following an accident when a patient was not monitored adequately. In the United States of America the adoption of minimal monitoring standards proposed by Eichhorn and colleagues (1986, Standards for patient monitoring during anaesthesia at Harvard Medical School) has reduced the frequency of complications of anaesthesia to less than one-fifth (from 0.16/10 000 cases to 0.031/10 000 cases, Eichhorn, 1989) and in some cases had allowed lower malpractice insurance premiums. The difficult working environment in the Charnley enclosure, the scale of surgery often undertaken and the advanced age of many orthopaedic patients add to the need for comprehensive monitoring.

Pulse oximetry and capnography have become the most important forms of monitoring and properly used would have prevented 69 per cent of complications of anaesthesia studied by the Closed-Claims Study Committee of the American Society of Anesthesiologists over the past five years. Both are non-invasive, simple to use and provide important information about gas exchange.

Whilst all anaesthetists observe a patient's colour, a pulse oximeter increases the acuity of the observation and allows earlier intervention as saturation falls. In a study in children (Cote *et al.*, 1988) found that an anaesthetist assisted by a pulse oximeter was consistently better at recognizing hypoxic episodes than a skilled colleague. Nevertheless, oximeters have technical limitations: the algorithm used by the manufacturer to process the electrical signal is confidential and differs from manufacturer to manufacturer resulting in large differences in bias and precision. An error of 3 per cent at a saturation reading of 93 per cent would mean the patient had a possible arterial oxygen tension of between 59 and 88 mmHg! (Clayton *et al.*, 1991). Particular errors may arise at high saturations caused by compression of readings due to the need for the software to avoid percentages greater than 100. This is important in neonates because of the need to ensure oxygenation yet avoid hyperoxic retinopathy. Inaccuracy increases at low saturations owing to the difficulty of calibration in human subjects. Further limitations are the response time and the difficulty in recording from cold or poorly perfused sites: Paulus (1989) recommends wrapping a paediatric warming blanket round the forearm as a simple means of increasing perfusion to a cold finger if the oximeter signal is weak. In addition oximeters may be affected by haemoglobinopathies, ambient light and electrocautery. The probe should be shielded from ambient light and the sampling site chosen as far as possible from the operation site. Long nails and nail varnish also introduce errors and Ralston *et al.* (1991) recommend that the probe should be mounted sideways on fingers to avoid this. The effects of change in pH or blood temperature at the sampling site are small and clinically negligible. Wavelength absorption due to skin pigmentation is cancelled out in the wavelength comparison of the oximeter and does not introduce error: pulse oximetry should be mandatory for all coloured patients because of the difficulty of recognizing cyanosis visually.

A capnograph provides incontrovertible evidence that the trachea has been intubated and not the oesophagus and that ventilation is adequate. This in turn means that the breathing system has been assembled correctly and if an automatic ventilator is in use that appropriate settings have been chosen. This reassurance is fundamental to good anaesthetic practice and essential if a circle breathing system is being used. Measurement of the fractional expired CO_2

concentration makes it possible to avoid massive overventilation of babies and elderly patients with resulting respiratory alkalosis and cerebral vasoconstriction.

The electrocardiogram should always be displayed and is most informative if a specific lead is adopted; lead CM5 has many advantages for operating theatre use. This lead uses one electrode over the manubrium sterni and a further electrode in the V5 position in the anterior axillary line (Blackburn *et al.*, 1967). There is minimal attenuation of the signal so that a clear display can almost always be achieved; P-waves are prominent which helps in the interpretation of arrhythmias and the lead in the V5 position picks up left ventricular ischaemia early (Prys-Roberts, 1981).

Arterial pressure is most conveniently measured using one of the many automatic non-invasive blood pressure devices now available. These may be programmed to record the blood pressure every 2 or 3 minutes and provide invaluable information. However, their accuracy has been questioned, they fail to make measurements when the pressure is low – the very time when a measurement is needed – and they are very sensitive to patient movement. This is a serious problem in an orthopaedic theatre where passive movement of the patient due to surgical manipulation is common.

In addition to the now widespread oscillotonometric devices the Finapres has been available since 1989 as an alternative non-invasive monitor of blood pressure. This uses a small finger plethysmograph cuff and is very compact and more resistant to transmitted vibration. A measured pressure is applied to the cuff such that the volume of the finger remains constant thus exactly balancing arterial pressure.

In a review of indirect and direct means of measuring the blood pressure Jones *et al.* (1992) found the updated Finapres 2300e more accurate than a Colin non-invasive blood pressure monitor but no substitute for an arterial line and direct measurement. In particular the Finapres was subject to growing inaccuracy with time (drift) and over-read diastolic and mean pressures throughout the range. Direct measurement of arterial pressure should therefore be considered when particular difficulty with a patient is expected, if the patient has cardiovascular disease, or when an operation is expected to cause major blood loss.

The patient's temperature should be monitored during all major procedures in the clean air enclosure or if the patient is a child: despite all attempts at warming, a fall in core temperature of 4 or 5 degrees is not uncommon. The rapid air flow in the enclosure gives rise to an appreciable chill effect and the relatively large surgical wounds provide an extensive area for heat loss by evaporation. Vasodilatation caused by inhalational anaesthesia, hypotensive agents or regional anaesthesia will contribute to cooling. Core temperature is most simply monitored in the operating theatre using an oesophageal temperature probe. Care should be taken to advance the probe well into the oesophagus until the thermistor tip lies at the level of the atria and thus records heart temperature. Pharyngeal readings may be distorted by the temperature of inhaled gas.

A running total of estimated blood loss must be maintained during all major orthopaedic procedures. The commonest error for a newcomer to orthopaedic anaesthesia is to underestimate blood loss which unlike in other surgery, continues throughout the operation: bleeding from bone is difficult to stop and wounds are often extensive. Resection of primary tumours of bone or the stabilization of secondary deposits in bone, major surgery of the back and the removal of loose or infected prostheses are all associated with heavy blood loss and should not be undertaken without replacement blood at hand. A simple estimation of loss based on 1⅓ (weighed loss on swabs + volume in the sucker) is adequate to plan replacements and to ensure that the anaesthetist does not get too far behind. For patients on cardiovascular blocking agents in whom compensation for loss is impaired, greater importance attaches to estimation of loss and early replacement of blood. In these patients it may be advisable to monitor central venous pressure as a guide to blood replacement.

The ideal arrangement for monitors is to have similar systems in the anaesthetic room and theatre so that monitoring may be established in the anaesthetic room for the induction of anaesthesia and then continued in theatre simply by transferring the leads to the theatre monitors. The same pattern of monitor in the plaster room and the recovery rooms allow similar subsequent transfers.

References

Allenby, F., Pflug, J. J., Boardman, L. and Calnan, J. S. (1973). Effects of external pneumatic intermittent compression on fibrinolysis in man. *Lancet*, **2**, 1412.

Blackburn, H., Taylor, H. L., Okamoto, N., Rautaharju,

P. M., Mitchell, P. L. and Kerkhoff, A. C. (1967). Standardization of the exercise electrocardiogram. A systematic comparison of chest lead configurations employed for monitoring during exercise. In M. J. Karvonen and A. J. Barry (eds), *Physical Activity and the Heart*. Thomas: Springfield, Ill., p. 101.

Bonnar, J. (1987). Coagulation effects of oral contraception. *American Journal of Obstetrics and Gynaecology*, **157**, 1042–8.

Brenkel, I. J. and Clancy, M. J. (1989). Total hip replacement and antithrombotic prophylaxis. *British Journal of Hospital Medicine*, **42**, 282–4.

Charnley, J. (1972). Postoperative infection after total hip replacement with special reference to air contamination in the operating room. *Clinical Orthopaedics and Related Research*, **87**, 167.

Clayton, D. G., Webb, R. K., Ralston, A. C., Duthie, D. and Runciman, W. B. (1991). A comparison of the performance of 20 pulse oximeters under conditions of poor perfusion. *Anaesthesia*, **46**, 3–10.

Cote, C. J., Goldstein, E. A., Cote, M. A., Hoaglin, D. C. and Ryan, J. F. (1988) A single blinded study of pulse oximetry in children. *Anaesthesiology*, **68**, 184–8.

Eichhorn, J. H., Cooper, J. R., Cullen, D. J., Maier, W. R., Philip, J. H. and Seaman, R. G. (1986). Standards for patient monitoring at Harvard Medical school. *JAMA*, **256**, 1017–20.

Eichhorn, J. H. (1989). Prevention of intraoperative anaesthesia accidents and related severe injury through safety monitoring. *Anesthesiology*, **7**, 572–7.

Flanc, C., Kakkar, V. V. and Clarke, M. B. (1969). Postoperative deep vein thrombosis: effect of intensive prophylaxis. *Lancet*, **1**, 477.

Hirsch, J. (1981). Prevention of deep vein thrombosis. *British Journal of Hospital Medicine*, **26**, 143.

Hoffman, A. A. and Wyatt, R. B. W. (1985). Fatal pulmonary embolism following tourniquet inflation. *Journal of Bone and Joint Surgery*, **67A**, 633–4.

Homi, J., Reynolds, J., Skinner, A., Hanna, W., and Sergeant G. (1979). General anaesthesia in sickle cell disease. *British Medical Journal*, **1**, 1599.

Johnson, R., Green, J. R., Charnley, J. (1977). Pulmonary embolism and its prophylaxis following the Charnley total hip replacement. *Clinical Orthopaedics and Related Research*, **127**, 123.

Jones, R. D. M., Brown, A. G., Roulson, C. J., Smith, I. D. and Chan, S. C. (1992). The upgraded Finapres 2300e: A clinical evaluation of a continuous noninvasive blood pressure monitor. *Anaesthesia*, **47**, 701–5.

Kakkar, V. V., Stamatakis, J. D. and Bentley, P. G., Lawrence, D., de Haas, H. and Ward, V. P. (1979). Prophylaxis for postoperative deep vein thrombosis. Synergistic effect of heparin and dihydroergotamine. *Journal of the American Medical Association*, **241**, 39.

Knight, M. T. N. and Dawson, R. (1976). Effect of intermittent compression of the arms on deep venous thrombosis in the legs. *Lancet*, **2**, 1265.

Laverick, M. D., Croal, S. A. and Mollam, R. A. B. (1991). Orthopaedic surgeons and thrombo-prophylaxis. *British Medical Journal*, **303**, 549.

Lawrence, D. and Kakkar, V. V. (1980). Graduated static external compression of the lower limb: a physiological assessment. *British Journal of Surgery*, **67**, 119.

Leyvraz, P. F., Bachmann, F., Hoek, J., Buller, H., Postel, M., Samama, M. and Vandenbroek, M. D. (1991). Prevention of deep vein thrombosis after hip replacement: randomized comparison between unfractionated heparin and low molecular weight heparin. *British Medical Journal*, **303**, 543–9.

Lidwel, O. M., Lowbury, E. J. L., Whythe, W., Blowers, R., Stanley, S. J. and Lowe, D. (1982). Effects of ultraclean air in operating rooms on deep sepsis in the joint after total hip or knee replacement: a randomized study. *British Medical Journal*, **2**, 10.

McKenna, R., Galante, J. and Bachman, F., Wallace, D. L., Kaushal, S. P. and Meredith, P. (1980). Prevention of venous thromboembolism after total knee replacement by high dose aspirin or intermittent calf and thigh compression. *British Medical Journal*, **280**, 514.

Morris, G. K. (1980). Prevention of venous thromboembolism. *Lancet*, **2**, 572.

Morris, G. K. and Mitchell, J. R. A. (1977). The aetiology of acute pulmonary embolism and the identification of high risk groups. *British Journal of Hospital Medicine*, **18**, 6.

Parker-Williams, J. and Vickers, R. (1991). Major orthopaedic surgery on the leg and thromboembolism. *British Medical Journal*, **303**, 531–2.

Paulus, D. A. and Monroe, M. C. (1989). Cool fingers and pulse oximetry. *Anesthesiology*, **71**, 168–9.

Planes, A., Vochelle, N. and Fagola, M. (1990). Total hip replacement and deep vein thrombosis. *Journal of Bone and Joint Surgery (Br)*, **72B**, 9.

Prys-Roberts, C. (1981). Cardiovascular monitoring in patients with vascular disease. *British Journal of Anaesthesia*, **53**, 767.

Ralston, C. A., Webb, R. K. and Runciman, W. B. (1991). Potential errors in pulse oximetry III: Effects of interference, dyes, dyshaemoglobins and other pigments. *Anaesthesia*, **46**, 291–5.

Robinson, G. E., Bounds, W., Mackie, I. J., Stocks, J., Burren, T., Machin, S. J. and Guillebaud, J. (1991). Changes in haemostasis after stopping the combined contraceptive pill: implications for major surgery. *British Medical Journal*, **302**, 269–71.

Salzman, E. W. and Hirsch, J. (1987). Prevention of venous thromboembolism. In Colman, R. W., Hirsch, J., Marder, V. J. and Salzman, E. W. (eds), *Haemostasis and Thrombosis: Basic Principles and Clinical Practice*, 2nd edn. Philadelphia, J. B. Lippincott, pp. 1252–65.

Sanderson, M. C. and Bentley, G. (1976). Assessment of wound contamination during surgery: a preliminary report comparing vertical laminar flow and conventional theatre systems. *British Journal of Surgery*, **63**, 431.

Seagroatt, V., Tan, H. S., Goldacre, M., Bulstrode, C., Nugent, I. and Gil, L. (1991). Elective total hip replacement: incidence fatality and short-term readmission rates in a defined population. *British Medical Journal,* **303,** 1431.

Spira, E., Katznelson, A., Czerniak, P. and Mikolajkow, A. (1965). Osseous blood circulation in the lower limb: animal and clinical experiments. *Israel Journal of Medical Sciences,* **1,** 573.

Stamatakis, J. D., Kakkar, V. V., Lawrence, D., Bentley, P. G., Nairn, D. and Ward, V. (1978). Failure of aspirin to prevent postoperative deep vein thrombosis in patients undergoing total hip replacement. *British Medical Journal,* **1,** 1031.

Wilke, S. (1992). Pulmonary embolism following lower limb exsanguination. *Today's Anaesthetist,* **58,** 58.

Chapter 2

Preoperative assessment

The concept of risk

Anaesthetic risk and surgical risk were linked by Bendixen (1978) thus:

$$\frac{\text{Anaesthetic risk}}{\text{Surgical risk}} = \text{Constant}$$

which is an expression of the risk/benefit concept. In general, orthopaedic surgical procedures are of low morbidity and mortality (except perhaps for massive surgery or spinal surgery) and thus the anaesthetic risk, to be acceptable, must also be small.

Frequently, anaesthetic deaths occur amongst patients undergoing routine elective procedures (Editorial, 1979) and failure of the anaesthetist to appreciate the importance of the patient's age, disease, present physical condition or the potential impact of the operative procedure involved is a major contributory factor to the outcome. In emergency surgery, preoperative preparation is, of necessity, limited by the time available, but preparation for elective surgery can be exhaustive and it may be argued that time spent in this way is time invested in greater safety.

Stages of preoperative assessment

Before coming to surgery there are 4 stages at which the physical condition and fitness of a patient may be assessed:

1. at surgical outpatients;
2. at an anaesthetic outpatient clinic;
3. at a pre-admission clinic;
4. at the anaesthetist's preoperative visit.

At each stage the aim must be to identify those patients who are unfit for surgery and require further preparation or treatment. If patients with significant pathology escape detection needless mortality and, morbidity will be incurred and if they are detected late then surgery must be postponed after admission with consequent disruption of operating schedules, waste of theatre time and disappointment for the patient. However, many elderly patients are extremely fit and require little special assessment. Farmers for example, are particularly prone to osteoarthritis of hips perhaps due to repeated heavy lifting or the early start of work before joints are mature (Croft *et al.*, 1992): yet they are usually extremely fit because of their vigorous life.

Surgical outpatients

Some form of effective screening of the patient's general condition and medical history must be adopted at surgical outpatients, and the anaesthetist can help at this stage by establishing guidelines of fitness for anaesthesia within the surgical unit and by being consistent. Attempts have been made to employ a simple questionnaire filled in by patients at their initial visit in order to detect those who pose particular problems (Ogg, 1976; Rollason and Hems, 1981). This plan has obvious advantages in that nothing is likely to be overlooked and medical time may be saved. However, devising a questionnaire understood by all patients has difficulties of its own; a simple improvement might be for an experienced staff nurse or sister to help the patient to complete the questionnaire and in doing so provide an immediate screen, picking out those who require further attention.

Frost (1976) reported experience of a preoperative assessment clinic run by anaesthetists and located close to surgical outpatients. All patients seen by a surgeon and scheduled for surgery were referred immediately to the anaesthetic clinic where they were seen by an anaesthetist. She found that in 6 per cent of patients admission had to be postponed because of unsuspected or uncontrolled disease: diabetes mellitus, arterial hypertension, anaemia, pregnancy or a recent upper respiratory tract infection. She also found that both preoperative stay and total hospital stay were significantly reduced and that she had ample opportunity for discussing anaesthetic procedures with patients away from the pressure of an imminent operation. For many orthopaedic patients, however, this seems extravagant of anaesthetists' time since the young and clearly fit patients do not need this elaborate preparation.

Necessary investigations can be ordered and carried out so that the results are available when the patient is later admitted to the ward, provided that the admission date is not too far removed.

Blood should be taken for sickle cell screening in all patients of African origin, including American negroes, and anyone of Greek, Italian, Caribbean or Latin American ancestry of whom suspicions of thalassaemia or sickle cell trait are raised by a suggestive family history, the presence of anaemia or jaundice or bone or joint lesions due to infarction or infection commonly found in sickle cell disease. The lack of haste allows more accurate identification of the haemoglobinopathy by cellulose acetate electrophoresis at pH 8.4–8.6, a turbidity solubility test and a range of other investigations rather than a hurried sickledex detection test immediately preoperatively (Scott and Castro, 1979).

The anaesthetic assessment clinic

At the Nuffield Orthopaedic Centre, surgeons are encouraged to refer patients with significant medical problems to the anaesthetic outpatient clinic and at the same time to order obvious investigations so that they are available when that patient is seen. In practice, fewer than 5 new patients per week are referred and these can all be seen within the month. The commonest causes for referral have been cardiovascular disease and chronic respiratory disease, with a third group of patients referred because of a multiplicity of problems rather than the severity of any single one.

When the patient is seen, a careful history is taken, looking particularly for details of functional impairment. With disabling diseases such as osteoarthritis, cardiovascular and respiratory symptoms frequently appear to have improved over the year or so before help was sought; this may be the result of distraction by pain or, more likely, increasing limitation of mobility has meant that a restricted exercise tolerance is less and less of a handicap. Where mobility or posture are affected, any relieving surgical procedure may need to be carried out on both sides; so any decision to proceed with surgery means not one but two operations.

The precise complaint is important: if pain is the major problem an attempt should be made to quantify it to set against possible operative risk. Does the pain disturb the patient's life? Does it wake him at night? How effective are the analgesic drugs? Any intolerance of analgesics through intestinal ulceration or bleeding is a powerful argument in favour of surgery since so little can otherwise be done to alleviate the pain. Non-steroidal analgesics are a significant cause of gastric morbidity: at endoscopy 25 per cent of patients have gastric ulcers and up to 60 per cent have erosions or microhaemorrhages. One to 2 per cent of all patients on non-steroidal anti-inflammatory drugs (NSAIDS) will have ulcers that bleed or perforate and these complications are not reduced by H_2-blockers. It is not yet clear whether patients with rheumatoid arthritis who are taking non-steroidal analgesics are particularly prone to gastric ulceration (Hawkey, 1990).

If reduced mobility is the main complaint the relative importance of this to the patient should be ascertained. For some, reduced mobility is a nuisance but does not restrict life, whilst for others it may imprison them in their home and lead to a progressive loss of independence.

The patient is then examined, with particular attention paid to the condition which prompted referral. In fact, much valuable information can be obtained by watching the patient walk into the examination room and subsequently his response to the effort of taking off his clothes and climbing onto the examination couch – a standard test for all patients, so that one can be compared with another. Observing the relative ease with which he can lie flat for the period of examination may be helpful in assessing the severity of cardiac symptoms and also the feasibility of using a technique of local anaesthesia for surgery.

Finally, the prospects for anaesthesia and surgery can be discussed with the patient. For some patients, the decision is clear – their physical condition is no barrier to careful anaesthesia (the majority of patients referred). For others, major surgery entails an unacceptable risk. There remains a small group for whom no easy decision is possible. At this point it is perhaps helpful to think through the proposed surgical procedure in order to identify specific areas of difficulty; the induction of anaesthesia with consequent fluctuations in blood pressure; competing techniques of anaesthesia; cardiovascular consequences of the use of bone cement; a period of postoperative immobilization; the effects of plastering, particularly hip spicas and plaster jackets.

Some estimate of added risk can then be put to the patient and the proposed operation discussed with him. A joint decision then usually follows: the pain or limitation of life is so great that even an added anaesthetic risk is well worth while; or the patient, until now not having appreciated the risk, is unwilling to proceed.

When the interview is over, letters are written to the referring surgeon and to the general practitioner. Too often, important information discovered by anaesthetists remains buried in their notes and relatively inaccessible to others. The general practitioner may wish to alter management and he may also be consulted by the patient seeking further explanation of what was said, or reassurance. The letter to the surgeon is an opportunity to make clear current anaesthetic practice; it always seems a pity when a patient is denied operation at surgical outpatients because of anaesthetic risk.

The pre-admission clinic

A further safeguard is the surgical pre-admission clinic where patients are seen a few days before admission (Robin, 1991). They are clerked and the original indications for surgery checked, necessary investigations are ordered and blood samples taken. An anaesthetist should be available to see those patients about whom doubt arises. The clinic permits later admission and a simplified admissions procedure saving hospital costs. Patients who have died or moved or simply fail to arrive are identified and expensive gaps in operating lists can be avoided. If abnormalities are detected in the investigations performed, admission can be intercepted and onward referral arranged, whilst new patients can be summoned for admission.

Inpatient assessment

The preoperative visit

Each patient should be seen the night before operation by his anaesthetist. This makes it possible to establish some rapport and to understand a patient's fears and wishes. With careful questioning the surgical case notes can be augmented with details of previous anaesthetics and of any anaesthetic difficulties in the family: the patient's current drug therapy can be checked. Recent investigation results should be inspected; ward urine tests, a haemoglobin estimation, plasma electrolytes and an up to date electrocardiogram. There is some debate about the value of routine preoperative investigations but the discipline of a preoperative protocol ensures that nothing is overlooked. This is especially important in a specialized unit where it is all too easy for attention to be concentrated on the orthopaedic lesion in prospect at the expense of any other pressing but unconnected problems. Many old people have not undergone a thorough medical examination for a very long time. Routine preoperative chest *X*-ray is no longer recommended by the Royal College of Radiologists (1989) unless there is a suspicion of malignancy (Fig. 2.1) or tuberculosis or the patient belongs to an ethnic group in which tuberculosis is more common than 1 per 1000. Chest *X*-ray should

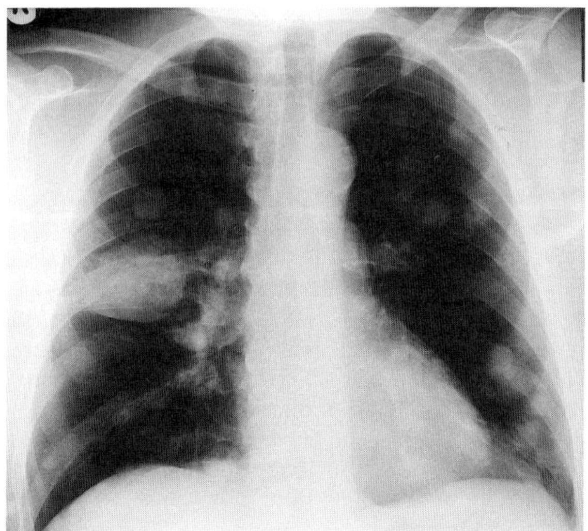

Fig 2.1 Chest *X*-ray of a patient with multiple metastases from an unknown primary tumour.

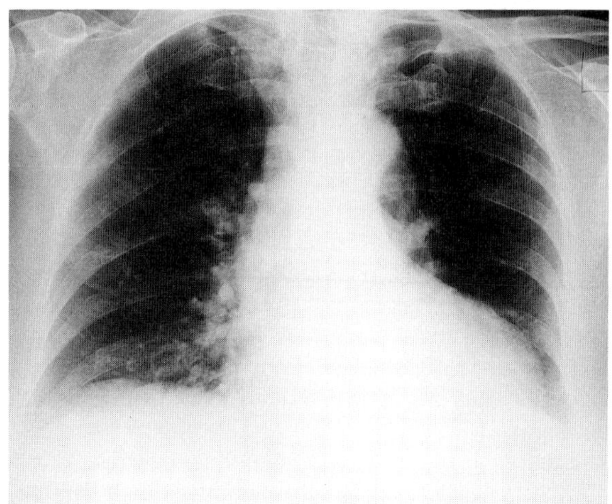

Fig 2.2 Chest *X*-ray showing right lower lobe bronchiectasis. The patient had a constant productive cough.

still be performed, however, where a clinical indication exists (Fig. 2.2). Finally, the proposed anaesthetic can be explained together with the means of postoperative pain relief.

Regrettably, however, this pattern represents an unattainable ideal in many units. In an unusually frank paper, Curran *et al.* (1985) surveyed current practice in one region and found that 22 per cent of anaesthetists saw fewer than 50 per cent of patients preoperatively, largely for organizational reasons.

The commonest reasons for which surgery is cancelled immediately preoperatively other than changed surgical indications are: unsuspected cardiovascular disease – much the most common of which are congestive cardiac failure, untreated hypertension, angina and myocardial ischaemia – disturbed renal or hepatic function and uncontrolled diabetes mellitus.

Clinical features of preoperative assessment

In this section prominence is given to those aspects giving rise to concern among the population presenting for orthopaedic surgery. More general consideration of medical problems can be found elsewhere (Corman and Bolt, 1979; Kaufman and Sumner, 1979).

In a landmark study of 1001 patients over 40 years of age admitted for general, orthopaedic, or urological surgery, Goldman and colleagues attempted to quantify cardiac risk factors preoperatively. They identified 8 criteria of prognostic importance by discriminant function analysis (Table 2.1) and for clinical use converted each discriminant function coefficient into a whole number to give a point weighting for each criterion. They went on to define 4 categories of risk into which individual patients might be fitted by adding up the total points for that patient (Table 2.2). Each rise in category represented a significant increment in cardiac risk. Thus only life saving surgical measures should be carried out if a patient scores more than 26 points, that specialist advice should be sought for patients scoring 13–25 points or with unstable angina or electrocardiographic changes suggestive of acute myocardial infarction, and that elective surgery should proceed only if a patient scores fewer than 13 points. This represents a finer and potentially more useful sieve than the American Society of Anesthesiologists' classification (Dripps *et al.*, 1961). This paper remains important as an

Table 2.1 Multifactorial index of cardiac risk

	Points
Gallop rhythm or elevated jugular venous pressure	11
Infarction if less than 6 months	10
Premature ventricular beats (more than 5 per minute)	7
Rhythm other than sinus rhythm	7
Age greater than 70	5
Emergency operation	4
Poor general condition	3
Tight aortic stenosis	3

Source: Reproduced, with permission, from Goldman et al. (1977).

Table 2.2 Frequency of complication and cardiac death

Points	Class	Life-threatening complications	Cardiac deaths
0–5	I	0.7%	0.2%
6–12	II	5%	2%
13–25	III	11%	2%
26+	IV	22%	56%

Source: Reproduced, with permission, from Goldman et al. (1977).

early example of an attempt to set a prediction rule. Prediction rules use several factors combined to derive a prognostic index which is better than using any one alone. The predictive factors should be easily reproducible to reduce interobserver variability, and clearly defined.

Ten years later the principal author reviewed experience with this classification (Goldman, 1987) and found it by and large consistent, although measurement of left ventricular function gave rise to difficulty, particularly the presence or absence of a third heart sound, whilst some important conditions such as angina and hypertension had occurred too rarely in the original series to allow proper assessment. Whilst exercise testing might improve predictability, this is clearly impractical in relatively immobile orthopaedic patients. Detsky *et al.* (1986) emphasized that the type of surgery influenced the risk; that body cavity surgery or prolonged surgery carried a greater risk than body surface surgery (i.e. almost all orthopaedic surgery).

Dirksen and Koller (1988) looked at cardiac predictors of death after non-cardiac surgery and ingeniously chose a population in which surgery was imperative thus disposing of the bias introduced when elective surgery is cancelled or postponed because of recognized cardiac risk. All the patients had suffered a myocardial infarct in the year previously and thus presented a variety of risk factors. Congestive cardiac failure was found to be a clear risk factor, as was multiple infarction. Recent myocardial infarction (within 3 months) was associated with a higher mortality, but this disappeared when the incidence of congestive cardiac failure was taken into account. The importance of this paper was to focus attention on ventricular function: congestive cardiac failure is evidence of poor function, however caused. In the case of those patients with multiple infarction, it is the degree of myocardial damage and ventricular impairment that is important rather than the history of infarction. Other factors such as stable angina and arrhythmias seemed to play only a minor part.

Measurement of ventricular ejection fraction in a cardiac department by two-dimensional echocardiography or nuclear imaging provides an objective index of ventricular function and is likely to become a useful clinical tool in preoperative assessment. An ejection fraction greater than 0.65 is reassuring; greater than 0.4 is marginal and less than 0.4 is unacceptable for elective surgery.

Mangano *et al.* (1992) studied 444 veterans who underwent elective non-cardiac surgery and left hospital in stable condition. Their results emphasized the long-term cardiac events which occur in this population. Eleven per cent had major cardiovascular complications during the 2-year follow-up period; cardiac death, non-fatal infarction, progressive angina requiring coronary artery surgery and unstable angina. Thirty per cent of these occurred within 6 months of surgery and 94 per cent within one year: 70 per cent of all adverse outcomes were preceded by early postoperative ischaemia. They identified three risk factors preoperatively; the presence of known vascular disease, a history of congestive heart failure, and known coronary artery disease. They also noted that patients who survived postoperative infarction or unstable angina had a 28-fold increase in the rate of subsequent cardiac complications in the following 6 months. In a further study of patients with known coronary artery disease 5 per cent of patients died in hospital after non-cardiac surgery (Browner *et al.*, 1992). Risk factors identified in this study were decreased renal function, a history of hypertension and severely limited activity. If 2 of these risk factors were present the mortality was 20 per cent, nearly 8 times higher than one alone. Half the deaths occurred more than 3 weeks after surgery and thus usually after hospital discharge, a point noted by Seagroatt *et al.* (1991) in consideration of the mortality of total hip replacement.

Myocardial ischaemia

Angina is a common symptom in elderly patients and if stable is not a significant risk. Unstable angina presents a similar risk to recent infarction and surgery should be postponed until satisfactory management of the angina has been achieved. Continuing angina following infarction suggests that the infarction is not complete and elective surgery would be unwise. Chung *et al.* (1988) found that although calcium channel blockers produced symptomatic relief of angina they did not protect against peri-operative ischaemia when compared with β blockers and recommended that a β blocker should be added to the drug regimen preoperatively.

Five major predictors for postoperative myocardial ischaemia were noted by Hollenberg *et al.* (1992) in reviewing the same series of veterans as Browner (Browner *et al.*, 1992). These were: left ventricular hypertrophy on electrocardiogram, a history of hypertension, diabetes mellitus, known coronary artery disease, and the use of digoxin. The risk of postoperative ischaemia increased progressively with the number of predictors present.

Painless myocardial ischaemia, so-called silent ischaemia, has attracted recent interest but its importance is not yet clear. Not uncommonly a routine preoperative ECG will reveal a previously unsuspected myocardial infarct which will clearly place the patient in the category of 'known coronary artery disease'.

Systemic hypertension

The border between normotension and hypertension is necessarily arbitrary but was set by the Joint National Committee in the United States (1984) as 140/90 and hypertension was classified as in Table 2.3 In 90–95 per cent of patients no cause can be found and this constitutes essential hypertension. In the remaining patients with secondary hypertension a specific cause can be found, most commonly renal disease. A series of important epidemiological studies (The Framingham Study, Kannel 1986, 1987) established that hypertension is not a necessary accompaniment of old age and that the risks in the elderly hypertensive did not differ from those in the younger hypertensive. The risks of hypertension were found to be better related to systolic pressure rather than diastolic pressures used more often in the past, and that variability of blood pressure was not a risk factor. The chief complications of hypertension are of stroke and ischaemic heart disease although the presence of other contributory factors such as smoking, obesity, diabetes mellitus and hyperlipidaemia is important. If there is damage to target organs, brain, heart or kidney, there is advanced disease and the likelihood of peroperative deterioration is correspondingly greater. Transient ischaemic attacks, stroke and renal failure represent a late stage of disease and are less common than ischaemic heart disease. Treatment should begin before target organ involvement since by then more than half of all cardiovascular clinical sequelae will have occurred! (Kannel, 1986). The level of blood pressure at which antihypertensive therapy should begin remains contentious (Borhani, 1987) but clinical trials have shown clear benefits in reducing the incidence of cardiac failure, stroke and renal failure. The evidence is less convincing for reduction of ischaemic heart disease.

Table 2.3 Classification of hypertension

Blood pressure diastolic	Category
<85	Normal
85–89	High normal
90–104	Mild hypertension
105–114	Moderate hypertension
>115	Severe hypertension
Systolic (when diastolic BP <90 mm Hg)	
<140	Normal
140–159	Borderline isolated systolic hypertension
>160	Isolated systolic hypertension

Source: Reprinted, with permission, from the Joint National Committee on Detection, Evaluation and Treatment of High Blood Pressure (1984).

Systemic hypertension as a surgical risk factor appears to have declined in importance since the classic work of Prys-Roberts, Foëx and others (Prys-Roberts *et al.*, 1971a, b, 1972) until omitted completely from the list of cardiac risk factors compiled by Goldman *et al.* (1977). In a study of the risks of general anaesthesia in the hypertensive patient, Goldman and Caldera (1979) reviewed the series of patients used for the earlier study and compared the complication rates and incidence of intraoperative hypotension amongst normotensive patients, mildly hypertensive patients on treatment and moderately hypertensive patients. They found that neither systolic or diastolic pressure measured preoperatively correlated with peroperative blood pressure lability; with the development of cardiac complications or postoperative renal failure. They concluded that elective surgery need not be delayed in order to achieve therapeutic control of blood pressure provided that:

1. the diastolic pressure is stable and not higher than 110 mmHg;
2. intraoperative and recovery room blood pressures are closely monitored.

Although this work is reassuring, of the patients studied, only 196 were hypertensive, none of them severely so. The experience is therefore small;

further, the overall incidence of postoperative renal failure (6 per cent) is worrying. One patient with a history of hypertension and a previous cerebrovascular accident had a second stroke postoperatively. This seems to be a not uncommon pattern: Beevers *et al.* (1973) found that the recurrence rate of strokes depended upon control of the blood pressure – that patients with a standing diastolic blood pressure greater than 100 mmHg had a three times greater chance of a second stroke.

Bedford and Feinstein (1980) noted that initial blood pressure recorded on admission to hospital was a better guide to the likely hypertensive response to stress than was the steady blood pressure recorded after a period of bed rest. Systemic hypertension therefore should not be disregarded because it settles later: it is an indication to search for other evidence of peripheral vascular, renal or cardiac disease. Coronary artery disease is the cause of death or serious morbidity in more than 60 per cent of all patients with established hypertension, and its course is only partially arrested by treatment of the hypertension (Berglund *et al.*, 1978).

In established treated hypertensives there is now agreement that drug therapy should be continued up to and including the morning of surgery to minimize the risk of a hypertensive response to stress-intubation or pain for example. Discontinuing drug therapy may additionally give rise to a rebound hypertension particularly if clonidine had been used.

The decision whether to proceed with elective surgery in an untreated hypertensive is often difficult. The guidelines given above by Goldman and Caldera are useful but should be considered in association with any other risk factors or evidence of target organ involvement when surgery should be postponed and expert advice sought. In all hypertensive patients serum potassium, urea and creatinine concentrations should be measured. Serum urea and creatinine are indicators of renal impairment albeit rather late, and provide a baseline measurement for postoperative management. Hypokalaemia caused by long-term diuretic therapy may predispose to peroperative ventricular dysrrhythmias (Freis, 1987), increase the requirement for suxamethonium and enhance the action of non-depolarizing relaxants. Acute hypokalaemia may be precipitated by respiratory alkalosis caused by incautious positive pressure ventilation.

The further management of hypertensive patients is considered in detail by Dagnino and Prys-Roberts (1989).

Heart block

Heart block is most frequently encountered in patients in their sixth and seventh decades. Although it is frequently due to a degenerative process affecting the conducting system, it may also be seen in younger patients following myocardial infarction and coronary heart disease, in myocardial inflammatory conditions and in myopathies and in certain drug intoxications. Although there may be a history of Stokes–Adams attacks, angina or heart failure, more commonly the patient is symptom-free, especially if his exercise tolerance is limited for other reasons, and heart block is only discovered as an incidental finding on the electrocardiogram. The problems associated with anaesthesia and heart block are reviewed by Wynands (1976), Simon (1977) and Foëx (1978). Preoperative management is simplified by the insertion of a temporary pacing wire percutaneously in all patients with symptoms and in those with an unstable rhythm. Precise indications for pacing remain controversial (Editorial, 1981) but those which meet general agreement are listed in Table 2.4.

Asymptomatic patients can be considered more conservatively. Temporary pacing is not without problems; the wire may become misplaced, particularly with patient movement, and cease pacing or the wire may penetrate the wall of the heart producing discomfort and a haemopericardium. This is usually marked by a loud pericardial rub close to the stethoscope. Further difficulty may arise in theatre.

During surgery, temporary pacemakers are particularly likely to be adversely affected by diathermy apparatus. If the pacemaker leads are left in position when the diathermy is in use, fibrillation currents will be induced in the pacing wire by radiation from the diathermy and ventricular fibrillation is likely to follow. This occurs even though the pacing box is

Table 2.4 Indications for insertion of a temporary pacemaker

Sinoatrial node dysfunction – sick sinus syndrome
Second-degree heart block – Möbitz type II
Third-degree heart block
Atrial fibrillation with a slow ventricular response
Bifascicular block

switched off. The best course is to proceed as follows: the pacing box should be left connected during the induction of anaesthesia and then removed, together with all extracorporeal leads (but left immediately available) before diathermy is used. Should the cardiac output be inadequate when the pacing box is switched off, prior to disconnection, then either surgery must proceed without using the diathermy or the present procedure should be abandoned and a permanent device implanted as a preliminary manoeuvre.

Fewer difficulties are encountered in patients in whom a permanent pacemaker has been implanted due to the improvements in shielding and input filters which have come about over the last few years. However, the output of demand pacemakers may be inhibited by signals arising from the diathermy and lead to periods of asystole when the diathermy is in use: all pacemakers are subject to heating of the implanted metal parts during sustained bursts of diathermy. If, as a result of this, burns occur of the ventricular wall at the tip of the pacing wire, the threshold may be raised and pacing cease. Reasonable precautions to be taken during anaesthesia and surgery for patients with a permanent pacemaker, as suggested by Rose *et al.* (1979) are: to position the diathermy indifferent electrode as far away from the pacemaker as possible; to limit the frequency and duration of use of diathermy to bursts of 1 second every 10 seconds; and to use direct monitoring of arterial pressure.

Anaemia

Anaemia is commonly encountered preoperatively in orthopaedic patients who may be elderly and taking an inadequate diet or who may have been ingesting regularly non-narcotic analgesics and anti-inflammatory agents likely to produce gastrointestinal bleeding. The significance of preoperative anaemia was reviewed by Gillies (1974), who found considerable support for a minimum acceptable haemoglobin concentration before anaesthesia of 10 g/dl, even though evidence of morbidity and mortality ascribable to anaemia is sparse; he noted the wisdom of accepting lower concentrations when they are the result of sickle cell disease, chronic renal failure or parasitic diseases. The actual concentration of haemoglobin is of less importance than the cause of an anaemia and a reason should be established during preoperative preparation. Eerola *et al.* (1980) found that in patients who had suffered a previous myocardial infarction a haemoglobin concentration of less than 12 g/dl appeared to contribute to the likelihood of reinfarction during or after operation.

Cardiovascular complications of Paget's disease

Cardiovascular complications may be found in Paget's disease, which is among the most common of chronic skeletal diseases, occurring in 3 per cent of all people over the age of 40. Its incidence increases with age, and patients usually present for surgery because of pathological fracture of a weakened long bone, with a neoplasm of bone or, most commonly, requiring hip replacement after collapse of the head of the femur.

Affected bone is hyperaemic, which was previously considered to be due to the development of arteriovenous anastomoses. Rhodes *et al.* (1972) demonstrated that, in the course of the disease, cancellous bone becomes replaced by coarse fibrous trabeculae threading a capillary bed of increased volume; they were not able to find any evidence of arteriovenous anastomoses. There is a fall in overall peripheral resistance, a rise in cardiac output and widening of the pulse pressure – the magnitude of these effects depending upon the volume of bone which has undergone change. Cardiac output may increase 2 or 3-fold if the disease is generalized, and eventually congestive cardiac failure results from the constant high output state. Howarth (1953) found that increased cardiac output occurred with at least 35 per cent skeletal involvement in the disease and with serum alkaline phosphatase titres greater than 315 i.u. (45 KA units) – the normal range being 21–92 i.u. (3–13 KA units).

Respiratory aspects of preoperative assessment

Although pulmonary complications are well recognized as a major cause of postoperative morbidity in general surgery and thoracic surgery, they are less troublesome following orthopaedic procedures: in general, the integrity and function of the chest are not impaired and means of pain relief are available which do not depend on frequent dosage with opiates. The principal exception is spinal surgery where pulmonary ventilation may be critically reduced by kyphoscoliosis, and careful evaluation is necessary before even minor procedures such as the fitting of a plaster jacket (spinal surgery is considered further in Chapter 4).

Specific disorders encountered amongst orthopaedic patients which may affect respiratory function include ankylosing spondylitis, rheurmatoid arthritis, myopathies and poliomyelitis. (Rheumatoid arthritis is considered further in Chapter 6.)

Ankylosing spondylitis

Patients with ankylosing spondylitis usually present scheduled for surgery of the hips or knees designed to achieve a more upright posture and greater mobility. They exhibit a restrictive ventilatory defect which is progressive with the disease and is caused by fusion and loss of movement at intervertebral and vertebrocostal joints. In 35 patients, Zorab (1962) found that vital capacity was reduced with severity of the disease, reaching a mean of 66 per cent of predicted value in the most handicapped; the lowest value was 38 per cent of predicted. There was no obstructive element and pulmonary compliance was normal. There was, however, an increase in residual volume due to fixation of the ribs in a position of inspiration. Progressively, ventilation becomes totally dependent on diaphragmatic function and any manoeuvre which puts that at risk (e.g. brachial plexus block by the interscalene or the supraclavicular route) should be avoided. In some cases, specific infiltration of the lungs occurs, with fibrosis of the upper lobes in particular – in the past often confused with pulmonary tuberculosis; Brown and Doll (1965) found a death rate from respiratory causes 2.5 to 3 times higher than average. Nevertheless, pulmonary ventilation is usually well maintained and chest infection well tolerated (Zorab, 1962). Early attempts to arrest progress of the disease by irradiation led to damage to haemopoietic tissue and resulting deaths from leukaemia and myelofibrosis (Brown and Doll, 1965). When assessing patients preoperatively, simple spirometry with a vitalograph is helpful in determining the degree of ventilatory defect and in plotting progress of the disease on subsequent admissions.

Fusion of cervical vertebral joints with fixation of the head and neck (Fig. 2.3) will make endotracheal intubation extremely difficult, and at the preoperative visit it is advisable to decide whether intubation will be required and to plan how to accomplish it. In practice, intubation is rarely necessary: the airway is surprisingly well maintained despite the loss of bony mobility and most procedures on the limbs can be carried out without endotracheal anaesthesia. If endotracheal intubation is required, blind nasal techniques may be successful but in difficult cases the intubating fibreoptic laryngoscope must be used. The technique of intubation by this method (Raj *et al.*, 1973; Wang *et al.*, 1976) is not easy and requires practice, the main difficulty being the tunnel vision enforced by the instrument. Lloyd (1980) finds that vision is improved if an assistant holds the tongue forward with a pair of lung-holding forceps. Difficulties in intubation are considered further in relation to rheumatoid arthritis (Chapter 6) and spinal disorders (Chapter 4). Other complications of the disease include aortic regurgitation and cardiomyopathy.

Poliomyelitis

New cases of poliomyelitis are now rare following the highly successful campaign of immunization, but there remains a large number of patients disabled to a greater or lesser extent. Of these, some continue to present for orthopaedic procedures such as tendon transplants and fusion of joints to minimize handicap and make the best use of remaining function. Usually only the less severely affected patients, who are mobile, are subjected to these procedures but they nevertheless demand careful assessment. There are two areas giving cause for concern: the patient's ventilatory capacity and laryngeal competence. It is easy to over-estimate the respiratory reserve since many patients who have recovered from poliomyelitis lead apparently normal lives despite a severely restricted vital capacity – often less than 1 litre. The frequency of previous respiratory infections and their severity should be ascertained and whether ventilatory support was required. Vital capacity is easily measured and the patients are well used to the measurement. If it is intended to use a local anaesthetic technique, it is important to be certain that the patient can lie flat comfortably for the duration of the surgical procedure. Those with

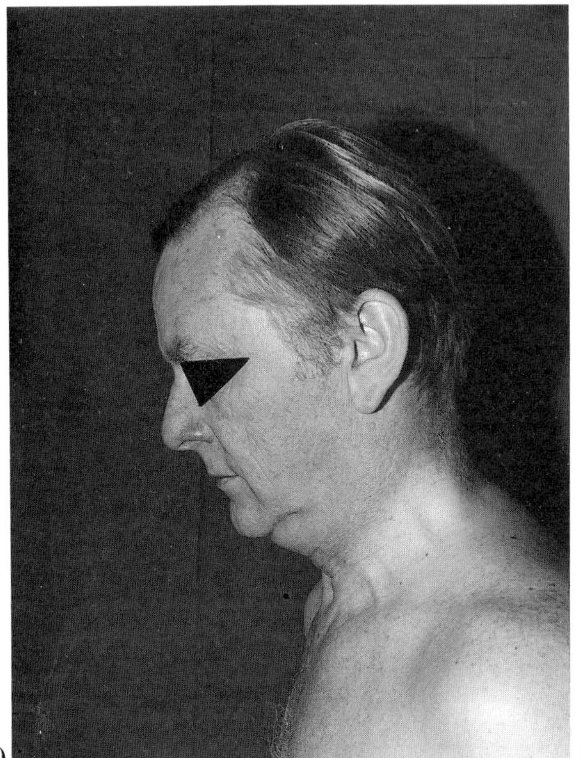
(a)

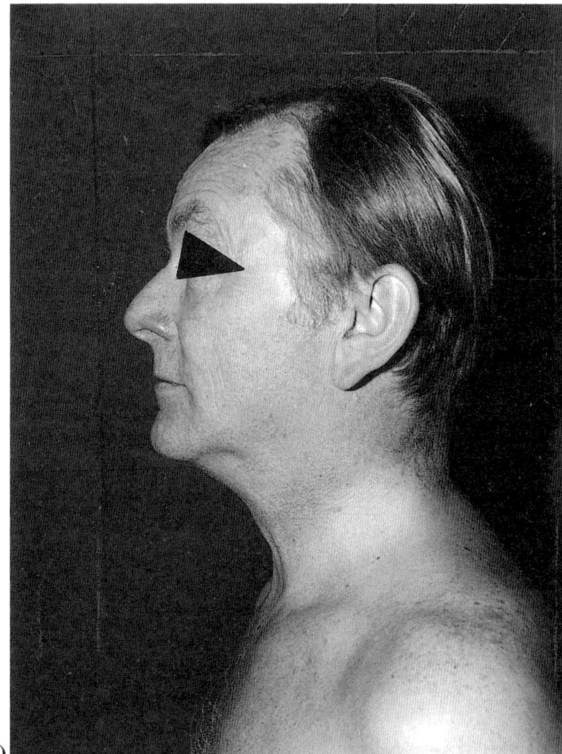
(b)

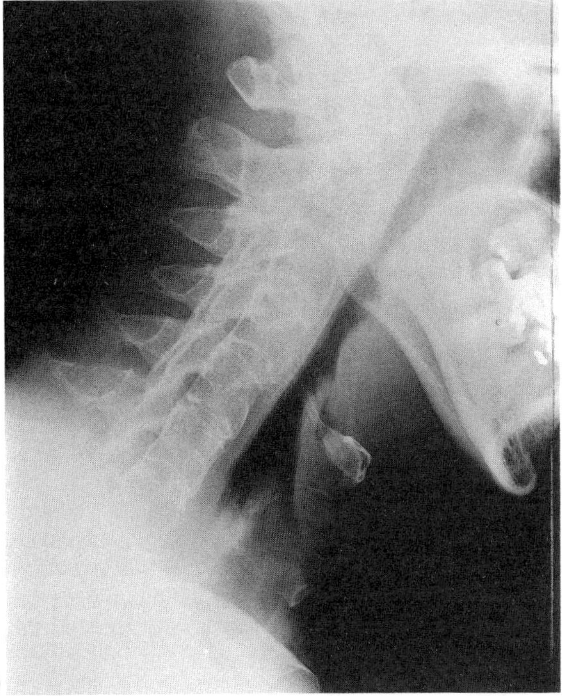
(c)

Fig 2.3 Ankylosing spondylitis: (a) full flexion of the neck; (b) full extension of the neck; (c) *X*-ray of the neck showing complete ankylosis of vertebral bodies. Despite the apparently normal appearance of this patient, lack of any movement of the neck would render endotracheal intubation extremely difficult.

bulbar symptoms usually have a permanent tracheostomy, but any history of a weak voice or aspiration of fluids is strongly suggestive and consideration should be given to endotracheal anaesthesia and careful reintroduction of oral fluids postoperatively.

Disorder of muscle

The inherited disorders of muscle – the dystrophies, the myotonias, glycogen storage diseases and the myopathies – are reviewed by Ellis (1980) and their investigation by Moosa (1974). Of these, patients suffering from myopathy or muscular dystrophy are most likely to be offered orthopaedic procedures. They frequently present for minor surgery to prevent recurrent dislocations of the patella or shoulder.

Muscular dystrophies vary in severity from mild late onset distal muscular dystrophy or ocular muscular dystrophy to the severe early onset Duchenne type. At the preoperative visit it is essential to obtain a clear understanding of the functional impairment of each patient, paying particular attention to ventilatory capacity and to myocardial performance, since in the early stages of muscle disorders diagnoses are often mistaken and corrected subsequently as new features become apparent. Patients with severe muscular dystrophy usually develop an obstructive cardiomyopathy which can be detected by the changes produced in the electrocardiogram and by right heart enlargement on chest *X*-ray. The electrocardiograph changes include a large R-wave in lead V1 and deep Q-waves in V4–6. T-wave inversion in the V leads is common and there may be a widening of the QRS complex with shortening of the PR interval. Right ventricular outflow obstruction predisposes to eventual heart failure. The diagnosis of severe muscular dystrophy is supported by finding a greatly increased resting serum creatinine phosphokinase (CPK) titre.

Congential myopthay is characterized by hypotonia and progressive weakness, and is usually distinguished in childhood. Skeletal abnormalities which acompany the myopathy include kyphoscoliosis, pigeon chest and pes cavus. The vital capacity is reduced both by the skeletal deformity and by the hypodynamic respiratory musculature. In addition, heart failure in childhood has been described. Malignant hyperpyrexia myopathy has been found amongst patients presenting for minor orthopaedic procedures (see Chapter 6).

Metabolic aspects of preoperative assessment

In addition to the routine testing of a patient's urine, a blood sample should be sent for biochemical screening tests from all patients scheduled for major surgery or in whom abnormality might be expected. Young women who might be pregnant should have a pregnancy test carried out on a sample of urine, since it is generally agreed that only emergency surgery should be performed during pregnancy (Pedersen and Finster, 1979).

The purpose of biochemical screening is to identify those patients with asymptomatic renal, hepatic or endocrine disease: hypercalcaemia may be found associated with myelomatosis, carcinomatous deposits in bone (not necessarily osteolytic), Paget's disease of bone or hyperparathyroidism.

Liver disease

Patients with unsuspected liver disease tolerate anaesthesia and major surgery badly, and detrimental postoperative changes in liver function occur which appear to be related to the extent of surgery. Whilst elective surgery clearly would not be contemplated in those with overt signs of active liver disease, the anaesthetist is frequently presented with 2 groups of patients in whom this is a possibility: those with a history of jaundice and normal liver function tests, and those with no history and abnormal liver function tests (Strunin, 1978).

Clinical biochemistry laboratories offer a battery of 'liver function tests' that include measurment of serum bilirubin concentration, alkalinephosphatase and aminotranserase activity, and serum albumin concentration. Additional investigations may include liver biopsy, computed tomography, ultrasonography and endoscopic cholangiography. In addition clotting factor activity may be measured and immunological tests undertaken for hepatitis antigen. Few of these tests are specific, alkaline phosphatase activity is increased in bone disease and aspartate aminotransferase after myocardial infarction while bilirubin and protein concentrations are affected by haemolysis and nutritional state. Further, the sensitivity of these tests (positive results in patients with disease) is low. Newer dynamic tests are assessed by Laker (1990) but appear to offer little to help the clinician.

Patients often give a history of earlier jaundice followed by complete recovery: the details should be elicited and in particular the relationship of the jaundice to any drugs taken at the time, general anaesthetic or blood transfusion. In the absence of an obvious cause, the most likely diagnosis is viral hepatitis; if liver function tests show no abnormality, then surgery may proceed. If the patient is a haemophiliac or has received blood products in the past a screening test for hepatitis B should be performed so that appropriate precautions can be taken (see also Chapter 6).

Less commonly, abnormal liver function tests are found on screening in the absence of overt symptoms: chronic hepatocellular disease may progress completely unsuspected by the patient. Its aetiology is largely unknown but chronic abuse of alcohol amongst older patients and chronic active viral hepatitis among younger patients are commonly recognized causes. Long-term abuse of alcohol may be revealed by estimation of a-glutamyl transferase and erythrocyte mean cell volume. In each case high values suggest a high alcohol intake (Papoz *et al.*, 1981).

Pugh *et al.* (1973) compiled a multifactorial index of the risk of surgery (Table 2.5). Only those patients at minimal risk should be considered fit for elective surgery.

When considering anaesthesia use the smallest number of drugs in the smallest possible dose. Premedication can be omitted and all central nervous system depressants kept to a minimum. Drugs which do not depend on the liver for detoxification and have a short half-life such as propofol should be preferred and local anaesthetic techniques chosen where possible, taking care not to exceed the toxic dose of lignocaine or marcain.

Renal disease

Screening tests for renal disease consist of urine testing and measurement of serum creatinine and urea concentrations. Whilst the urea concentration correlates better with the physical signs of uraemia, creatinine concentration is the better indication of glomerular filtration rate (GFR). The production of creatinine is relatively constant for any given individual as an end product of muscle metabolism; since creatinine production is dependent on muscle mass, higher levels are found in muscular athletes than in small immobile individuals. Because production of creatinine is steady, any change in its excretion caused by a change in GFR is reflected in a rise in serum creatinine concentration to a new equilibrium level. Kassirer (1971) suggested that this relationship is entirely predictable and that a 50 per cent reduction in GFR will double the serum creatinine concentration. The interpretation of borderline concentrations of creatinine is helped by measurement of the GFR by creatinine clearance. It is common, partiuclarly in the elderly, to find mildly elevated blood urea concentrations in blood samples taken early in the morning after the fluid restriction of the night.

With age renal function declines; the glomerular filtration rate falls, there is a reduction in tubular secretion and reabsorption and renal blood flow decreases. After the age of 50 renal abnormalities begin to appear and all kidneys show some abnor-

Table 2.5 Estimate of surgical risk in liver disease

	Minimal risk	Moderate risk	Severe risk
Bilirubin (μmol/l)	25	25–40	40
Serum albumin (g/l)	35	28–35	28
Ascites	None	Controlled	Poorly controlled
Encephalopathy	None	Minimal	Coma
Nutrition	Excellent	Good	Wasted
Operative mortality (portasystemic shunting)	0%	9%	53%

Source: Data from Pugh et al. (1973).

mality of function after 80. Reduced renal function may therefore compound other systemic disease in the elderly and has important implications for antibiotic therapy. Alternatives should be sought for nephrotoxic antibiotics such as the aminoglycosides and plasma concentrations monitored routinely if potentially disastrous vestibular nerve toxicity is to be avoided. Ototoxicity may be potentiated if the patient is taking frusemide or ethacrinic acid (Brit Nat Formulary, March 1992) and these drugs should not be used concurrently.

Conclusion

Patients no longer die during anaesthesia but in the days and weeks which follow. Any assessment of fitness must consider not only the immediate procedure but also recovery and rehabilitation. A good surgical result may be prejudiced by the patient's apathetic mental state; coexistent illness; disuse changes and obesity resulting from immobility. Precarious social circumstances may ultimately prevent discharge from hospital. Rehabilitation in such patients may require many resources and the active help and involvement of a department of geriatric medicine. Results might be improved if those patients who suffered peri-operative cardiovascular complications in particular were followed up and treated more aggressively than is currently the practice (Mangano *et al.*, 1992).

References

Bedford, R. F. and Feinstein, B. (1980). Hospital admission blood pressure: a predictor for hypertension following endotracheal intubation. *Anesthesia and Analgesia*, **59**, 367.

Beevers, D. G., Fairman, M. J., Hamilton, M. and Harpur, J. E. (1973). Antihypertension treatment and the course of established cerebral vascular disease. *Lancet*, **1**, 1407.

Bendixen, H. (1978). Risks in anaesthesia. Paper read to the Nuffield Department of Anaesthetics, Oxford.

Berglund, G., Wilhelmsen, L. and Sannerstedt, R. (1978). Coronary heart disease after treatment of hypertension. *Lancet*, **1**, 1.

Borhani, N. O. (1987). Left ventricular hypertrophy, arrhythmias and sudden death in systemic hypertension. *American Journal of Cardiology*, **60**, 131–81.

British National Formulary (1992). March.

Brown, W. M. D. and Doll, R. (1965). Mortality from cancer and other causes after radiotherapy for ankylosing spondylitis. *British Medical Journal*, **2**, 1327.

Browner, W. S., Li, J. and Mangano, D. T. (1992) In-hospital and long-term mortality in male veterans following noncardiac surgery. *JAMA*, **268**, 228–32.

Chung, F., Houston, P. L., Cheng, D. C. H., Lavelle, P. A., McDonald, N., Burns, R. J. and David, T. E. (1988). Calcium channel blockade does not offer adequate protection from perioperative myocardial ischaemia. *Anesthesiology*, **69**, 343–7.

Corman, L. C. and Bolt, R. J. (1979). Medical evaluation of the preoperative patient. *Medical Clinics in North America*, **63**, 1335.

Croft, P., Coggon, D., Cruddas, M. and Cooper, ?. (1992). Osteoarthritis of the hip: an occupational disease in farmers. *British Medical Journal*, **304**, 1269–72.

Curran, J., Chmielewski, A. T., White, J. and Jennings, A. M. (1985). Practice of preoperative assessment by anaesthetists. *British Medical Journal*, **291**, 391–3.

Dagnino, J. and Prys-Roberts, C. (1989). Strategy for patients with hypertensive heart disease. *Clinics in Anesthesiology*, **3**, 261–89.

Detsky, A. S., Abrams, H. B., Forbath, N., Scott, J. G., Hilliard, J. R. (1986). Cardiac assessment for patients undergoing non-cardiac surgery. *Archives of Internal Medicine*, **146**, 2131–34.

Dirksen, A. and Kjoller, E. (1988). Cardiac predictors of death after non-cardiac surgery evaluated by intention to treat. *British Medical Journal*, **297**, 1011–13.

Dripps, R. D., Lamont, A. and Eckenhoff, J. E. (1961). The role of anaesthesia in surgical mortality. *Journal of the American Medical Association*, **178**, 261.

Editorial (1979). Anaesthetic deaths. *British Medical Journal*, **1**, 2.

Editorial (1981). The pacing industry. *British Medical Journal*, **282**, 703.

Eerola, M., Eerola, R., Kaukinen, S. and Kaukinen, L. (1980). Risk factors in surgical patients with verified preoperative myocardial infarction. *Acta Anaesthesiologica Scandinavica*, **24**, 219.

Ellis, F. R. (1980). Inherited muscle disease. *British Journal of Anaesthesia*, **52**, 153.

Foëx, P. (1978). Preoperative assessment of patients with cardiac disease. *British Journal of Anaesthesia*, **50**, 15.

Freis, E. D. (1987). Diuretic induced hypokalaemia. The debate over its relationship to cardiac arrhythmias. *Postgraduate Medicine*, **81**, 123–9.

Frost, E. A. M. (1976). Outpatient evaluation: a new role for the anesthesiologist. *Anesthesia and Analgesia*, **55**, 307.

Gillies, I. D. S. (1974). Anaemia and anaesthesia. *British Journal of Anaesthesia*, **46**, 589.

Goldman, L., Caldera, D. L., Nussbaum, S. R., Southwick, F. S., Krogstad, D., Murray, B., Bume, D. S.,

O'Malley, T. A. (1977). Multifactorial index of cardiac risk in non-cardiac surgical procedures. *New England Journal of Medicine*, **297**, 845–50.

Goldman, L. and Caldera, D. L. (1979). Risks of general anaesthesia and elective operation in the hypertensive patient. *Anesthesiology*, **50**, 285.

Goldman, L. (1987). Multifactorial index of cardiac risk in noncardiac surgery: ten-year status report. *Journal of Cardiothoracic Anaesthesia*, **1**, 237–44.

Hawkey, C. J. (1990). Non-steroidal anti-inflammatory drugs and peptic ulcers. *British Medical Journal*, **300**, 278–84.

Hollenberg, M., Mangano, D. T., Browner, W. S., London, M. J., Tubau, J. F. and Tateo, I. M. (1992). Predictors of postoperative myocardial ischaemia in patients undergoing noncardiac surgery. *Journal of the American Medical Association*, **268**, 205–9.

Howarth, S. (1953). Cardiac output in osteitis deformans. *Clinical Science*, **12**, 271.

Joint National Committee on Detection, Evaluation and Treatment of High Blood Pressure (1984). *Archives of Internal Medicine*, **144**, 1045–57.

Kannel, W. B. (1986). Hypertension. Relationship with other risk factors. *Drugs*, **31**, suppl. 1, 1–11.

Kannel, W. B. (1987). Status of risk factors and their consideration in antihypertensive therapy. *American Journal of Cardiology*, **59**, 80A–90A.

Kassirer, J. P. (1971). Clinical evaluation of kidney function–glomerular function. *New England Journal of Medicine*, **285**, 385.

Kaufman, L. and Sumner, E. (1979). *Medical Problems and the Anaesthetist. Current Topics in Anaesthesia, No. 4*. Edward Arnold, London.

Laker, M. F. (1990). Liver function tests. *British Medical Journal*, **301**, 250–51.

Lloyd, E. L. (1980). Fibreoptic laryngoscopy for difficult intubation. *Anaesthesia*, **35**, 719.

Mangano, D. T., Browner, W. S., Hollenberg, M, Li, J. and Tateo, I. M. (1992). Long-term cardiac prognosis following noncardiac surgery. *JAMA*, **268**, 233–9.

Moosa, A. (1974). The investigation of neuromuscular disease in early childhood. *British Journal of Hospital Medicine*, **12**, 166.

Ogg, T. W. (1976). Assessment of preoperative cases. *British Medical Journal*, **1**, 82.

Papoz, L., Warner, J. M., Pequignot, G., Eschwege, E., Claude, J. R. and Schwarz, D. (1981). Alcohol consumption in a healthy population: relationship to gamma-glutamyl transferase activity and mean corpuscular volume. *JAMA*, **245**, 1748–51.

Pedersen, H. and Finster, M. (1979). Anaesthetic risk in the pregnant surgical patient. *Anesthesiology*, **51**, 439.

Prys-Roberts, C., Greene, L. T., Meloche, R. and Foëx, P. (1971a). Studies of anaesthesia in relation to hypertension, haemodynamic consequences of induction and endotracheal intubation. *British Journal of Anaesthesia*, **43**, 531.

Prys-Roberts, C., Meloche, R. and Foëx, P. (1971b). Studies of anaesthesia in relation to hypertension. Cardiovascular responses of treated and untreated patients. *British Journal of Anaesthesia*, **43**, 122.

Prys-Roberts, C., Foëx, P., Greene, L. T. and Waterhouse, T. D. (1972). Studies of anaesthesia in relation to hypertension IV. The effect of artificial ventilation on the circulation and pulmonary gas exchange. *British Journal of Anaesthesia*, **44**, 335.

Pugh, R. N. H., Murray-Lyon, I. M., Dawson, J. L., Pietroni, M. C. and Williams, R. (1973). Transection of the oesophagus for bleeding varices. *British Journal of Surgery*, **60**, 646.

Raj, P. P., Forestner, J., Watson, T. P., Morris, R. E. and Jenkins, M. T. (1973). Techniques for fiberoptic laryngoscopy in anaesthetics. *Anesthesia and Analgesia*, **53**, 798.

Rhodes, B. A., Greyson, N. D., Hamilton, C. R., White, R. I., Giargiana, F. A. and Wagner, H. N. (1972). Absence of arteriovenous shunts in Paget's disease of bone. *New England Journal of Medicine*, **287**, 686.

Robin, P. E. (1991). Preadmission clinics. *British Medical Journal*, **302**, 532.

Rollason, W. N. and Hems, G. (1981). Preoperative assessment for outpatient anaesthesia. *Annals of the Royal College of Surgeons of England*, **63**, 45.

Rose, S. D., Corman, L. C. and Mason, D. T. (1979). Cardiac risk factors in patients undergoing noncardiac surgery. *Medical Clinics of North America*, **63**, 1271.

Royal College of Radiologists (1989). *Making the best use of a Department of Radiology. Guidelines for Doctors*. RCR, London.

Seagroatt, V., Tan, H. S., Goldacre, M., Bulsbrode, C., Nugent, I. and Gil, L. (1991). Elective total hip replacement: incidence fatality and short-term readmission rates in a defined population. *British Medical Journal*, **303**, 1431.

Scott, R. B. and Castro, O. (1979). Screening for sickle cell haemoglobinopathies. *Journal of the American Medical Association*, **241**, 1145.

Simon, A. B. (1977). Preoperative management of the pacemaker patient. *Anesthesiology*, **46**, 127.

Strunin, L. (1978). Preoperative assessment of the patient with liver dysfunction. *British Journal of Anaesthesia*, **50**, 25.

Wang, J. F., Reeves, J. G. and Corssen, G. (1976). Use of the fiberoptic laryngoscope for difficult tracheal intubation. *Alabama Journal of Medical Sciences*, **13**, 247.

Wynands, J. E. (1976). Anesthesia for patients with heart block and artificial pacemakers. *Anesthesia and Analgesia*, **55**, 626.

Zorab, P. A. (1962). The lungs in ankylosing spondylitis. *Quarterly Journal of Medicine*, **31**, 267.

Chapter 3

Anaesthesia for Surgery of the limbs

Introduction: anaesthesia for elderly patients

In elderly patients declining hepatic and renal function effectively extend the half-life of many drugs, particularly central nervous system depressants and non-depolarizing relaxants; tubocurare, pancuronium and alcuronium (Kent and Hunter, 1991). When relaxants are used, it is better to wait for a sign of movement before giving an increment rather than give them regularly. The number of drugs used should be kept to a minimum and dosages made as sparing as possible. Care should be taken to maintain hydration and preserve renal function without overloading the patient: it may be necessary to use a central venous catheter as a guide to fluid administration.

Hypothermia

The elderly are vulnerable to hypothermia and heat is lost during surgery for many reasons; the low ambient temperature; the chill factor of the air flow in the Charnley enclosure; ventilation of the lungs with cold, dry gases; drug induced vasodilatation and administration of cold intravenous fluids. Ip Yam and Carli (1990) found that heat loss in ventilated patients undergoing hip replacement was minimized if the inspired gas was humidified and warmed to 40°C but that there was little value in using a condenser humidifier alone. Measures can be taken to conserve heat with careful draping and the use of an aluminized overblanket but means of adding heat such as a heated water blanket or 'ripple mattress' inevitably cause localized burns. A device which blows warmed air under a sealed patient drape is effective ('Bair Hugger', Actamed, Wakefield, UK) and has little potential for harm provided core temperature is monitored throughout. Infused fluids should be warmed.

Positioning

Positioning on the table must be accomplished gently and all supports padded: superficial nerves at the elbow and the neck of the fibula must be free from compression. Great care should be taken to support the patient's neck during turning to avoid inadvertent injury.

Postoperative confusion

Anaesthesia in the elderly is often followed by mental confusion which is difficult to manage and occasionally may be long lasting and disabling. Many factors are relevant; the drugs administered, minor cerebral hypoperfusion and cerebral hypoxia, but very little work has been done in this area: the work done is often flawed and seldom involves a trained psychologist. Flatt *et al.* (1984) found impaired mental function after general anaesthesia in elderly patients with some failing to regain their preoperative performance 6 weeks after surgery. Hovorka (1982) considered the psychometric deterioration after general anaesthesia to be due to cerebral vasoconstriction caused by overventilation and hypocapnia. However Jhaveri (1989) found that hyperventilation to a mean $_{p}CO_2$ of 2.9 kPa in 30 subjects over 60 years of age produced no detectable impairment to a range of psychometric tests. Despite this study, which involved only superficial surgery (cataract surgery) of short duration, it is preferable to ensure normocapnia during ventilation and to avoid cerebral vasoconstriction.

There is a growing feeling that unsupplemented regional anaesthesia is the most benign technique available in terms of postoperative mental changes and that each drug added will impair the result a little. However, it is asking a great deal of many patients to lie still for 2 hours during hip replacement and the building noises involved may be unpleasant: some supplementation is usually necessary, although often very small doses will suffice. Premedication is usually not necessary if the anaesthetist has won the patient's confidence but, if needed, a benzodiazepine in minimal dosage or pethidine 25–50 mg with an anti-emetic given intramuscularly are suitable (White, 1980). There is no need for antisialogogues with modern anaesthetic agents unless it is intended to use ketamine. Hyoscine is well known to cause confusion in patients over 60, whilst atropine and, to a lesser extent, glycopyrronium may exacerbate arrhythmias (Mirakhur *et al.*, 1978). Mixtures of drugs may give unpredictable results; for example, the combination of diazepam with a potent analgesic, which is popular as a means to provide suitable conditions for minor surgery, may sometimes lead to respiratory arrest.

Suppression of the hormonal response to surgery

The neuroendocrine response to major surgery such as joint replacement or resection of a malignancy may complicate the postoperative period with hyperglycaemia, fluid and sodium retention and loss of potassium resulting from substrate mobilization and tissue catabolism. The hormonal changes may also predispose to venous thromboembolism. Many different approaches have been tried to minimize these metabolic changes including high dose opiate anaesthesia (Hall, 1980); peri-operative heat conservation during surgery (Carli and Itiaba, 1986) infusion of insulin (Woolfson *et al.*, 1979) and all have claimed some success. However, if a regional block is included in the technique of anaesthesia, along with sedation or accompanied by full general anaesthesia, then these changes may be bypassed.

Brandt *et al.* reported in 1978 marked attenuation of the postoperative catabolic response to surgery if epidural anaesthesia was employed. In a further paper Brandt *et al.* (1979) found that rises in plasma renin, aldosterone, and cortisol concentrations brought about by the stress of hysterectomy in a control group were completely suppressed in a trial group which received epidural anaesthesia. Engquist *et al.* (1980) found that secretion of adrenaline in response to surgical stress was abolished by epidural blockade. Postoperative protein breakdown in elderly patients undergoing hip surgery was specifically studied by Christensen *et al.* (1986) who found that excretion of muscle protein breakdown products remained at the preoperative level after hip replacement if epidural anaesthesia was used compared with a marked increase after general anaesthesia: a similar finding was reported by Vendrinne and colleagues (1989) after colonic surgery under epidural anaesthesia. Similarly, secretion of cortisol remained at resting levels during hip replacement when epidural anaesthesia was used but more than doubled in a comparable group during surgery with general anaesthesia (Carli and Emery, 1990). Interestingly, in this study no difference in postoperative protein catabolism was found between groups but epidural anaesthesia was used only for the duration of surgery and intramuscular papaveretum was used for analgesia postoperatively. There is thus a clear benefit in continuing epidural blockade into the postoperative period, something which emerges from many other papers.

Surgery of the lower limb

Surgery of the lower limb may involve correction of congenital deformities (see Chapter 7); lengthening or shortening procedures in adolescents with growth abnormalities; resection of musculo-skeletal malignancy; osteotomy and realignment of bone to treat osteoarthritis, or replacement of destroyed joints with a prosthesis. The femur and tibia are also common sites for osteomyelitis the management of which may require the drilling or deroofing of an abscess cavity or removal of a sequestrum. The surgery thus covers all age ranges but the most difficult problems are amongst the elderly patients presenting for osteotomy or joint replacement.

The success of joint replacement has changed the face of orthopaedic surgery and created enormous unsatisfied demand. Over 50 000 hip replacements per year are now performed in the United Kingdom (Clift and Rowley, 1992) compared with 17 000 in 1978. Patients who receive a hip replacement have a better than 90 per cent chance of the prosthesis lasting 12–15 years (Harrold, 1982) so that the operation can be offered to younger patients at an earlier stage of disease with the real prospect of abolishing pain and improving mobility. However, patients who are under 30 at operation do less well: 54 per cent of joint replacements fail within 5 years (Harrold, 1982). In these patients, therefore, other procedures such as osteotomy are offered first in order to buy time, relieve symptoms and postpone joint replacement.

Some problems remain, however. There is controversy over whether the prosthesis should be cemented into bone or be uncemented and rely on better fit for security: uncemented prostheses require more exacting technique at insertion in order to gain the best possible fit between prosthesis and bone. In general, uncemented prostheses are preferred for younger patients who are likely later to need a revision operation. Continuing research is examining the bone-prosthesis interface in order to improve the union. Some prostheses have a porous surface into which bone can grow (Fig. 3.1) whilst others are coated in bone mineral, hydroxyapatite, in order to encourage bone ingrowth (Thomas, 1990).

The success rate of knee replacement has increased steadily over the last decade to rival that of hip replacement and is now able to relieve pain in 95 per cent of patients and increase function in 90 per cent. This improvement has occurred with the adoption of resurfacing procedures rather than wholesale joint replacement (Fig. 3.2). Hinged prostheses and prostheses with long intramedullary stems are now being used much more selectively. Resurfacing of the joint with condylar replacements also reduces the sacrifice of bone stock at operation and makes possible later revision procedures. Knee replacement is particularly effective in young patients with severe rheumatoid arthritis where a condylar replacement may be expected to last 15 years in 90 per cent of patients (Noble *et al.*, 1987). The risk of deep vein thrombosis and pulmonary embolus is greater than with hip replacement (Stulberg *et al.*, 1984) possibly because both knees are commonly operated on at the same time.

For surgery of the lower limb there are many advantages in the use of regional anaesthesia for those patients who are suitable, and much of this section will consequently be given over to a discussion of epidural and spinal anaesthesia.

(a) 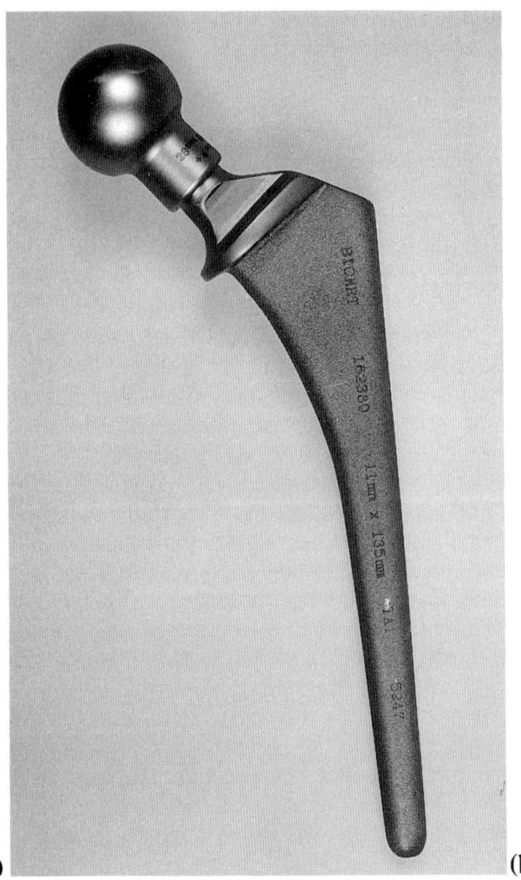

(b) 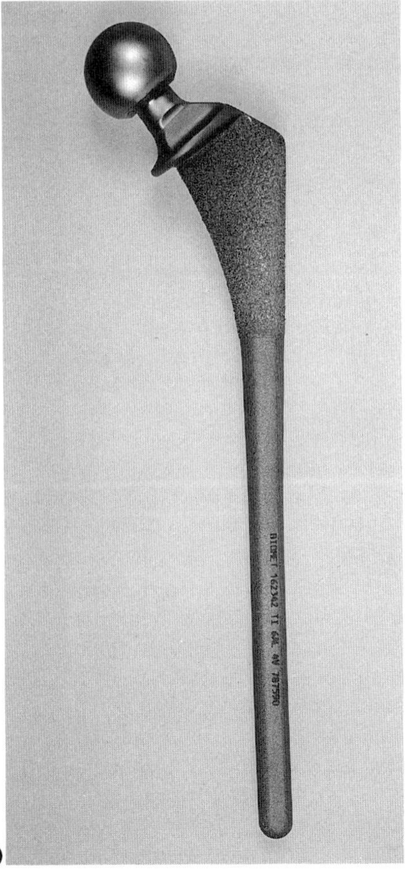

Fig 3.1(a) Femoral prosthesis; plain shaft. (b) Femoral prosthesis; porous coated shaft.

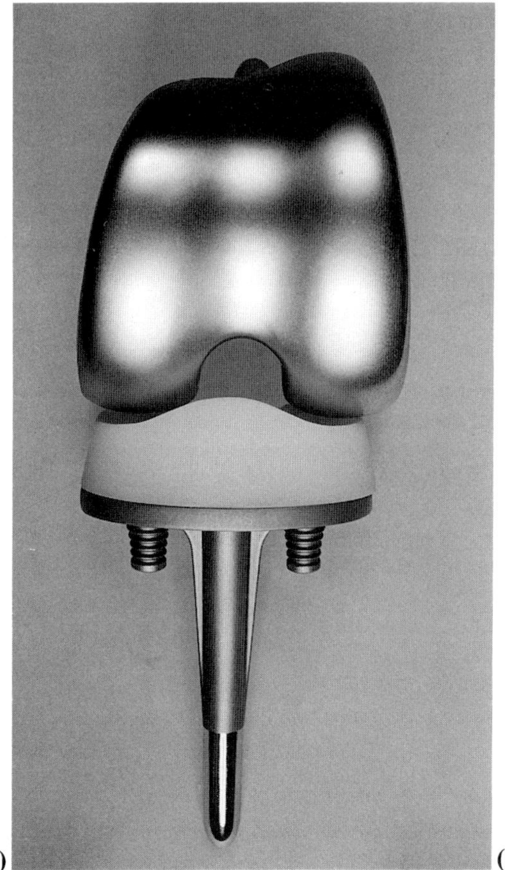
(a)

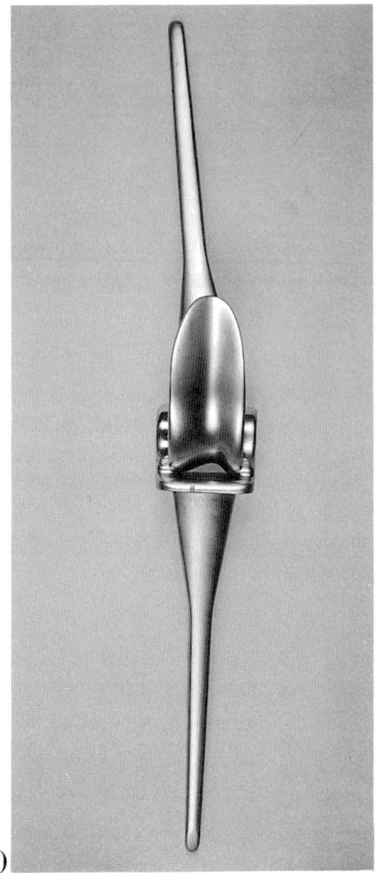
(b)

Fig 3.2(a) Knee replacement; condylar prostheses. (b) Knee replacement; hinge prosthesis.

Regional blocks and general anaesthesia

> One important advance (in hip replacement surgery) has been the introduction of regional anaesthesia, which has decreased the incidence of deep vein thrombosis and pulmonary embolism by two-thirds when compared with general anaesthesia.
>
> (Clift and Rowley, 1992)

This quotation probably overstates the case but nevertheless evidence has been accumulating over the past decade that spinal and epidural blocks reduce the incidence of deep vein thrombosis (see Table 3.1). There are 3 suggested means by which this might occur; an increase in leg blood flow with less stasis; blockade of sympathetic-mediated increases in clotting factors; and an antithrombotic effect of local anaesthetic agents themselves.

Circulatory changes with epidural anaesthesia

Sympathetic blockade resulting from epidural anaesthesia leads to dilatation of arteries and veins in the dermotomes supplied by the blocked sympathetic efferent fibres. There may be compensatory vasoconstriction elsewhere. Modig *et al.* (1980) compared the circulation in the legs of patients receiving general anaesthesia and regional anaesthesia: they found that calf blood flow and venous capacity were lower in patients during general anaesthesia and significantly lower again when measured 3 hours postoperatively. In 3 of the 8 patients receiving general anaesthesia venous capacity was so low postoperatively that thrombus formation could be presumed. Davis *et al.* (1989) found an enhanced rate of blood flow in the legs and decreased venous compliance in patients who had spinal anaesthesia for total hip replacement. They concluded that the augmented blood flow contributed to the improvement in incidence of deep vein thrombosis in these patients. The

Table 3.1 Incidence of deep vein thrombosis in published series comparing general anaesthesia (GA) with regional anaesthesia (RA)

Study	Number	Joint	Detection	Block	GA (%)	RA (%)	P
Modig et al. (1981)	30	Hip	Venography	Epidural	73	20	0.05
Thornburn et al. (1980)	85	Hip	Venography and fibrinogen	Spinal	54	29	0.05
Sharrock et al. (1991)	541	Knee	Venography	Epidural	64	48	0.001
Jorgensen et al. (1991)	39	Knee	Venography	Epidural	59	18	0.002

circulation in the legs thus becomes hyperdynamic during epidural or spinal anaesthesia with reduced blood transit time, in contrast to conditions during general anaesthesia when the circulation in the legs is sluggish, particularly if venous pressure is forced up by positive pressure ventilation of the lungs.

Despite venodilatation with epidural and spinal blocks, venous pooling is reduced, provided drainage is maintained with a small degree of head-down tilt, which also reduces venous ooze from the operation site and thus improves operating conditions. Venous return to the heart is preserved and therefore cardiac output is maintained or even shows a modest increase (German *et al.*, 1979).

Changes in coagulation with epidural anaesthesia

There is a complicated series of changes in blood coagulation factors associated with the stress response to surgery which are difficult to investigate because of the considerable individual variation. During surgery enhanced fibrinolysis occurs whilst factor VIIIC and VIIIRAg concentrations decrease initially, due to consumption, and then increase. There is also evidence of platelet activation. These changes reach a peak of hypercoagulability about the fifth postoperative day marked by prolonged euglobulin clot lysis time, increased platelet count and increased platelet coagulant activity (Walsh *et al.*, 1976). Bredbacka *et al.* (1986) found that the stress-induced increase in factor VIII complex activity in patients who underwent hysterectomy with epidural anaesthesia was attenuated compared with women who had general anaesthesia. Davis *et al.* (1987) showed that spinal anaesthesia for hip replacement was associated with a fall in thrombin generation index (TGI) during surgery compared with a rise in a comparable group which received general anaesthesia, but by the fifth day TGI had risen to markedly increased levels in both groups: factor VIIIRAg remained at baseline values in the spinal anaesthesia group as long as the spinal was effective, before climbing sharply to match levels found in the general anaesthesia group. Factor VIII responses correlate closely with adrenaline concentration and are blocked by propranolol (Small *et al.*, 1984), which suggests that this response is mediated by the sympathetic nervous system. Activation of the sympathetic nervous system during surgery is blocked by epidural or spinal anaesthesia: Engquist *et al.* (1980) found that epidural blockade of afferent (and efferent) pathways during and after hysterectomy, inhibited the secretion of adrenaline seen in patients subjected to hysterectomy under general anaesthesia. The role of sympathetic blockade with regional anaesthesia in the modification of the haemostatic response to surgery remains unclear but there is at least a suggestion that it plays a beneficial part.

Anti-platelet effects of local anaesthetic agents

Local anaesthetic agents themselves have properties which may offer some further protection against thrombus formation: Luostarinen *et al.* (1981) demonstrated that lignocaine, and to a lesser extent, bupivacaine, reduced platelet aggregation and reduced adhesion between blood cells and vessel walls after microvascular injury. This work provided an explanation for the earlier observation of Cooke (1977) that infusion of lignocaine intravenously after hip replacement to provide analgesia appeared to reduce the incidence of deep vein thrombosis. When the infusion was stopped, the rate of deep vein thrombosis returned to that of the control group.

Although regional anaesthesia reduces the incidence of venous thromboembolism, it remains an appreciable hazard and it is important that effective adjuvant forms of prophylaxis are employed, particularly some form of anticoagulation.

The effect of epidural and spinal anaesthesia on blood loss

There is little doubt that operative blood loss is reduced when a regional block is used. Modig and Karlstrom (1987) measured blood loss during hip replacement using 3 techniques of anaesthesia; epidural block with sedation; intubation and spontaneous respiration with halothane; intubation with non-depolarizing relaxant and automatic ventilation of the lungs with fentanyl supplementation. Blood loss was measured intraoperatively and postoperatively for the first 24 hours. In the epidural group intraoperative blood loss was 17 per cent lower than the inhalation group and 38 per cent lower than the ventilated group. Postoperative loss was also significantly lower in the epidural group than in the other two groups which had a similar loss. These results are in agreement with many other published studies (Modig and Malmberg, 1975; Modig *et al.*, 1980; Hole *et al.*, 1980; Chin *et al.*, 1982). Modig (1988) ascribed the reduction in blood loss to the lower arterial blood pressure, lower central venous pressure and lower peripheral venous pressure. There was, therefore, less arterial bleeding from the wound and notably less venous oozing. Thus the requirement for blood transfusion was reduced with a consequent reduction in cost and risk of homologous blood transfused. Many patients now wish to avoid blood transfusion if this is possible. At the least, it is easier to delay transfusion until the recovery room where a mismatched transfusion is easier to detect.

Effect of regional anaesthesia on cementing of prostheses

There is also evidence that cementing technique is improved with epidural or spinal anaesthesia. Loosening is now the commonest cause of failure of a prosthesis and results from mechanical failure at the bone-cement interface. If bleeding occurs from the cancellous bone surface during cementing it leads to lamination of the cement and reduces the strength of the bone-cement bond by up to 50 per cent (Bannister *et al.*, 1988). When regional anaesthesia was used, the rate of bleeding from the bone surface was half that associated with general anaesthesia. Bannister *et al.* (1988) concluded that if general anaesthesia were to be used it would be desirable to use induced hypotension. Ranawat *et al.* (1991) assessed the quality of the cement-bone interface from postoperative radiographs in patients who underwent hip replacement under general anaesthesia and under regional anaesthesia. The quality of the bond was significantly better in the regional anaesthesia group and the authors argued that the hypotension recorded in the regional anaesthesia group had facilitated the entry of cement into the bone.

Available evidence suggests then that epidural or spinal anaesthesia is the technique of choice for elective surgery of the lower limb. If a regional block is impractical, an alternative technique based either on simple inhalational anaesthesia or automatic ventilation of the lungs must be used depending on the patient's clinical state and the length of the procedure proposed. In either case consideration should be given to controlling the blood pressure to reduce blood loss and improve cementing.

Techniques of epidural and spinal anaesthesia

Techniques for establishing epidural caudal and spinal blockade are already familiar and in widespread use. At the Hospital for Special Surgery, New York, for example, the use of regional blocks increased sharply from 1985 onwards until now virtually every patient receives either a spinal or an epidural block (Fig. 3.3).

By simple extrapolation from experience with

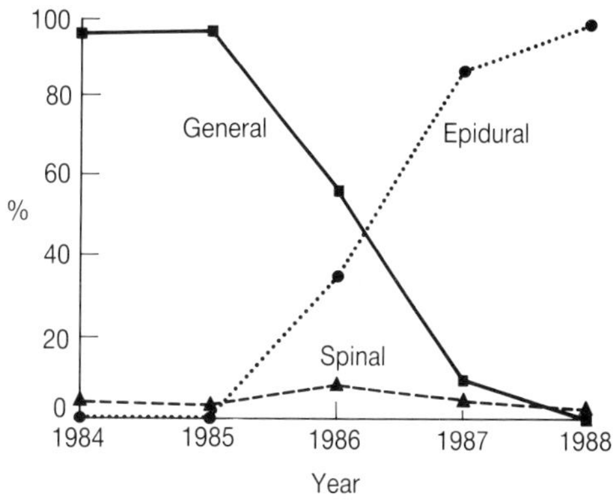

Fig 3.3 The percentage of patients who received general, epidural or spinal anaesthesia for total knee arthroplasty at the Hospital for Special Surgery, New York. Reprinted with permission.

spinal blocks it is best to perform an epidural or caudal block with the patient positioned with the side to be operated on dependent. In practice, however, the difference in level of block achieved on the dependent side when compared with the upper side has been unimpressive. Grundy *et al.* (1978) found that on the upper side the onset of analgesia took a mean of 2 minutes longer and its extent was 2 spinal segments less. There was, however, an important difference in the duration of the block: that on the dependent side lasted about 75 minutes longer. Thus the benefit of positioning a patient for epidural puncture with the side to be operated on underneath is virtually confined to the difference in the duration of the block between the two sides. If an epidural catheter is inserted the difference can easily be overcome and patients who find it too painful to lie on one particular side can have their epidural lying on the other. Great pain in a hip to be revised strongly suggests that the joint is infected.

The age of the patient is an important factor in determining the dosage of local anaesthetic required. Bromage (1962) noted that the dosage required to block a single segment diminished in a linear manner from 20 = 80 years of age. Such a clear pattern was not found by Park *et al.* (1980) who also related dosage to height: below 40 years of age the dose required was 0.69 ml/segment per metre of height and above 40 years of age 0.62 ml/segment per metre of height, with no further decline. This discrepancy is probably explained by the different methods of investigation. Bromage used a varying volume of agent whilst Park and colleagues used a constant volume of 20 ml and measured the varying result. Since local anaesthetic is lost from the epidural space through intervertebral foramina, the greater the dose injected, the greater will be the dose requirement per segment. Park and colleagues also found that the patient's height was a significant factor, but this of course tends to diminish with age – in their study from 1.79 m at 20 years to 1.71 m at 80 years – so that by giving results per unit of height, Park and colleagues were in fact eliminating a factor which changes with age but was not germane to their argument. In practice the range of dosage is from 8–20 ml of bupivacaine. If there is concern about the age or fitness of the patient a catheter can be inserted and the appropriate dose built up in increments of say 5 ml which allows progressive cardiovascular compensation to occur and cushions the effect upon the blood pressure. Epidural anaesthesia has no advantage in that catheter techniques are familiar and their hazards known: spinal catheters have become available but are expensive and the risk of infection rises when the dura is breached.

Although kyphoscoliosis in the patient may present a relative contraindication to epidural or spinal block – and it is unwise to plan to use epidural anaesthesia without inspecting the patient's back – epidurals are frequently carried out in such individuals (Carlson *et al.*, 1978). Surprisingly frequently, minor degrees of kyphoscoliosis are present and epidural puncture will be difficult if this is not recognized. A plain AP radiograph of the lumbar spine will show the amount of anatomical distortion but usually the lower lumbar vertebrae, approaching the sacrum, are in increasingly normal alignment so that the epidural space can be entered at L3–4 or L4–5 level. When most elderly patients are positioned for an epidural the apparent midline of the skin droops below the anatomical midline because the skin is loose and baggy so the anatomical features must be determined by palpation before inserting the needle.

Complications of epidural and spinal anaesthesia

Accidental dural puncture is seldom a problem provided it is recognized: it is usually revealed by a free flow of cerebrospinal fluid from the needle. Rotation of the epidural needle (i.e. drilling motion) and aspiration of the needle may promote puncture and should be avoided (Hollway and Telford, 1991).

Orthopaedic patients are usually immobilized in bed for 24–48 hours after operation to prevent dislocation of a prosthesis or awaiting 'cure' of a plaster so that spinal headaches even after a dural tap with a 16 swg Tuohy needle are very uncommon. If the dura is pierced then a suitable dose of heavy bupivacaine perhaps with morphine added for postoperative analgesia, should be injected and the block converted to a spinal block.

Complications and difficulties with central neural blockade continue to be reported and there is no doubt that care and constant vigilance are the price of using the techniques safely. Many difficulties arise from the superimposition of general anaesthesia when profound falls in blood pressure may occur, followed rapidly by cardiac arrest. Autonomic blockade is more extensive than sensory block, indeed there is an incidence of Horner's syndrome with lumbar epidural anaesthesia (Mohan and Potter, 1975; Evans *et al.*, 1975) due to blockade of cervical sympathetic fibres. This must be anticipated when performing the block and considered when the general fitness of patients for surgery is being assessed.

It is preferable to carry out the block with the patient awake and responsive since the complications of hypotension, accidental intravascular injection or total spinal block are more quickly recognized. All usual monitoring should be connected throughout.

Hypotension

Hypotension occurs surprisingly quickly after epidural injection of bupivacaine: at 2 minutes the blood pressure had fallen by 12 per cent (Kerkkamp and Gielen, 1991) and went on to fall by 21 per cent at 20 minutes in fit young patients, before recovering. In the same study, however, if ropivacaine was injected the changes occurred more slowly reaching a maximum at 20 minutes with a fall in pressure of only 12 per cent. Ropivacaine is a new aminoamide long-acting local anaesthetic and initial trials suggest it has less cardiotoxicity than bupivacaine (Arthur *et al.*, 1988) on a dose for dose basis and also that it possesses vasoconstrictive properties (Kopacz *et al.*, 1988). With its benign effects on the circulation, ropivacaine could become a very useful drug for epidural anaesthesia.

It has been customary to preload patients with a litre of crystalloid solution before carrying out a spinal or epidural block in order to prevent systemic hypotension, but there is no evidence that this is effective in the elderly (Coe, 1990) and it may even cause pulmonary oedema. Hypotension can be minimized by using the smallest dose of bupivacaine consistent with the block required, by giving this dose in increment over 20 minutes and by delaying induction of general anaesthesia as long as possible. Undue arterial hypotension should be treated by a sympathomimetic venoconstrictor either ephedrine in 3 mg aliquots intravenously or, if the tachycardia is undesirable because of ischaemic heart disease, then methoxamine, a pure α-agonist, 1–2 mg intravenously.

Intravascular injection

Intravascular injection of local anaesthetic is the most common cause of adverse reactions in epidural anaesthesia (Covino, 1978) and is difficult to detect with a small volume test – dose. It may be recognized if blood leaks from the needle after puncture. It is better therefore to leave the needle open for a moment before connecting a syringe for injection of the drug and then passing the catheter. Similarly, cerebrospinal fluid runs more easily through the needle than the catheter and is more easily seen. Verniquet (1980) found a substantial reduction in the frequency of vessel puncture in obstetric patients if the dose of local anaesthetic was injected directly through the epidural needle rather than indirectly through the catheter. Similar findings were reported by Mannion *et al.* (1991) who found that dural vessel puncture occurred less often if the catheter were preceded by 10 ml of saline through the needle. The fluid injected creates a space for the catheter which is usually easier to thread as a result.

Spinal anaesthesia

Subarachnoid block has few disadvantages in orthopaedic anaesthesia and is more certain for procedures below the knee than caudal extradural anaesthesia: it is also more rapid in onset. Since postspinal headache is seldom a problem, there is less need to use a fine needle and in many elderly patients a 22 swg needle is required to pierce thickened spinal ligaments. Even a needle of this gauge is deflected in its path by the bevel (Drummond and Scott, 1980) by about 1 mm for each 1 cm travelled. Thus with the bevel facing laterally to avoid shearing longitudinal fibres of the dura the needle is progressively forced away from the midline. Drummond and Scott showed that this effect was reduced if an introducer was used or if the needle was whistle tipped.

Dense spinal anaesthesia of long duration may be obtained by using hyperbaric bupivacaine 0.5 per cent: Chambers *et al.* (1982) found that the mean duration of analgesia after 2 ml of 0.5 per cent in 8 per cent dextrose was more than 3 hours and almost 4 hours when a volume of 3 ml was used. The onset of analgesia was slow and took 20 minutes to be complete. Plain bupivacaine is hypobaric at body temperature and so could be used to block the upper side with the patient in the lateral position. However, the spread of solution is unpredictable and the upper limit of the block variable from patient to patient (Cameron *et al.*, 1981).

Supplementation of regional anaesthesia

After the block is established and checked, with pain free movement of the arthritic joint and demonstration of a sensory level, general anaesthesia can be induced. Smaller induction and maintenance doses of anaesthetic agents will be required owing to the hypotension produced by the block and to the depressant effects upon the central nervous system of plasma concentrations of lignocaine or bupivacaine.

For most patients light anaesthesia with an infusion of propofol intravenously is all that is necessary for the period of surgery. Because of the epidural, smaller infusion rates are needed than the regimen recommended by Roberts *et al.* (1988). Induction by infusion occurs over 2 or 3 minutes at a rate of 6 mg/kg/hr, and for maintenance a little over half that rate is required. The infusion can be delivered from any standard infusion pump which should preferably have a separate venous cannula (Fig. 3.4). If the propofol is fed into the intravenous line, the latter should be protected by a non-return valve which prevents the propofol from backing-up the giving set in the event of an obstructed infusion (Fig. 3.5). The delivery site should be in view at all times.

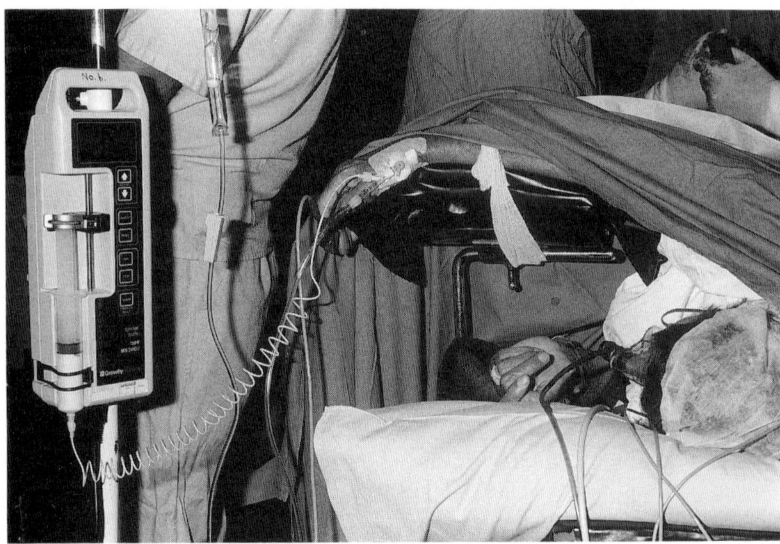

Fig 3.4 Intravenous sedation with propofol. Arrangement of pump (left) and intravenous line.

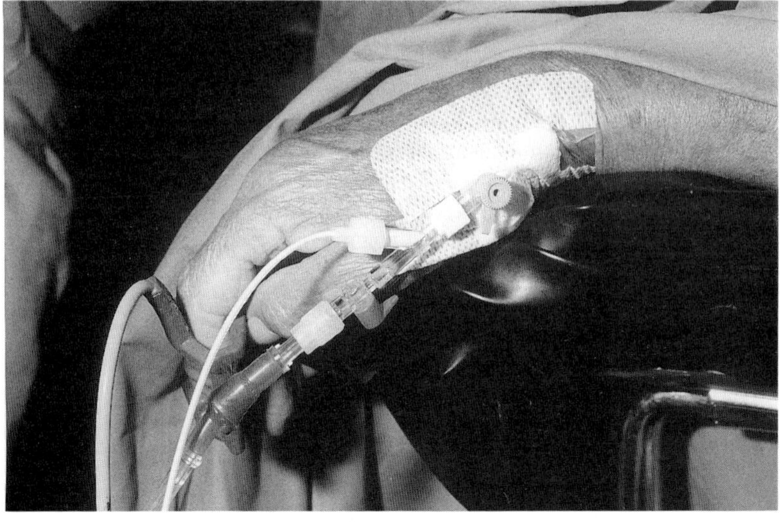

Fig 3.5 Intravenous sedation with propofol. Non-return valve Y connector joining propofol and intravenous infusions.

Infusion pumps are still at an early stage of development and one should be chosen with adequate alarms to warn of an obstructed line and the end of the infusion since either of these events will allow the patient to wake up. Disposable syringes are lubricated for single use only and the resistance of the syringe rises if it is refilled and used again: some infusion pumps cannot deal with the added resistance whilst others will simply alarm. A second full syringe should be immediately available to exchange for the empty one: if time is spent refilling the original syringe, the patient may become too light.

The patient should breathe added oxygen from a polythene mask and bubble tubing. There is seldom any need to intubate the trachea or even use a laryngeal mask: many operations are performed with the patient in the lateral position and maintenance of the airway requires no special measures. If the patient is supine, there may be a tendency for airway obstruction to occur: this can be resolved with the gentle insertion of a soft nasopharyngeal airway. To save time, the patient can be positioned on the table ready for surgery as induction proceeds. Intubation and deeper anaesthesia are necessary only if it is decided to ventilate the patient or if there is a history of regurgitation or hiatus hernia.

Propofol (di-isoprophyl phenol as a 1 per cent emulsion in 10 per cent soya bean oil, 1.2 per cent egg phosphatide and 2.5 per cent glycerol) is a near perfect agent in these circumstances. Low-dose infusion with the patient breathing oxygen enriched air preserves cardiovascular stability, even in the elderly (Claeys *et al.*, 1988), and permits very rapid recovery at the end of the operation. Normal mental function is usually quickly restored and the post-operative period is marked by a freedom from nausea. Induction by bolus dosage in elderly patients causes a fall in blood pressure of 35 per cent (Larsen *et al.*, 1988) and may increase myocardial ischaemia in patients with coronary artery disease (Otteni *et al.*, 1987). If a bolus is given, it should be given slowly and in reduced dosage of 1–1.5 mg/kg.

Induced hypotension

Hypotensive techniques of anaesthesia have been employed for surgery of the pelvis, hip and upper femur where tourniquets cannot be used to create a satisfactory surgical field and to reduce blood loss (Lawson *et al.*, 1976; Vazeery and Lunde, 1979). The hypotension is usually achieved either by central neural blockade or by using specific hypotensive agents such as sodium nitroprusside (SNP) labetalol or trimetaphan or by inhaled anaesthetic agents. It is not clear that blood loss is directly related to blood pressure: other factors such as venous pressure are also important. The advantages of induced hypotension must be weighed against the risk for any particular patient and the techniques used with care in the elderly. If SNP is used, the toxic dose must not be exceeded – this was found by Vesey *et al.* (1976) to be 1.5 mg/kg – and the body temperature must be monitored since the widespread vasodilatation and the inhibition of cellular metabolism brought about by quantities of cyanide released from SNP are likely to lead to hypothermia (Vesey and Cole, 1975). Any hypotensive infusion should be withdrawn gradually towards the end of surgery to avoid rebound hypertension associated with increased plasma renin concentrations (Khambatta, 1979) and to allow the surgeon to complete haemostasis as the wound is closed. Any prophylactic antibiotics must be given before the hypotensive phase since there is evidence that penetration of the drug into bone at low blood pressures is impaired.

Anaesthesia for specific operations

Hip replacement

A particular problem posed by replacement of the hip joint is the use of polymethylmethacrilate cement to secure the acetabular and femoral prostheses and to act as a grouting agent. Commonly there is a fall in arterial pressure following insertion of bone cement and this fall is greater after insertion into the femoral shaft. Whilst the fall in arterial pressure is usually slight and transient, on occasion it is precipitate and severe. The cement is cold-curing methylmethacrilate supplied in two packs: an ampoule of liquid monomer and a sterile package of finely powdered methylmethacrilate polymer. The two are mixed under sterile conditions with the evolved vapour ducted away until the semifluid mass acquires the consistency of dough. Liquid monomer is known to be cytotoxic; when injected into dogs, it causes hypotension, tachycardia and a large increase in cardiac output associated with peripheral vasodilatation

(Peebles *et al.*, 1972; Ellis and Mulvein 1973). The cement consistency should therefore be as stiff as possible before insertion so that little monomer remains. The reaction is exothermic and the mix rapidly becomes hot.

Although it is possible that, in some cases, absorption of liquid monomer from the operation site is the cause of the observed hypotension, it seems more likely that air embolism observed in up to 30 per cent of patients is the dominant clinical event (Ngai *et al.*, 1974; Michel, 1980). After reaming the femur, an air space is created and venous sinuses are opened: this space is then closed with a plug of hot cement and finally the femoral prosthesis is driven into the space to exclude all air. Although an attempt is made to vent the cavity with a fine polythene tube, this has been shown to have little effort on intramedullary pressures which may rise to 1900 mmHg (Phillips *et al.*, 1971).

Significant falls in PaO_2 lasting up to 30 minutes have also been found following insertion of methylmethacrilate cement (Park *et al.*, 1973; Turnbull *et al.*, 1974; Modig and Malmberg, 1975). Modig and Malmberg (1975) also reported an increase in pulmonary vascular resistance following impaction of the femoral prosthesis. They suggested that crushed femoral medullary contents including fat were injected into the pulmonary circulation in addition to air as microemboli lodging chiefly in the better-perfused dependent pulmonary vascular bed. This caused local pulmonary vasoconstriction with a resulting increase in pulmonary vascular resistance and disturbance of ventilation-perfusion relationships. Methylmethacrilate cement is a fat solvent and may even predispose to fat embolism by mobilizing fat from the marrow of the femur.

In order to improve distribution of cement within the femoral cavity many surgeons now use a cement gun to inject cement into the femur, beginning at the bottom and layering the cement up the cavity. This has the effect of displacing the contained air and reduces the incidence of air embolism (Evans *et al.*, 1989). Evans and colleagues also noted further episodes of air embolism occurring when the leg was straightened as the joint was reduced at the end of surgery.

Blood pressure should be monitored closely during the insertion of bone cement into both acetabulum and femur as supportive measures may be required if a steep fall in pressure does occur. It is important not to be behind with blood and fluid replacement at this stage since this is likely to compound any cardiovascular changes: if nitrous oxide is being used, it should be withdrawn from 10 minutes before femoral cementing and additional oxygen given. This will reduce rather than expand an air embolus and counter the hypoxaemia which follows insertion of the femoral prosthesis.

Uncemented prostheses seem to be free of these problems but the surgery takes longer because of the greater precision required and the blood loss is correspondingly higher. Some centres have adopted 'hybrid' total hip arthroplasties consisting of a press-fit acetabulum (i.e. uncemented) and a cemented press-fit femoral component. This is to overcome the inevitable compromise that arises because press-fit components cannot be produced in sizes to fit everyone. Compression with these femoral components is likely to be greater when cemented than with components intended to be used with cement. Watson and Stulberg (1989) reported 4 cases of severe fat embolism after such arthroplasties. In each case, respiratory failure and cerebral confusion developed soon after recovery from anaesthesia. Tachycardia and pyrexia were accompanied by pulmonary oedema and all developed petechial skin rashes. Two of the cases required artificial ventilation for 3 and 4 days. These authors considered that epidural anaesthesia had contributed to the development of fat embolism because of the low venous pressure and increased venous capacitance.

Total knee replacement

Owing to the greater biomechanical complexity of the knee, a wide range of replacement prostheses has been developed. Knee replacements differ not so much in minor detail but more in matters of fundamental conception, and experience in their use is still being accumulated. At present most patients receive surface replacements and hinges or constrained replacements are reserved for the more severely affected joints of older patients.

The problems of heavy blood loss and systemic absorption of air or debris are usually bypassed, since most knee replacements are carried out with an arterial tourniquet in place. However, Harris (1970) reported a case of cardiac arrest when the tourniquet was deflated and debris, fat or air gained access to the systemic circulation. No tourniquet is used when the patient has peripheral vascular disease and then haemodynamic changes are found similar to those that occur with hip replacement, if marrow cavities are reamed and cemented. Mean overall blood loss was a little more than 2 units (Berman *et al.*, 1988) and was greater when the femur was reamed. Commonly both knees are replaced together as patients tolerate it well and rehabilitation time is reduced. Postoperative pain, however, is very severe.

Long-term complications of joint replacement

The chief complications of joint replacement are dislocation, loosening, infection and mechanical failure. Most of these require revision arthroplasty which is becoming an ever more common operation. Some surgeons now find that half of all hip replacements are revisions (Wroblewski, 1990) and that proportion is likely to increase.

Dislocation usually occurs early and is the least serious problem. Artificial joints all employ the surrounding tissues to hold the joint surfaces in apposition, so that until the cut and divided tissues have repaired, the joint can dislocate easily. This is most likely to happen in the restless or confused patient in whom it is impossible to maintain the joint in its most stable position. Continuing epidural anaesthesia makes restless movement less likely but the reduced muscle tone increases the likelihood of dislocation during nursing procedures – lifting onto a bedpan, for example. Early dislocation is treated by reduction under light general anaesthesia, which may need supplementation with a depolarizing muscle relaxant to allow the surgeon to overcome muscle tone. A plaster hip spica is then applied to prevent further movement and allow healing to take place. Late dislocation or recurrent dislocation usually occurs because of incorrect placing of one or other of the components and requires full operative revision.

Loosening is the commonest complication and presents as increasing pain and instability, often following a fall. It is confirmed by demonstrating movement on *X*-ray screening with 'telescoping' of the femoral component and is treated by the replacement of one or both prostheses. Loosening always raises the suspicion of infection in the joint.

Infection is the most serious complication and the most to be feared since it too often condemns the patient to years of pain and an unsatisfactory result after a great deal of surgery. Current management is aggressive with removal of the infected prosthesis and its replacement using gentamycin impregnated cement. Initial results are good with a 91 per cent success rate at 2 years. Slightly better results are achieved by a 2-stage procedure with removal of the prosthesis, a 3 to 6 week course of antibiotics and reimplantation carried out 3–12 months later. If this is not possible, usually because of loss of bone, the patient is left with an excision arthroplasty (Girdlestone's operation) and a pain-free though unstable and short leg. Excision arthroplasty is associated with heavy blood loss because of the large potential space left afterwards which cannot be closed and the amount of blood loss is easily underestimated. Infection at the knee may be followed by further replacement, arthrodesis and finally amputation.

Patients presenting for these operations are often in intense pain and systemically ill with intermittent fevers and anaemia due to toxic suppression of bone marrow. They cannot be positioned adequately for spinal or epidural anaesthesia whilst awake. Their intake of powerful analgesics may have led to hepatic enzyme induction and to tolerance of narcotic analgesic supplements administered during anaesthesia. The procedure itself takes longer because of the need to remove the components and all the old cement and blood loss is consequently greater. The operations are expensive with costs due to investigations, antibiotic cover, antibiotic impregnated cement, use of non-standard prostheses longer hospital stays and a greater use of consumable items. It all adds up to an argument to cut no corners with primary joint replacement!

The trend is towards creating centres specializing in revision procedures with experience of advanced bone grafting techniques, custom made components and sophisticated microbiological advice available in order to achieve the best results.

There are a number of reports of implants becoming infected by blood stream spread of organisms arising in distant sites. A review of 43 cases gave the recognizable source of infection as skin 46 per cent; dental 15 per cent; urinary tract 13 per cent; and gastrointestinal tract in 2 per cent (Maderazo, 1988). Particularly at risk were patients who were medically compromised with rheumatoid arthritis, diabetes mellitus or who were immunosuppressed. Provision of antibiotic cover for patients who have a prosthetic joint and undergo other procedures likely to cause a bacteraemia remains controversial. Until conclusive data are available one report recommends prophylactic phenoxymethylpenicillin or erythromycin in all patients (Nelson *et al.*, 1990).

Mechanical failure is becoming less common as

the design and material of prostheses improve. In the hip (where experience is greatest) it is usually the intramedullary stem of the femoral prosthesis which fractures across, especially in active men. The removal of the distal fragment from the femoral shaft can be extremely difficult, usually requiring a window to be opened in the distal femur to allow the impacted terminal portion to be knocked out from below.

The replacement of painful, stiff or deformed joints is now commonplace: the implants are reliable and dramatically successful. The challenge is how to cope with success?

Surgery of the upper limb

The surgery of the upper limb divides into a series of small operations performed on the hand and forearm such as carpal tunnel release, fasciectomy, trigger finger release and tenolysis, and larger repair procedures such as joint replacement of wrist, elbow or shoulder or following major trauma to the hand and arm. Many of the smaller operations can be performed as day cases under either regional anaesthesia or light general anaesthesia and are considered elsewhere (Day Surgery – Chapter 9, Regional Anaesthesia – Chapter 8). Techniques of anaesthesia for the large procedures consist largely of regional anaesthesia supplemented with general anaesthesia as for the lower limb.

Microsurgical techniques

The search for better functional results of surgical repair after trauma has drawn heavily upon microsurgical techniques and linked orthopaedic surgeons more closely to their plastic surgery colleagues. Experience with microsurgical repair of nerve trunks and minute vessels had led on to free skin transfer, the transfer of more complex myocutaneous flaps for immediate skin cover of traumatic skin defects and finally to complete replantation of severed parts. The operating microscope offers perfect illumination and magnification of the surgical field up to 25 or 40 times, making possible better alignment of small structures – nerves and vessels which may be sutured accurately using 10/0 sutures specially developed for the purpose.

Complete cover of a traumatic skin defect can be achieved in one operation by using a skin or a myocutaneous transfer; earlier it was necessary to raise pedicle grafts in a series of operations transferring a skin flap to its intended site whilst always preserving a vascular supply through the pedicle. A skin transfer consists of an area of skin complete with its vessels of supply and drainage, which is sutured into a new site: arterial and venous anastomoses are carried out to existing vessels. The skin transfer may be taken from the inguinal region where, drawing upon skin folds, adequate skin closure is easily achieved. Myocutaneous transfers consist of a muscle with its vascular supply and overlying skin, and are similarly used to provide skin cover of a large defect. Although there are many suitable donor sites (and more are constantly being devised for specific applications) the latissimus dorsi provides a large flap with a vascular supply composed of vessels 2 mm or more in diameter. This makes it easier to work on and more reliable. Minimal functional deficit is left after transfer because of the overlap of function of neighbouring muscles. The latissimus dorsi also has a particularly long vascular pedicle which makes vascular anastomosis easier. Bone from one or two ribs can also be incorporated in the flap because the pedicle of latissimus dorsi anastomoses with intercostal vessels, and this has been used for replacing part of the mandible, for example. The cutaneous innervation of some flaps may be preserved and reconnected to provide innervated skin cover which is particularly useful for covering skin defects of the hand or foot. Suitable donor sites are from the thigh (using tensor fascia lata and the lateral cutaneous nerve of the thigh) or a deltoid flap from the shoulder complete with its neurovascular pedicle. The nerve may then be sutured to a sensory nerve at the recipient site. These procedures take many hours unless two surgical teams are available – one to prepare the donor site and one to prepare the skin defect – but complete cover is thus obtained with one operation and the patient's time in hospital and away from work is minimized.

Sustained attempts have been made to anastomose divided nerve, with mixed results (Dickson, 1978). Better anatomical continuity can be achieved if the cut ends are dissected into individual fascicles to be matched and sutured; it is hoped that there will thus be less confusion of motor, sensory and autonomic fascicles, and greater chances of nerve regeneration and recovery of function. In the proximal part of the course of a nerve individual fascicles are constantly changing position, so matching and repair are technically more difficult and the result is correspondingly poorer; better results are obtained with more peripheral nerve injuries. There is debate about the optimum time to carry out nerve repair, but if repair is delayed, the period of degeneration of the limb is lengthened which allows muscle atrophy to occur and, after 9 months, dissolution and loss of sensory nerve endings, principally Meissner's corpuscles, now thought to be responsible for discriminant sensation (Dellon, 1981). The repair should be as atraumatic as possible, avoiding lengthy mobilization of the cut ends which tends to devascularize the nerve trunk; meticulous intraneural haemostasis is required to prevent the formation of an intraneural haematoma. In practised hands, correct interfascicular matching is achieved for about 90 per cent of bundles (Millesi, 1977). Detailed dissection is eased by the use of an arterial tourniquet. When there is loss of nerve substance, interfascicular nerve grafting may be carried out using, commonly, the sural nerve whose loss gives rise only to a mild hypoaesthesia behind the lateral malleolus at the ankle or other similarly relatively unimportant sensory nerves (e.g. the medial cutaneous nerve of the forearm, the lateral cutaneous nerve of the thigh and the posterior cutaneous nerve of the forearm).

Anaesthesia for nerve repair, skin transfers and myocutaneous flaps

These procedures are lengthy, taking up to 8 hours; anaesthesia must be planned with this in mind. For nerve repair there are no additional special requirements, but for skin and myocutaneous transfers consideration throughout anaesthesia must be given to the preservation of perfusion through the graft. Regional anaesthesia alone is seldom possible because the donor and recipient sites may be widely separated and epidural anaesthesia is not popular because of the difficulty of being certain that perfusion is always adequate. During anaesthesia, blood pressure should be maintained and hypotension avoided at all costs; blood replacement should run a little ahead of loss so that the circulating blood volume is always preserved. All blood transfused should be warmed and filtered. a-Adrenergic blocking agents may be used in cautious increments to secure dilatation of vessels supplying the flap, and some surgeons advocate that isoxsuprine, a further vasodilator, be given during the completion of the anastomoses. Circulating blood volume must be adequate at this point to ensure that the increase in vascular capacity does not cause hypotension.

Automatic ventilation of the lungs is to be preferred to spontaneous ventilation for the longer procedures, which may last all day, but care must be taken to ensure that a respiratory alkalosis is not induced with resultant vasoconstriction. Ventilation should be adjusted to give a normal or even a slightly elevated $PaCO_2$, which should be checked frequently during the procedure either by blood gas analysis or by the use of an end tidal CO_2 analyser. The patient's body temperature must be carefully maintained so that vasoconstriction of skin vessels triggered by a fall in body temperature does not occur; a warming blanket should be used under the patient and heat conserved by an aluminized space blanket; skin and core temperatures should be monitored throughout anaesthesia. It may be necessary to reposition the patient between raising the flap and suturing it in position if both sites are not readily accessible at once. Two tourniquets may be in use on separate limbs and these should be deflated one at a time if circulatory stability is to be maintained. When sections of rib are removed, although efforts are made not to pierce the pleura, this is almost inevitable and it is preferable to drain the chest postoperatively.

Replantation of severed parts

The combining of these techniques of repair of nerves and small vessels of supply is being used increasingly in the replantation of parts of limbs severed by trauma. Major centres of replantation have developed, such as those at Munich and Louisville, Kentucky, and the results reported are encouraging; centres that perform 20 or more replantations per year are obtaining 80 per cent or better success rates (Urbaniak, 1979). The initial problem of maintaining viability of the replant has thus largely been overcome and the chief problem remaining is that of the relative success of the nerve repair and the functional result, but this too is improving. Severed parts of both upper and lower limbs have been replanted, but efforts have concentrated upon the upper limb where both the functional result and the cosmetic appearance are more important. Replants have ranged in size from parts of a digit to a hand and even whole limbs.

Deterioration in a severed part begins with loss of

its blood supply and proceeds more rapidly in active tissue such as muscle than in skin, bone or tendon. Thus a hand or limb is more susceptible to ischaemia than is a digit. If stored at just above 0°C, a digit may successfully be replanted after 24 hours whilst in the hand increasingly poor results follow 12 hours' cool ischaemia. There is, however, adequate time after trauma to move a patient to a regional replant centre for surgery following preoperative preparation. With small replants the problems are essentially those of the local repair; with larger replants the volume of ischaemic muscle replanted is greater, so systemic problems arise from myoglobin released by deteriorating muscle (which may precipitate acute renal failure) and metabolic acidosis caused by systemic release of accumulated lactic acid when venous anastomoses are completed.

Indications for replantation

Detailed indications vary from centre to centre, but those generally recognized are as follows:

1. When the patient is a child, much higher success rates are obtained for all replants. The functional results are also better than in adults, and children have less trouble with contractures and joint stiffness.
2. If the thumb is involved, the contribution of the thumb to hand function is so great that, even if the final result is a fixed post for a thumb with poor sensation, then it is worth proceeding.
3. Without digits the hand is almost useless and so an attempt will be made to replant multiple amputated fingers.

In addition, if the thumb or fingers are destroyed, substitutes may be fashioned from the great toe (the thumb) and the second and third toes.

Strong contraindications are: the presence of other major injuries or illness; other injuries to the same limb; extensive tissue damage to the part during amputation with crushing or degloving. In addition, previous surgery at the site adds discouraging technical difficulty. The best results therefore are obtained with a clean amputation in a young patient, and those over 60 are not usually considered for replantation procedures.

Surgical procedure

After dissecting out the structures in the stump and the severed part, the bone is shortened to facilitate adequate debridement and to avoid tension on subsequent anastomoses. Firm bony union should then be obtained by wiring or plating. Usually tendon repair is undertaken before the vascular anastomoses, unless the ischaemia time is long, followed by nerve repair and then skin closure. Whilst restoration of the circulation to the part is essential for its survival, tendon and nerve repair are vital for its function and later surgical procedures may be undertaken to modify or improve function. It is essential that a good arterial inflow through the anastomoses be obtained, but just as important is adequate venous drainage (in the ratio, arteries/veins, 1:2) without which pressure in the part rises, flow falls off and the vessels eventually thrombose. The surgery takes between 4 hours for a simple digital replant and up to 20 hours for a major limb replantation. Details of the surgical procedure are given by O'Brien (1977) and Urbaniak (1979).

Anaesthesia

Preoperative preparation

Preoperative preparation must include a rigorous search for any unrelated hidden injury, particularly in the chest or abdomen, before committing the patient to lengthy surgery. Chest X-ray, electrocardiogram and baseline estimation of serum electrolytes, urea, creatinine, myoglobin, lactate, haemoglobin, packed cell volume and blood gases and pH should be obtained. An estimate of the volume of blood already lost should be made and blood cross-matched for transfusion.

Anaesthetic technique

As with the previous repair procedure, provision must be made for anaesthesia of long duration. The patient should be placed on a padded water circulation (Ripple) mattress with facilities for warming and covered with an aluminized space blanket; a urinary catheter should be passed so that hourly urine output may be measured. Almost all authorities prefer regional anaesthesia (O'Brien, 1977; Urbaniak, 1979; Kleinert and Jupiter, 1981) because of the vasodilation resulting from sympathetic blockade which renders vascular anastomoses easier and improves blood flow through the part. In addition, sedation or light general anaesthesia are used for adult patients and general anaesthesia for chil-

Table 3.2 Monitoring for major replantation procedures

Cardiovascular	Electrocardiogram Arterial pressure from an indwelling arterial cannula Central venous pressure	
Body temperature	Oesophageal Skin (against warming blanket)	
Urine output	Hourly urine production	
Respiration	end-tidal $F\text{ECO}_2$ or respirometer	
Metabolic	Serum electrolytes Urea and creatinine lactate Myoglobin	1. immediately after arterial anastomosis from limb venous return 2. 3 hours later

dren under 12 years. Because the surgery might outlast a one-shot brachial block, even when bupivacaine is used, there is much to be said for a catheter technique as described in Chapter 9. This would further allow continuation of the sympathetic block into the postoperative period and the provision of excellent analgesia. During protracted surgery, comprehensive monitoring (Table 3.2) is mandatory in order to follow cardiovascular and metabolic variables. It is essential that perfusion of the replanted part is never compromised, so blood should be transfused against the central venous pressure to maintain the circulating blood volume; since most patients are young, slight overtransfusion is preferable to undertransfusion. Mircofiltration and warming of transfused blood are advisable to preserve body temperature and to reduce any risk of anastomoses or small vessels becoming clogged with debris. Body temperature must be monitored to ensure that no significant fall or rise occurs. Children in particular may easily become hyperthermic when adequate measures are taken to conserve heat in a warm operating theatre.

Bleeding during surgery should be controlled using a padded pneumatic tourniquet on the limb, which may be deflated and inflated many times during the course of the procedure to provide a surgical field free of blood. This is preferable to using clips directly on vessels which may traumatize them and prejudice the success of an anastomosis.

When the arterial anastomosis is complete and before beginning the venous anastomoses, the torniquet should be released and the part allowed to bleed freely from the veins. This sweeps debris and metabolites out of the capillary bed of the part and reduces the amounts which will enter the systemic circulation when all the anastomoses are complete. This involves rapid blood loss of up to 2 units, which must be replaced immediately.

Drugs to improve blood flow

Various regimens have been suggested for intraoperative heparin, dextran and aspirin, but as confidence has grown in anastomotic techniques so dependence upon drugs has diminished. Heparin in particular is rarely given for replantation of clean amputations, as the benefits are marginal and it has several disadvantages: it may provoke haemorrhage from other injuries; there may be uncontrolled bleeding from the replant, requiring further transfusion with the possibility of rebound clotting in the vascular repairs. In avulsion injuries or where flow is marginal, heparin 3000–5000 i.u. may be given as the first arterial anastomosis is completed, followed by 1000 i.u. hourly (Urbaniak, 1979). Postoperatively, aspirin 300 mg may be given once every 3 days and dextran 40 infused over 12 hours daily for the first 3 days.

Postoperative care

The postoperative management is crucial to success and has been carefully reviewed by Bright and Wright (1979). Meticulous monitoring of the transplanted part is necessary to ensure that thrombosis or failure of a microvascular anastomosis is detected early and the patient returned to theatre so that the vessel can be re-explored. Up to one-third of patients require repeat surgical procedures. Dressings should be arranged so that the colour of the transplanted part is easily visible. The skin temperature should be monitored, both of the part and of a control digit; a discrepancy greater than 2 or 3°C suggests poor perfusion. Other monitoring which may be used includes photoplethysmography and transcutaneous measurement of capillary blood PO^2.

Urine output should be monitored, and patients who have undergone replantation of larger parts should have daily estimation of serum myoglobin and lactate for the first 3 days in addition to electrolyte urea and creatinine.

Pain relief is important since pain or anxiety provokes a rise in sympathetic tone, with constriciton of proximal vessels of supply and reduced blood flow thorugh the replant. In addition, denervation of vessels in the part may lead to denervation sensititivity to circulating catecholamines and profound vasoconstriction (Bright and Wright, 1979). Patients should be sedated with chlorpromazine 25 mg 8-hourly and generous pain relief provided if a regional block is not in use. The patient should be strongly discouraged from smoking, since the vasoconstriction which accompanies it can be enough to sacrifice the replant.

References

Arthur, G. R., Feldman, H. S. and Covino, B. G. (1988). Comparative pharmacokinetics of bupivacaine and ropivacaine, a new amide local anaesthetic agent. *Anesthesia and Analgesia*, **67**, 1053–8.

Bannister, G. C. and Miles, A. W. (1988). The influence of cementing technique and blood on the strength of the bone-cement interface. *Engineering Medicine*, **17**, 131–3.

Berman, A. T., Geissele, A. E. and Bosacco, S. J. (1988). Blood loss with total knee arthroplasty. *Clinical Orthopaedics*, **234**, 137–8.

Brandt, M. R., Fernandes, A., Mordhorst, R. and Kehlet, H. (1978). Epidural anaesthesia improves postoperative nitrogen balance. *British Medical Journal*, **1**, 1106.

Brandt, M. R., Olgaard, K. and Kehlet, H. (1979). Epidural analgesia inhibits the renin and aldosterone response to surgery. *Acta Anaesthesiologica Scandinavica*, **23**, 267.

Bredbacka, S., Blomback, M., Hagnevik, K., Irestedt, L. and Raabe, N. (1986). Peroperative changes in coagulation and fibrinolytic variables during abdominal hysterectomy under epidural or general anaesthesia. *Acta Anaesthesiologica Scandinavica*, **30**, 204–10.

Bright, D. S. and Wright, S. (1979). Postoperative management in replantation. In J. R. Urbaniak and D. S. Bright (eds), *American Academy of Orthopaedic Surgeons Symposium on Microsurgery: Practical Use in Orthopaedics*. Mosby, St Louis, Miss, p. 83.

Bromage, P. R. (1962). Spread of analgesia solutions in the epidural space and their site of action; a statistical study. *British Journal of Anaesthesia*, **34**, 161.

Cameron, A. E., Arnold, R. W., Ghoris, M. W. and Jamieson, V. (1981). Spinal analgesia using bupivacaine 0.5% plain: variation in extent of the block with patient age. *Anaesthesia*, **36**, 318.

Carli, F. and Emery, P. W. (1990). Intra-operative epidural blockade with local anaesthetics and postoperative protein breakdown associated with hip surgery in elderly patients. *Acta Anaesthesiologica Scandinavica*, **34**, 263–6.

Carli, F. and Itiaba, K. (1986). Effect of heat conservation during and after major abdominal surgery on muscle breakdown on elderly patients. *British Journal of Anaesthesia*, **58**, 502–7.

Carlson, D. W., Engelman, D. R. and Bart, A. J. (1978). Epidural anesthesia for cesarian section in kyphoscoliosis. *Anesthesia and Analgesia*, **57**, 125.

Chambers, W. A., Littlewood, D. G., Edstrom, H. H. and Scott, D. B. (1982). Spinal anaesthesia with hyperbaric bupivacaine: effects of concentration and volume administered. *British Journal of Anaesthesia*, **54**, 75.

Chin, S. P., Abou-Madi, M. N., Eurin, B., Witvoet, J. and Montagne, J. (1982). Blood loss in total hip replacement: extradural v. phenoperidine analgesia. *British Journal of Anaesthesia*, **54**, 491.

Christensen, T., Waaben, J., Lindeburg, T., Vesterberg, K., Vinnan, E., Kehlet, H. (1986). Effect of epidural analgesia on muscle aminoacid pattern after surgery. *Acta Chirurgica Scandinavica*, **152**, 407–11.

Claeys, M. A., Gepts, E. and Camu, F. (1988). Haemodynamic changes during anaesthesia induced and maintained with propofol. *British Journal of Anaesthesia*, **60**, 3–9.

Clift, B. A. and Rowley, D. I. (1992). Hip replacement surgery. *British Journal of Hospital Medicine*, **47**, 273–9.

Coe, A. J. (1990). Is crystalloid preloading useful in spinal anaesthesia in the elderly? *Anaesthesia*, **45**, 241–3.

Cooke, E. D., Lloyd, M. J., Bowcock, S. A. and Pilcher, M. F. (1977). Intravenous lignocaine in prevention of deep venous thrombosis after elective hip surgery. *Lancet*, **ii**, 797–9.

Covino, B. G. (1978). Systemic toxicity of local anaesthetic agnets. *Anesthesia and Analgesia*, **57**, 387.

Davis, F. M., Laurenson, V. G., Gillespie, W. J., Foate, J. and Seagar, A. D. (1989). Leg blood flow during total hip replacement under spinal or general anaesthesia. *Anaesthesia and Intensive Care*, **17**, 136–43.

Davis, F. M., McDermott, E., Hickton, C., Wells, E.,

Heaton, D. C., Laurenson, V. G., Gillespie, W. J. and Foate, J. (1987). Influence of spinal and general anaesthesia on haemostasis during total hip arthroplasty. *British Journal of Anaesthesia*, **59**, 561–71.

Dellon, A. L. (1981). *Evaluation of sensibility and reeducation of sensation in the hand*. Williams and Wilkins, Baltimore, Maryland, p. 65.

Dickson, R. A. (1978). Nerve repair. *British Journal of Hospital Medicine*, **20**, 295.

Drummond, G. B. and Scott, D. H. T. (1980). Deflection of spinal needles by the bevel. *Anaesthesia*, **35**, 854.

Edde, R. R. and Deutsch, S. (1977). Cardiac arrest after interscalene brachial plexus block. *Anesthesia and Analgesia*, **56**, 446.

Ellis, R. H. and Mulvein, J. (1973). Cardiovascular effects of methylmethacrilate. *Anesthesiology*, **38**, 102.

Engquist, A., Fog-Muller, F., Christiansen, C., Thode, J., Vester-Anderson, T., Nistrup, Madsen, S. (1980). Influence of epidural analgesia on the catecholamine and cyclic AMP responses to surgery. *Acta Anaesthesiologica Scandinavica*, **24**, 17.

Evans, J. M., Gauci, C. A. and Watkins, G. (1975). Horner's syndrome as a complication of lumbar epidural block. *Anaesthesia*, **30**, 774.

Evans, R. D., Palazzo, M. G. A. and Ackers, J. W. L. (1989). Air embolism during total hip replacement: comparison of two surgical techniques. *British Journal of Anaesthesia*, **62**, 243–7.

Flatt, J. R., Birrell, P. C. and Hobbes, A. (1984). Effects of anaesthesia on some aspects of mental functioning of surgical patients. *Anaesthesia and Intensive Care*, **12**, 315–24.

German, P. A. S., Roberts, J. G. and Prys-Roberts, C. (1979). The combination of general anaesthesia and epidural block 1: The effects of sequence of induction on haemodynamic variables and blood gas measurements in healthy patients. *Anaesthesia and Intensive Care*, **7**, 229–38.

Grundy, E. M., Rao, L. N. and Winnie, A. P. (1978). Epidural anaesthesia and the lateral position. *Anesthesia and Analgesia*, **57**, 95.

Hall, G. M. (1980). Fentanyl and the metabolic response to surgery. *British Journal of Anaesthesia*, **52**, 561–3.

Harris, N. H. (1970). Cardiac arrest and bone cement. *British Medical Journal*, **3**, 523.

Harrold, A. J. (1982). Outlook for hip replacement. *British Medical Journal*, **1**, 139.

Hole, A., Terjesen, T. and Breivik, H. (1980). Epidural versus general anaesthesia for total hip arthroplasty in elderly patients. *Acta Anaestheiologica Scandinavica*, **24**, 279.

Hollway, T. E. and Telford, R. J. (1991). Observations on deliberate dural puncture with a tuohy needle: depth measurements. *Anaesthesia*, **46**, 722–4.

Hovorka, J. (1982). Carbon dioxide homeostasis and recovery after general anaesthesia. *Acta Anaesthesiologica Scandinavica*, **26**, 498–504.

Ip Yam, P. C. and Carli, F. (1990). Maintenance of body temperature in elderly patients who have joint replacement surgery. *Anaesthesia*, **45**, 563–5.

Jhaveri, R. M. (1989). The effects of hypocapnic ventilation on mental function in elderly patients undergoing cataract surgery. *Anasthesia*, **44**, 635–40.

Jorgensen, L. N., Rasmussen, L. S., Nielsen, P. T., Leffers, A. and Albrecht-Best, ?. (1991). Antithrombotic efficacy of continuous extradural analgesia after knee replacement. *British Journal of Anaesthesia*, **66**, 8–12.

Kent, A. P. and Hunter, J. M. (1991). The pharmacodynamics of alcuronium in the elderly. *Anaesthesia*, **46**, 271–4.

Kerkkamp, H. E. M. and Gielen, M. J. M. (1991). Cardiovascular effects of local anaesthetics. *Anaesthesia*, **46**, 361–5.

Khambatta, H. J., Stone, J. G. and Khan, E. (1979). Hypertension during anaesthesia on discontinuation of sodium nitroprusside induced hypotension. *Anesthesiology*, **51**, 127.

Kleinert, H. E. and Jupiter, J. B. (1981). Replantation – an overview. In: *Clinical Trends in Orthopaedics*. Thieme-Stratton: New York.

Kopacz, D. J., Carpenter, R. L. and Mackey, D. C. (1988). Ropivacaine constricts cutaneous blood vessels. *Anesthesiology*, **69A**, 343.

Larsen, R., Rathgeber, J., Bagdahn, A., Lange, H. and Rieke, H. (1988). Effects of propofol on cardiovascular dynamics and coronary blood flow in geriatric patients. A comparison with etomidate. *Anaesthesia*, **43**, suppl., 25–31.

Lawson, N. W., Thompson, D. S., Nelson, C. L., Flacke, J. W. and North, E. R. (1976). Sodium nitroprusside induced hypotension for supine total hip replacement. *Anesthesia and Analgesia*, **55**, 654.

Luostarinen, V., Evers, H., Lytikainen, M. T., Sceinen, A. and Wahlen, A. (1981). Antithrombotic effects of lidocaine and related compounds on laser induced microvascular injury. *Acta Anaestheiologica Scandinavica*, **25**, 9.

Maderazo, E. G., Judson, S. and Pasternak, H. (1988). Late infections of total joint prostheses: a review and recommendations for prevention. *Clinical Orthopaedics*, **229**, 131–42.

Mannion, D., Walker, R. and Clayton, K. (1991). Extradural vein puncture – an avoidable complication. *Anaesthesia*, **46**, 585–7.

Millesi, H. (1977). Interfascicular grafts for repair of peripheral nerves of the upper extremity. *Orthopaedic Clinics of North America*, **8**, 387.

Mirakhur, R. K., Clarke, R. S. J., Elliott, J. and Dundee, J. W. (1978). Atropine and glycopyrronium premedication. *Anaesthesia*, **33**, 906.

Michel, R. (1980). Air embolism in hip surgery. *Anaesthesia*, **35**, 858.

Modig, J. (1988). Regional anaesthesia and blood loss. *Acta Anaestheiologica Scandinavica*, **32**, suppl. 89, 44–8.

Modig, J. and Karlstrom, G. (1987). Intra- and postoperative blood loss and haemodynamics in total hip replacement when performed under lumbar epidural versus general anaesthesia. *European Journal of Anaesthesiology*, **4**, 345–55.

Modig, J. and Malmberg, P. (1975). Pulmonary and circulatory reactions during total hip replacement surgery. *Acta Anaesthesiologica Scandinavica*, **19**, 219.

Modig, J., Malmberg, P. and Karlstrom, G. (1980). Effect of epidural versus general anaesthesia on calf blood flow. *Acta Anaestheiologica Scandinavica*, **24**, 305.

Modig, J., Hjelmstedt, A., Sahlstedt, B. and Maripuu, E. (1981). Comparative influences of epidural and general anaesthesia on deep venous thrombosis and pulmonary embolism after total hip replacement. *Acta Chirurgica Scandinavica*, **147**, 125–30.

Mohan, J. and Potter, J. M. (1975). Pupillary constriction and Ptosis following caudal epidural analgesia. *Anaesthesia*, **30**, 769.

Nelson, J. P., Fitzgerald, R. H., Jaspers, M. T., Little, J. M. (1990). Prophylactic antimicrobial coverage in arthroplasty patients. *Journal of Bone and Joint Surgery (Am)*, **72**, 1.

Ngai, S. H., Stinchfield, F. E. and Triner, L. (1974). Air embolism during total hip arthroplasty. *Anesthesiology*, **40**, 405.

Noble, J., Hodgkinson, J. P., Brabu, K. J. and Potts, H. (1987). The total condylar knee replacement: a robust and reliable prosthesis. In J. Noble and C. S. B. Galasko (eds), *Recent Developments in Orthopaedic Surgrey*. Manchester University Press, Manchester, pp. 274–82.

O'Brien, B. (1977). *Microvascular Reconstructive Surgery*. Churchill Livingstone, Edinburgh and London.

Otteni, J. C., Steib, A., Freys, G., Beller, J. P. and Curzola, U. (1987). *Haemodynamic Effects of Propofol and Thiopentone during Induction of Anaesthesia in Patients of ASA Class III and IV*. International Symposium Royal College of Physicians, London.

Park, W. Y., Balingit, P., Kenmore, P. I. and Macnamara, T. E. (1973). Changes in arteral oxygen tension during total hip replacement. *Anesthesiology*, **39**, 642.

Park, W. Y., Massingale, M., Kim, S. I., Poon, K. C. and Macnamara, T. (1980). Age and spread of local anesthetic solutions in the epidural space. *Anesthesia and Analgesia*, **59**, 768.

Peebles, D. J., Ellis, R. H., Stride, S. D. K. and Simpson, B. R. J. (1972). Cardiovascular effects of methylmethacrilate cement. *British Medical Journal*, **1**, 349.

Phillips, H., Cole, P. V. and Lettin, A. W. F. (1971). Cardiovascular effects of implanted acrylic bone cement. *British Medical Journal*, **3**, 460.

Ranawat, C. S., Beaver, W. B., Sharrock, N. E., Maynard, M. J., Urquhart, B. and Schneider, R. (1991). Effect of hypotensive epidural anaesthesia on acetabular cement-bone fixation in total hip arthroplasty. *Journal of Bone and Joint Surgery (Br)*, **73B**, 779–82.

Roberts, F. L., Dixon, J., Lewis, G. T. R., Tackley, R. M. and Prys-Roberts, C. (1988). Induction and maintenance of propofol anaesthesia. A manual infusion technique. *Anaesthesia*, **43**, suppl., 14–17.

Sharrock, N. E., Haas, S. B., Hargett, M. J., Urquhart, B., Insall, J. N. and Scuderi, G. (1991). *Journal of Bone and Joint Surgery*, **73A**, 502–6.

Small, M., Tweddel, A. C., Rankin, A. C., Lowe, G. D., Prentice, C. R. and Forbes, C. D. (1984). Blood coagulation and platelet function following severe exercise: effects of beta-adrenergic blockade. *Haemostasis*, **14**, 262.

Stulberg, B. N., Insall, J. N., Williams, G. W. and Ghelman, B. (1984). *Journal of Bone and Joint Surgery (Br)*, **66A**, 194–201.

Thomas, K. A. (1990). Biomechanics and biomaterials of hip implants. *Current Opinion in Orthopaedics*, **1**, 28–37.

Thorburn, J., Louden, J. R. and Vallance, R. (1980). Spinal and general anaesthesia in total hip replacement: frequency of deep vein thrombosis. *British Journal of Anaesthesia*, **52**, 1117–21.

Turnbull, K. W., Berezowsky, J. L., Poulsen, J. B. and Root, L. S. (1974). General anaesthesia and total hip replacement. *Canadian Anaesthetists Society Journal*, **21**, 546.

Urbaniak, J. R. (1979). Replantation of amputated parts – technique, results and indications. In J. R. Urbaniak and D. S. Bright (eds), *American Academy of Orthopaedic Surgeons Symposium on Microsurgery: Practical Use in Orthopaedics*. Mosby, St Louis, Miss, p. 64.

Vazeery, A. K. and Lunde, O. (1979). Controlled hypotension in hip joint surgery. *Acta Orthopaedica Scandinavica*, **50**, 433.

Vendrinne, C., Vendrinne, J. M., Guiraud, M., Patricot, M. C. and Bouletreau, P. (1989). Nitrogen sparing effect of epidural administration of local anaesthetics in colon surgery. *Anesthesia and Analgesia*, **69**, 354–9.

Verniquet, A. J. W. (1980). Vessel puncture with epidural catheters: experience with obstetric patients. *Anaesthesia*, **35**, 660.

Vesey, C. J. and Cole, P. V. (1975). Nitroprusside and cyanide. *British Journal of Anaesthesia*, **47**, 1115–16.

Vesey, C. J., Cole, P. V. and Simpson, P. J. (1976). Cyanide and thiocyanate concentration following sodium nitroprusside infusion in man. *British Journal of Anaesthesia*, **48**, 651.

Walsh, P. N., Rogers, P. H., Marder, V. J., Gagnatelli, G., Escovitz, E. S. and Sherry, S. (1976). The relationship of platelet coagulant activities to venous thrombosis following hip surgery. *British Journal of Haematology*, **32**, 421.

Watson, J. T. and Stulberg, B. N. (1989). Fat embolism associated with cementing of femoral stems designed for press-fit application. *Journal of Arthroplasty*, **4**, 133–7.

White, D. G. (1980). Anaesthesia in old age. *British Journal of Hospital Medicine*, **24**, 145.

Woolfson, A. M. J., Heatley, R. V. and Allison, S. P. (1979). Insulin to inhibit protein catabolism after surgery. *New England Journal of Medicine*, **300**, 14–18.

Wroblewski, B. M. (1990). Introduction. In *Revision Surgery in Total Hip Arthroplasty*. London, Springer Verlag.

Chapter 4

Anaesthesia for spinal disorders

Neil Schofield

General considerations

Preoperative assessment and management

The preoperative visit by the anaesthetist is particularly valuable to the patient when spinal surgery is planned. The prospect of any operation causes anxiety but only a few other fields of surgery are as emotive as major spinal procedures. The need to explain to the patient many aspects of the anaesthetic and their care before and after surgery is increasingly recognized and required. Patients respond well to the anaesthetist's explanations and reassurances. It may be considered unnecessary to premedicate some people and others may request that it is avoided. Many, however, are likely to remain apprehensive and will benefit from preoperative night sedation and subsequent premedication if these are not contraindicated.

Premedicant drugs should be prescribed according to the anaesthetist's usual practice, except in cases where there are particular reasons to change. Patients may prefer oral premedication, and a combination of a sedative, a hydrogen ion antagonist and a promoter of gastric emptying is often favoured. Spinal surgery may result in a painful period postoperatively, and the use of narcotic analgesic premedication may give an indication of the patient's susceptibility to such drugs and aid initial postoperative prescribing. Care in the prescribing of sedative drugs may sometimes be necessary, especially after recent head injury or where the cervical spine is unstable. In the latter instance, the deliberate use of an antisialogogue may be helpful in preventing the accumulation of secretions during induction and avoiding suction at this stage. In other patients who have been injured analgesics will have already been used and their response to them be known.

There are many special considerations in anaesthesia for spinal surgery. Most relate either to the condition for which surgery is planned or are associated with its development and aetiology. Instability and restriction of permitted movement may influence the approach to intubation, long-standing thoracic deformity affects circulatory and respiratory reserve and the ability of the patient to have exercised normally, and injuries rarely affect the spine in isolation.

The spinal condition may be part of a more generalized disease process. Some patients are treated for the associated spinal abnormalities of congenital disorders where the most striking problems are cranial or facial deformity. Some have neuromuscular disorders, either congenital or acquired, many of which are progressive and causes widespread weakness. Those who have Duchenne muscular dystrophy (Brownwell *et al.*, 1983) may progress to severe myocardial insufficiency and instability (see Chapter 7) There is an association between deformity secondary to neuromuscular disorders and malignant hyperpyrexia or rhabdomyolisis (Miller *et al.*, 1978; Boltshauser *et al.*, 1980; Brownwell *et al.*, 1983; Leatherman and Dickson, 1988).

Spinal surgery may be needed in neurofibromatosis, and deformity may occur with mesenchymal disorders, such as osteogenesis imperfecta, Marfan's syndrome, homocysteinuria or Ehlers-Danlos syndrome. The mucopolysaccharidoses and bone dysplasias can have spinal manifestations, as may metabolic disorders such as rickets or the endocrine disturbances associated with pituitary, thyroid or adrenal disease.

Pyogenic or cold tuberculous bone destruction may occur, and deformity is relative common from tumours within the spinal canal, in the bones of the spine or arising in organs adjacent to the spine. Many of these are remarkably vascular.

The spine, being a load-bearing structure, is also very vulnerable to degenerative disease of many kinds, as well as rheumatoid, Paget's disease and ankylosing spondylitis. It is commonly affected by the irritative lesions of discitis and disc prolapse (Moe *et al.*, 1978; Leatherman and Dickson, 1988).

The preoperative investigations required for most patients are dictated by their age, clinical history and the surgery proposed. The anaesthetist's normal requirements are appropriate to spinal surgery. Special consideration needs to be given to those with thoracic deformity, especially if it is long-standing, and to those whose primary condition is known to have significant associations for anaesthesia. In major corrective surgery, the loss of a large volume of blood should be anticipated and, if appropriate, the patient assessed for suitability for a hypotensive anaesthetic technique.

The effects of associated non-spinal injuries and their management up to the time of surgery must be considered in post-traumatic surgery. Difficulty with intubation should be anticipated especially in those whose cervical spine is involved (Wood and Lawler, 1992) or who have craniofacial anomalies. The atlanto-occipital instability associated with Down syndrome should be remembered (Stein *et al.*, 1991).

Where major corrective surgery is proposed, the team approach is essential involving support from experienced nurses and physiotherapists from the earliest opportunity (Sawyer, 1983; Brosnan, 1991; Brown and Seltzer, 1991; Dartyka, 1991). The patient needs to be confident in the support and continuity of care that is planned and to understand the whole treatment programme.

Thoracic deformity

In numerical terms operations for correction of scoliosis are predominantly performed in childhood (see Chapter 8) or into early adulthood. The cardiorespiratory complications (Bjure and Nachemson, 1973) of long-standing kyphosis or kyphoscoliosis are, however, much more likely to be of concern in the adult patient presenting for anaesthesia. Lung volumes are decreased and a restrictive pattern is seen on pulmonary function testing. To this are added the mechanical inefficiency of the deformed thoracic cage and relative splinting of the diaphragm as scoliosis develops (Bergofsky, 1979; Jones *et al.*, 1981). The patient may become unable to cough effectively as vital capacity falls, and eventually progressive alveolar hypoventilation and atelectasis occur with consequent blood gas changes and pulmonary hypertension (Zorab, 1977).

The total lung capacity (TLC) and vital capacity (VC) are reduced in parallel (Shannon *et al.*, 1970; Bjure and Nachemson, 1973) until the deformity becomes very severe, when vital capacity is greatly reduced. The reduction in vital capacity is related to the severity of the deformity in idiopathic scoliosis (Riseborough, 1973; Westgate and Johnson, 1971) and a relative sparing of residual volume may be seen (Bjure and Nachemson, 1973). Intra-pulmonary airways obstruction is not a feature of kyphoscoliosis (Bjure and Nachemson, 1973; Secher-Walker *et al.*, 1979), but occasionally grossly deformed patients may have extrathoracic obstruction of the trachea due to obliquity of the thoracic outlet. Absolute values of forced expiratory flow measurements are reduced owing to the acquired mechanical inefficiency of the thorax and abdomen (Bergofsky, 1979). The onset of airways closure may encroach upon the functional residual capacity (FRC) more commonly and at a younger age than in normal subjects (Bjure and Nachemson, 1973).

Abnormal distribution of ventilation and perfusion is not usually apparent in the supine position, but when sitting there is a shift in perfusion towards the upper zone, particularly on the side of the concavity, probably due to a decrease in vertical height of the lung (Shannon *et al.*, 1970). As the deformity worsens, ventilation and perfusion abnormalities affect both lungs as their vertical height is reduced (Riseborough, 1973). More specifically, ventilation may be reduced at the level of greatest deformity (Secher-Walker *et al.*, 1979). In younger patients very severe deformity may be present before ventilation/perfusion (V/Q) ratios are upset, and in these cases basal blood flow may be impaired (Bjure and Nachemson, 1973).

A degree of arterial hypoxemia is common (Shannon *et al.*, 1970; Secher-Walker *et al.*, 1979) but a rise in carbon dioxide tension is confined to severe cases. Early cases may have a slight reduction in carbon dioxide tension (Secher-Walker *et al.*, 1979). Small changes in pulmonary perfusion pressure occur which are inversely related to systemic arterial oxygenation and are rarely abnormal at rest, but they may become so during exercise. This tendency becomes greater as lung size diminishes (Sneerson, 1977).

Measurements of pulmonary diffusing capacity (transfer factor) show a reduction in accordance with the patient's clinical respiratory impairment, but these are in the normal or high normal range when related to lung volume and expressed as transfer coefficients (Prime, 1977), except in those with severe respiratory difficulty who have developed hypercapnia. The absolute values of transfer factor can be improved temporarily by assisting ventilation in patients with normal transfer coefficient, suggesting that at this stage irreversible lung changes are not widespread (Bergofsky, 1979). These findings may be accounted for by the changes in perfusion of the lungs.

The preoperative assessment of cardiopulmonary impairment and its significance primarily depends on a careful history with special emphasis on cardiorespiratory tolerance. In many patients it will be clearly adequate, but in others respiratory function tests should be performed. They should include forced expiratory spirometry and the measurement of the subdivisions of lung volume and of transfer factor. As standard tables for predicting the normal values for these measurements rely on the subject's sex, age, height and weight, there is some difficulty in deciding which values should be used for comparative purposes, each laboratory having its own method of estimating the patient's stature in the absence of scoliotic deformity, such as the use of arm span. The results of pulmonary function tests are best viewed as a whole in conjunction with the anaesthetist's clinical impression of the patient. If the overall picture is of clinically significant reduction in respiratory tolerance with over 40 per cent reduction in pulmonary function test results, then respiratory difficulties may be experienced in the postoperative period (Westgate and Johnson, 1991). Surgery should be undertaken only in such cases where facilities exist for postoperative ventilation. Arterial gas tensions should be measured if any impairment of respiratory function is considered likely. Electrocardiography is essential as a baseline investigation in all those with significant deformity or proposed thoracic surgery. Patients in whom cardiac impairment is suspected or whose condition has an association with cardiac disease should be considered for referral to obtain a cardiological opinion on the severity of the impairment and the optimal treatment.

The effects of surgery and correction of kyphoscoliosis are variously reported. In the immediate postoperative period, lung volumes and maximum expiratory flow rates may be further reduced by as much as 30 per cent. This worsening of lung function is particularly important in patients with moderate or severe preoperative impairment. The possibility of elective postoperative ventilation should be considered if preoperative respiratory function tests are reduced by more than about 40 per cent from predicted values (Westgate and Johnson, 1971), though practice suggests more severely affected patients can often be managed without ventilation.

In the longer term, the reports of improvement or deterioration in cardiopulmonary function are conflicting. An improvement in lung and forced expiratory at 1–3 years after operation for scoliosis irrespective of the severity of deformity treated has been reported (Lindh and Bjure, 1975; Carstens *et al.*, 1991). Other have found little overall change in lung volumes (Lamalre *et al.*, 1971; Riseborough, 1973; Zorab *et al.*, 1979; Westgate and Johnson, 1991), though spinal fusion usually arrests deterioration in pulmonary function and may result in a small increase in systemic oxygenation (Mole *et al.*, 1978). In addition, there is the important psychological benefit of a good cosmetic result, together with improved mobility in the more severely affected patient.

Difficult intubation

Anticipation of difficulty in intubation is essential. It is obvious in conditions affecting the face and neck but severe thoracic deformity can be equally difficult, nor are those admitted for spinal surgery exempt from problems which may occur in any patient. Bull-necked individuals, the obese, those with high arched palates, protuberant or diseased teeth, and some with restricted mouth opening have all caused anaesthetists to have moments of panic.

Intubation aids must be available and are best assembled in a single portable container for easy access should unanticipated intubation difficulties occur. These aids may include a variety of soft-tipped and malleable endotracheal tube introducers, straight and left-handed laryngoscope blades, obtusely fitting (polio) blades, a Huffman's prism, and suitable sized nasopharyngeal airways and nasotracheal tubes. In addition, a needle and catheter suitable for transcricothyroid puncture or a commercial cricothyrotomy kit and a preassembled system for connection to the anaesthetic machine or oxygen outlet should be included. On rare occasions, the method described by Waters (1963) for passing a retrograde catheter from the larynx to the mouth via a transcricothyroid route may be helpful, though it is not without its difficulties (Akinglini, 1979).

More recently, fibreoptic instruments have become increasingly available. Taylor and Towey in 1972 (Taylor and Towey, 1972) described the use of a fibreoptic bronchoscope, over which an endotracheal tube is placed prior to inserting the instrument. Fibreoptic equipment has developed considerably and is much more readily available since that time. An intubating laryngoscope may be used with topical or general anaesthesia. The use of a fibreoptic instrument is especially valuable when extension of the head on the neck is contraindicated or impossible, but considerable experience in handling the equipment should be gained before attempting a difficult intubation by this method.

The anaesthetic used when intubation is to be attempted in a potentially difficult case is the individual anaesthetist's choice. The more difficult cases may warrant the use of topical anaesthesia and awake intubation, either blind through the nose or with the aid of a fibreoptic instrument. Topical anaesthesia for the nose and pharynx may be achieved with a combination of sprays, nasal drops and lozenges. Vasoconstriction of the nasal mucosa is helpful. Transcricothyroid topical anaesthetic injected after a full inspiration should reach the vocal cords and larynx. A similar approach may be made to orotracheal intubation using fibreoptic or conventional laryngoscopy. Oropharyngeal anaesthesia may be obtained by lozenges and sprays, or topical application in the classic manner using Krause's forceps.

Most cases, however, are suitable for general anaesthesia, which is usually more acceptable to patient and anaesthetist alike. Inhalational or intravenous induction followed by deepening of the anaesthetic breathing spontaneously and judicious topical anaesthesia may be favoured in some cases. Frequently, however, the easiest technique is to use intravenous induction via a secure venous access, to check that the lungs can be inflated by mask, and then to administer a short-acting agent which provides profound relaxation. On these occasions where depolarizing relaxants are contraindicated, blind or fibreoptic intubation may be attempted under general anaesthesia with spontaneous respiration. The use of carbon dioxide to stimulate respiration in those who can respond adequately may be helpful to blind intubation, as may intravenous doxapram (Davies, 1968). Intubation may also be attempted under ketamine anaesthesia (MacClennan and Robertson, 1981), permitting more prolonged efforts to be made, though salivation can be inconvenient. If great difficulty is anticipated, security of oxygenation can be established using a small cricothyrotomy device before induction of anaesthesia.

Once the patient is intubated, the anaesthetist may employ any subsequent anaesthetic sequence for maintenance purposes, but must bear in mind that the cause of the difficulty in intubation may equally affect the immediate postoperative period. Extubation with the patient fully awake will overcome most problems, but may not be desirable in those with residual cervical spinal instability. When it is known that the patient's airway is not difficult to maintain, extubation while fully anaesthetized and breathing spontaneously may be an acceptable approach provided that adequate recovery facilities are available.

In those few patients with potentially extreme problems of intubation, and especially when a series of surgical procedures are planned, consideration of elective tracheostomy should be made. It may be necessary to perform the tracheostomy under local anaesthetic.

Equipment and monitoring

Only a few items of equipment need special consideration in anaesthesia for spinal surgery. Save for some manipulations of the spine, most cases require intubation for security of the airway, as accessibility is much reduced once the patient is positioned on the operating table. Because intraoperative access to the airway is so limited, an endotracheal tube designed to resist obstruction, such as an armoured or Oxford pattern tube, should be used. In addition, to minimize the risk of occlusion of its distal end by the tracheal wall due to the position of the head and neck, an additional lateral perforation in the wall of the tube in the longer portion of the oblique tip is desirable. The endotracheal tube must be securely fixed in place, as adjustment or replacement may be impossible during the operation.

Surgery on the spine tends to be prolonged and intermittent positive pressure ventilation (IPPV) is usual, especially as the position of the patient on the table may not be conducive to adequate spontaneous respiration. Various devices have been used to support the prone patient and minimize the adverse respiratory and circulatory effects of abdominal and consequent inferior vena caval compression. They also help avoid an accentuated lordosis. These vary from combinations of firm and soft pads and pillows, through sculptured foam blocks to purpose-designed supporting frames (Relton and Hall, 1967; Martin, 1978; Wayne, 1984).

Since 1986 recommended standards for minimum monitoring during anaesthesia have received increasing attention (Eichhorn *et al.*, 1986; *Recommendations for Standards . . .*, 1988) and should apply to all spinal patients. In particular the electrocardiograph, peripheral oxygen saturation and end tidal carbon dioxide levels should be measured. As access to the patient after surgery has started is often restricted, a ventilator disconnection alarm or expired volume monitor is very desirable as is breathing circuit oxygen analysis. Automatic non-invasive blood pressure measurement is adequate except when major corrective or transthoracic surgery is undertaken.

As the surgical approach to the spine is through relatively vascular tissues, blood loss can at times be large. The anaesthetist's access to drip sites may be almost as restricted as his access to the airway, so a well and securely positioned venous cannula of good size is essential. Where replacement of more than 2 units of blood is anticipated, facilities for warming of the blood should be included. When very large blood losses are likely, the use of equipment to permit the saving and re-infusion of autologous blood may be considered (Flynn *et al.*, 1982) and even the blood which accumulates in closed drainage receivers postoperatively may be used later (Flynn *et al.*, 1991).

If extensive corrective spinal surgery is proposed, insertion of a central venous catheter may be considered, and intra-arterial blood pressure measurement is virtually essential. In choosing a site for introducing a central catheter, the anaesthetist must be aware of the patient's ultimate position on the operating table and the need for good fixation of the catheter. The antecubital route may be preferable to the internal jugular or subclavian. Similarly, the site of arterial cannulation should be chosen with final positioning in mind. The radial artery is usually the first choice, provided Allen's test is negative indicating adequate ulnar collateral circulation. A false negative result is unusual (Husum and Berthelsen, 1981). The dorsalis pedis or brachial artery may be considered as an alternative.

In any surgery where the position of the patient on the table is other than supine, thought should be given to the arrangement of anaesthetic and monitoring equipment. In major spinal cases, it should also be given to the surgeon's preferred approach and the usual theatre routine in order to avoid placing equipment in a position awkward for the surgical team or inaccessible to the anaesthetist. It may be found convenient, especially in some cervical and thoracic cases, to manage the anaesthetic from the side or foot of the patient. ECG electrodes, diathermy connections and the like must avoid all possible sites of surgery, as an unforeseen bone graft may be needed. Again, whatever monitoring is attached to the patient must remain so.

Spinal cord monitoring

In corrective spinal surgery and in some cases when fractures are stabilized or manipulated or the cord is decompressed, there is an increasing requirement to monitor spinal cord function. Traditionally this has been achieved by performing the 'wake-up' test which was introduced in association with scoliosis surgery by Stagnara (Vauxelle *et al.*, 1973).

Most anaesthetic techniques are variations on balanced anaesthesia. A simple method is neuroleptanaesthesia following narcotic premedication. Droperidol, fentanyl, thiopentone and tubocurarine are used at induction of anaesthesia, suxamethonium being added to the sequence when difficulty in intubation is anticipated or at the anaesthetist's preference. The patient is ventilated with nitrous oxide and oxygen, and increments of fentanyl are given at 20-minute intervals or by infusion whilst curare is given half-hourly. Any hypotensive technique may be added to this regimen if necessary though halogenated inhalational agents are best avoided. When wake-up is anticipated (Leatherman and Dickson, 1988), the timing of fentanyl and curare increments is adjusted to leave about 30 minutes before wake-up. In order to arouse the patient, the nitrous oxide is turned off and oxygen flow increased. At the same time, minute ventilation is decreased to allow the systemic carbon dioxide tension to rise. One eye of the patient is exposed and observed as an indicator of return of consciousness, and the patient instructed to move his toes. It usually takes 3–5 minutes to achieve this. Rarely, small increments of naloxone are required to encourage arousal. As soon as movement of both feet has been observed, double the incremental doses of fentanyl and curare are given, together with an additional increment of droperidol. It is very unusual to have to reverse the neuromuscular blockade.

Similar techniques using increments of morphine and nitrous oxide/oxygen ventilation are widely used, (Hall *et al.*, 1978; Abott and Bentley, 1980) and satisfactory wake-up has been achieved using a background of trichloroethylene 0.2 per cent or other vapours and incremental fentanyl. Carbon dioxide may be added to speed awakening, and diazepam administered at its conclusion to aid amnesia (Abbott and Bentley, 1980). The observation of the return of spontaneous respiration before attempting wake-up may be used to prevent awareness while the patient is still paralysed (Hall *et al.*, 1978). Alternatively, a peripheral nerve stimulator can be used (Waldman *et al.*, 1977). The patient's ability to cooperate in the test can be confirmed by asking for hand movement prior to eliciting responses in the feet (Hall *et al.*, 1978). The introduction of etomidate and later propofol has increased the spectrum of available techniques, though etomidate is no longer used for continuous infusion. Propofol combined with alfentanyl administered by infusion offers a readily reversible anaesthetic combination used with air or conventional nitrous oxide/oxygen ventilation (Gokel *et al.*, 1991).

The object of the variations in technique is to permit controlled awakening of the patient to a level allowing cooperation, but the patient should suffer no pain and preferably not remember the event. Postoperative recall was not reported by patients when the neuroleptic technique described had been used, nor has it with similar techniques used in other centres (Leatherman and Dickson, 1988).

The wake-up test technique must allow a repeat test to be performed in two circumstances. First, when no functional impairment has occurred, further correction of the deformity may be possible after a short interval as some loss of tissue tension occurs, and the surgeon may wish to re-assess cord function after distraction. Alternatively, absent or impaired function on initial testing may recover over a few minutes or if distraction has been released. Further attempts at lesser degrees of correction may be made (Waldman *et al.*, 1978). In these circumstances, nitrous oxide may be reintroduced between the periods where patient cooperation is required.

A need to monitor cord function throughout surgery, and the limitations of the wake-up test to one or two attempts during an operation, has led to the development of spinal cord monitoring using evoked potential recordings. Most commonly sensory evoked potentials are evoked distal of the area of surgery and recorded centrally, but methods have also been developed to evoke and monitor motor responses (Owen *et al.*, 1991).

The principle of sensory evoked potentials is to apply a recurring electrical stimulus to the afferent pathway. As the voltage to be recorded centrally is very small in relation to background noise from muscular and other activity, the centrally conducted potentials resulting from a large number of stimulating impulses are summed. A waveform emerges and the background noise is minimized. The primary measurements are of the latent period to the first peak of the summed evoked potentials and the magnitude of this peak. An increase in latency of 10 per cent and a reduction in peak magnitude by 50 per cent are usually considered to be significant indication of cord function impairment (Ben David, 1988; Nash and Braun, 1989). There are, however, many other measurements which can be made from the evoked potential waveforms and the subject is still developing (Friedman and Grundy, 1987; Nash and Braun, 1989).

The usual stimulation sites for sensory evoked potential monitoring are the peroneal or posterior tibial nerves for thoracolumbar surgery and ulnar or median for cervical work. Surface or percutaneous electrodes are often used, or epidural electrodes may be introduced by Tuohy needle preoperatively or under direct vision during surgery. Similarly, recording electrodes may be attached to the skin over spinous processes or into them percutaneously, attached over the sensory cortex, or introduced epidurally in the cervical region. The equipment must be suitable for use with surgical diathermy.

Experience with a system for somatosensory or somatocortical evoked potential recording is essential to obtain reproducible results in any particular hospital location. Positive, that is abnormal results, do correlate with cord dysfunction postoperatively or at the wake-up test in about 70 per cent of cases, but the incidence of false positive and false negative results is fairly high (Dawson *et al.*, 1991). The former cause anxiety to the surgical team but no harm to the patient unless the surgical procedure is significantly modified as a result. False negatives may be associated with permanent neurological deficit which is not detected until recovery from anaesthesia. Motor evoked potentials may be less susceptible to false results and be expected to correlate better with the wake-up test or clonus test (Ben David, 1988; Hoppenfield *et al.*, 1991). The simple criteria for abnormality are similar to those for sensory evoked potentials. Stimulation may be instituted over the cortical motor areas, either electrically or magnetically, or electrically over the upper spinal column. Recording electrodes are inserted into or attached to skin over suitable muscles or major nerved peripherally (Ben David, 1988; Dvorak *et al.*, 1990; Owen *et al.*, 1991).

The wake-up test is still advised as an adjunct to spinal cord function monitoring, especially to confirm a positive result (Dawson *et al.*, 1991). Baseline recordings should be obtained after stable anaesthesia has been established so that changes secondary to surgical intervention can be observed. Anaesthetic agents, particularly halogenated hydrocarbons (Calancie *et al.*, 1991), may impair evoked potentials as may nitrous oxide (Kalkman *et al.*, 1990, 1991) and extradural lignocaine (Loughnan *et al.*, 1990). Propofol and alfentanyl anaesthesia appears to inhibit the potentials less than do opiates with nitrous oxide (Kalkman *et al.*, 1990, 1991a, 1991b).

The cervical spine

Preoperative management

All patients who are to undergo surgery of the cervical spine require preoperative assessment by the anaesthetist. The cause of the disorder and its local and remote associations are of obvious importance. In addition, any patient may have an unrelated condition of concern to the anaesthetist (see Chapter 2). Spinal injuries tend to occur in industrial or road traffic accidents, particularly involving motorcyclists, and so involve a younger group of patients than do some other orthopaedic procedures. Infective lesions occur more commonly in developing communities and likewise tend to affect younger people. Surgery for the sequelae of degenerative disorders does, however, involve more elderly patients (Crockard and Ransford, 1991).

Specific points of interest to the anaesthetist include the stability of the cervical spine, any neurological impairment associated with the condition, and evidence of cardiovascular instability where cord function is compromised. In cases of trauma, the results of head and faciomaxillary injuries should be evaluated. Conditions which result in symptoms of cord compression at cervical level but without gross cord dysfunction or spinal instability such as disc protrusion, canal stenosis and cervical spondylosis tend not to cause the anaesthetist many problems. As always, the ease or otherwise of intubation must be assessed, including the degree of mouth opening and the state of the teeth as well as symptoms arising from head position, especially in those with spondylosis. Where surgical removal of tumour tissue or an infected area is contemplated, the anaesthetist should again be aware of more generalized associations of the disease, particularly pulmonary and renal. Current therapy should be noted and modified if necessary for the peri-operative period.

Operative procedures which may be undertaken following injury to the cervical spine include the application of a skull calliper or halo for traction, manipulation, open reduction of a fracture or spinal decompression by either the anterior or posterior approach (Leatherman and Dickson, 1988). The treatment of degenerative disorders may require either the anterior or the posterior approach in order to achieve adequate removal of the compressive element or access for stable fixation. Prior to the definitive surgery, these patients too may need a halo to be attached if the cervical spine is unstable. Operations for conditions associated with the cervical spine such as division of the sternomastoid muscle for torticollis or removal of a cervical rib may also be undertaken. It is important that the anaesthetist is aware of the intended position of the patient and the surgical approach to be used.

Premedication for patients about to undergo surgery of the cervical spine should follow the anaesthetist's normal practice except when there is a specific indication to modify the agents used. In some patients care must be taken in the use of any sedative drug. These include patients with spinal instability, recent head injury, compromised airway or major trunk trauma, but individual assessment is the only means of deciding which patients may safely be given sedative or narcotic premedication. Where difficulty in intubation is anticipated, the deliberate reduction of salivary secretion is helpful because coughing or the need for suction during induction is at least an irritation to the anaesthetist and at most may cause cord damage where the spine is unstable. In the presence of clinical cord damage, atropine may reduce the incidence of reflex bradycardia during anaesthesia (see Chapter 11).

Anaesthesia

Attachment of skull calliper or halo

Traction apparatus is used to assist or maintain the reduction and stability of cervical fractures and dislocations, and is applied under local anaesthesia, usually by the orthopaedic surgeon. Local infiltration of all layers, including the periosteum, is required at each fixation site. Traction apparatus may occasionally be applied as part of a procedure under general anaesthesia. If a halo is to be attached, the anaesthetist must allow sufficient mobility in his connection of the anaesthetic circuit to the patient to allow the surgeon adequate access.

Manipulative reduction of fractures

When general anaesthesia is required by a surgeon to facilitate reduction of a cervical fracture, it should provide some diminution in neck muscle tone. During induction of anaesthesia, full appropriate monitoring should be used. The possibility of difficulty in intubation is always present where freedom to move the head and neck is restricted, and should be anticipated (see section on 'Difficult intubation'). The surgeon's opinion on the stability of the spine should be sought, and if instability is a significant factor, he should be present and responsible for the head and neck position during induction of anaesthesia. In general, the patient's head may be placed on pillows, depending on the most stable position for the fracture, and traction applied usually at about 20° to the horizontal with a chin/occipital halter, which is held by the surgeon during induction of anaesthesia (Bedbrook and Hardcastle, 1991). In most injuries the head may be gently extended on the partly flexed neck, with the surgeon's consent, to assist intubation, though published information on safe positioning is limited.

Where difficulties with maintenance of the airway are anticipated, it may be prudent to employ an inhalational induction. Normally, however, an intravenous induction through a secure venous access followed by a short acting muscle relaxant which produces profound relaxation is easier, though depolarizing relaxants may have to be avoided if a high cord lesion is present. In addition, respiratory function in the quadriplegic patient is impaired by lack of trunk muscle tone even when diaphragmatic innervation is intact, and pulmonary oedema may occur because of trauma, fluid load, autonomic nervous imbalance or myocardial damage following crush injury.

The means of maintenance of anaesthesia is open to choice, but an intravenous technique with IPPV providing for rapid awakening is suitable for most cases and is indicated where there is a history of recent head injury. Otherwise inhalational anaesthesia provides the simplest technique and suitable reduction in muscle tone. Once the patient is adequately anaesthetized and has a secure airway, the surgeon may begin the manipulation. Maintenance of reduction if required is usually by skull traction which may be attached before or after manipulation. Extubation should be smooth and coughing prevented if at all possible.

Anterior approach to cervical spine

The anterior approach through the neck provides access to the vertebral bodies for spinal fusion, and for removal of disc or tumour, or for drainage of infection (Crockard and Ransford, 1991; Hamblen, 1991). Occasionally the odontoid is approached transorally (Merwin *et al.*, 1991) but this route is more likely to be encountered in neurosurgical centres. Cervical fusion may be indicated in post-traumatic instability, or to stabilize the spine after surgery for neoplasm or infection, in degenerative disease or after extensive laminectomy. The cervical spine may also be fused when progressive nerve root or cord compression occurs in cervical spondylosis. The anaesthetist must be wary of possible spinal instability and anticipate difficulties in intubation (Calder, 1987; Crockard and Ransford, 1991; Wood and Lawler, 1992).

During surgery the patient is supine with some head-up tilt and the head rotated away from the side of the incision. The surgery involves considerable handling of the structures in the neck anteriorly and the anaesthetic technique should anticipate the effects of position and surgery. Vagal reflexes, tracheal distortion and occasionally blood loss, especially when tumour is excised, may require attention. Intermittent positive pressure ventilation is usually preferred to spontaneous respiration owing to the length of surgery and the possible advantages of a higher mean intrathoracic pressure in minimizing venous air embolism in the head-up position. In quadriplegic patients, muscle relaxants are rarely required to permit IPPV, and restitution of adequate spontaneous ventilation may be difficult after their use. In most cases the anaesthetic circuit will approach the patient over his head, but the anaesthetic and monitoring equipment may be sited where convenient.

Posterior approach to cervical spine

The cervical spine may be approached from the posterior aspect after generous infiltration of the area with local anaesthetic solution (Magnaes and Hauge, 1980; Hamblen, 1991). Procedures such as laminectomy in patients with cervical spondylosis may be performed this way, though patients do experience arm and leg pain and sensations akin to electric shocks.

More commonly, general anaesthesia is employed. Procedures undertaken include decompression of spinal and nerve root canals and spinal fixation and fusion often following trauma (Bedbrook and Hardcastle, 1991; Hamblen, 1991). Where surgery is for decompression, there are normally no specific difficulties for the anaesthetist save those secondary to any degree of denervation distal to the level of cord compression, except when the compression is associated with instability of the spine. Instability of the cervical spine presents a number of difficulties in intubation and handling of the patient during positioning.

Maintenance of anaesthesia may be achieved with either intravenous or inhalational agents, and muscle relaxants used to facilitate IPPV except when contraindicated. In the prone position, some head-up tilt and moderate degree of hypotension may be helpful to the surgeon, while in the sitting patient the avoidance of hypotension may be more relevant. Suitable supports are required to minimize abdominal compression in the prone patient, and the head may be supported on a horseshoe or fixed in a calliper attached to the table. The arrangement of anaesthetic and ancillary equipment will depend on the theatre routine adopted for the type of case (Martin, 1978).

Good access to a vein is required which may be improved for drug administration by adding an extension tube or remote injection catheter. Blood loss should not be so great nor so rapid as to make a warming coil mandatory. Non-invasive blood pressure, ECG and peripheral oxygen saturation should be monitored, but arterial cannulation is not necessary provided that the general arrangement of the patient on the table does not preclude reasonable access by the anaesthetist. End tidal carbon dioxide measurement is usual in prone patients.

The sitting position for cervical surgery is more favoured in neurosurgical than in orthopaedic units. It has the advantage of easy surgical access and good operating conditions, especially a relatively blood-free field. For the anaesthetist it presents some problems not encountered in recumbent patients, especially the effects of IPPV and posture on blood pressure and the possibility of air embolism.

At the end of surgery, relative instability of the cervical spine may still be present, and care must be exercised in handling the patient during extubation. External support of the neck may be applied or continued after the surgery is complete. If problems of stability are anticipated, an anaesthetic technique which provides a rapid but smooth recovery might be favoured.

Postoperative management

In most cases where operations have been performed on the cervical spine, some form of mechanical restriction such as pillows or bean bags are placed upon movements of the neck in the immediate postoperative period. The increasing use of internal fixation aids stability. Restricted movement helps to reduce pain, but analgesia may still be required. Great care must be taken in administering narcotic analgesia to patients with cord lesions, as respiratory depression or sleep apnoea may be induced. Non-narcotic analgesics can be very effective. Active treatment of nausea is essential because vomiting, especially if violent, may cause dislocation of an unstable spine. Intravenous fluids should be continued until oral fluids are being taken adequately and further blood replacement is no longer necessary. Postoperative ileus is not a major problem in cervical surgery though it may occur in patients with other injuries. Pharyngeosophageal perforation has been reported and usually presents early in the postoperative course though late perforation does occur (Kelly *et al.*, 1991).

Patients recovering from anterior cervical surgery should be observed for airway difficulties or neck swelling especially if several vertebrae have been operated upon (Emery *et al.*, 1991).

The thoracic spine

The disorders of the thoracic spine which attract surgical attention are similar to those affecting the cervical region, with the addition of kyphosis and scoliosis. Surgical treatment may be undertaken for fractures, dislocations, and degenerative or compressive lesions which may affect spinal cord and nerve roots or be confined to bone or soft tissue. The aetiology of the condition has less bearing on the anaesthetist's approach than it does in surgery of the cervical spine, mainly because the operative site is more remote from the airway. This is not to suggest that the anaesthetist need not be fully aware of the general sequelae of the patient's disease. The cervical spine may also be involved. There may be respiratory impairment and long-term cardiopulmonary changes, and when the spine has been fractured the remainder of the trunk is unlikely to have entirely escaped injury.

The procedures available to the surgeon in treating disorders of the thoracolumbar spine include the open and closed reduction of fractures, decompression of the spinal canal and nerve roots, removal of tumour mass, attachment of traction apparatus and spinal fusion. The approach to spinal fusion may be made from anteriorly or posteriorly at any level, and may be used in the treatment of tumours and infections of vertebral bodies, and of fractures and kyphoscoliosis. Fusion with correction of deformity is most commonly performed in children and young adults, but can take place later in life (see General considerations: Thoracic deformity, and Paediatric, Chapter 7).

Preoperative management

The anaesthetic assessment of the patient's general status and, in cases of trauma, the effects of the overall management of the injuries received should take place as usual (see General considerations). In cases where the injury has resulted in an unstable spinal fracture, the anaesthetist should be familiar with the traction arrangement and the operating mechanism of the bed, and determine whether the traction is to be maintained during induction. Induction of anaesthesia is usually performed on the bed to avoid an additional move (Whitesides and Shah, 1976; Wang *et al.*, 1979). The premedication prescribed in these cases will depend on the patient's general condition and on specific problems associated with the injuries, and is often omitted.

Patients for whom spinal decompression is planned and whose condition results from infection or neoplasm may have involvement of sites other than the spine. In general, these will not much affect the anaesthetist though they may necessitate special care in turning or positioning the patient. Only rarely will surgery be undertaken in the presence of active pulmonary infection or pulmonary neoplasia. Involvement of the liver to a degree producing hepatic insufficiency would nearly always exclude the patient from surgical treatment long before the stage of anaesthetic assessment, as would significant renal disease.

Scoliosis surgery is dealt with in Chapter 8. The physiological changes and some peri-operative problems of patients with kyphoscoliosis are discussed earlier in this chapter.

Anaesthesia

Closed reduction of thoracic fracture dislocation

Any anaesthetic technique which provides sufficient reduction in muscle tone to permit satisfactory manipulation may be employed. Limitations of choice may be imposed by a degree of paralysis, which might exclude the use of depolarizing relaxants or cause respiratory difficulties due to weakness of the trunk muscles. If the patient has recently been unconscious, control of respiration and end tidal carbon dioxide levels should be considered.

A chin/occipital halter or other apparatus may be awkward to manage, though in most cases this can be released for anaesthesia, with the surgeon's consent. The possibility of ileus and inadequate gastric emptying should be remembered, as well as that of intrathoracic damage especially to the lungs and pleura. In the presence of established quadriplegia, cardiovascular instability may occur (see Chapter 11) and a lesser degree of vasomotor instability might be expected in paraplegic patients. The patient is usually supine for the attempted reduction, with the fracture site over the break in the table.

Anterior approach to thoracic spine

The spine is approached from the front for some decompression procedures, for access to a vertebral body, or for the more extensive access required for spinal mobilization and fusion (Dwyer, 1973; Leatherman and Dickson, 1988). The anterior resection and mobilisation and subsequent fixation by the Dwyer or Zielke (Leatherman and Dickson, 1988; Trammel *et al.*, 1991) techniques may be part of a two stage procedure. The second stage is posterior fixation and fusion by Remmington or Lagren type equipment. If Cotrel–Dubousset fixation is used posteriorly anterior fixation may not be needed as it is more rigid than the other systems (Leatherman and Dickson, 1988).

Premedication may follow the anaesthetist's normal practice. The choice of anaesthetic depends on the surgeon's technique and the level at which the vertebral bodies have to be exposed. If correction of spinal deformity is planned, spinal cord monitoring with the possibility of a wake-up test should be considered (see General considerations). If wake-up is not required, any suitable combination of anaesthetic agent, analgesic and relaxant may be used.

Most frequently, a left thoracotomy is performed in order to avoid the liver if an abdominal extension of the incision is needed, though the right-sided approach may be favoured for the upper thoracic spine. When the left side is to be opened and a semi- or full lateral position used, the patient should be suitably positioned over the bridge on the operating table. The ipselateral arm should be supported. A double-lumen endobronchial tube is an advantage if access to the upper or mid-thoracic vertebral bodies is required. The design of double-lumen tube should be that most familiar to the anaesthetist. Whether a right- or left-handed tube is used is not important, though positioning of a left-sided tube is less critical and slight displacement during positioning of the patient is less liable to compromise ventilation. In cases where a low left thoracotomy or thoraco-abdominal incision is to be made, the left lung may be retracted rather than collapsed and a standard or kink-resistant endotracheal tube used.

Arterial cannulation is essential for intrathoracic surgery for both blood pressure measurement and blood gas analysis. The heart, aorta and vena cava may all be handled and the spleen or kidney mobilized. Central venous pressure monitoring should also be established. Blood loss may be considerable and facilities for warming transfused blood should be available (Gardner, 1970). For vascular lesions autologous transfusion equipment may be considered (Flynn *et al.*, 1982) If anterior surgery is part one of a 2-stage mobilization and fixation, the planned timing of the second stage may influence the total blood replacement administered. The ECG and peripheral oxygen saturation should as usual be monitored. An oesophageal stethoscope and temperature probes to the patient and between the patient and warming blanket may also be used.

Posterior approach to thoracic spine

Surgical access to the posterior aspect of the thoracic spine is relatively easy and most surgery is performed in a prone position with carefully positioned supports. Occasionally a sitting position may be used for upper thoracic work especially if the cervical region is to be exposed as well.

Some procedures can be carried out under extensive local anaesthetic infiltration or epidural anaesthesia but most require full anaesthesia with tracheal intubation and most of these IPPV. The choice of anaesthetic technique is not important unless constrained by the need for peri-operative assessment of spinal cord function (see General considerations) or to induce relative hypotension to reduce blood loss.

The anaesthetist's access to the patient may be very limited after surgery has started and security of all anaesthetic, intravascular and monitoring equipment connections is vital. If extensive surgery is proposed and especially if hypotensive anaesthesia is to be used, intra-arterial pressure measurement is virtually essential and central venous pressure measurement should equally be considered. If cardiopulmonary function is severely compromised, a pulmonary artery balloon catheter is indicated if surgery is still appropriate. Postoperative intensive therapy facilities are necessary for such patients.

The blood loss during posterior spinal instrumentation can be considerable and should be anticipated. Losses up to 150 per cent of circulating volume have been reported in scoliosis surgery, though 15–25 per cent is more usual (Gardner, 1970; Abott and Bentley, 1980). Saline infiltrations with or without added adrenaline have been used to reduce losses, though careful positioning and hypotensive anaesthesia are the most effective means (Bennett and Abbott, 1977).

When hypotension is to be induced, the best means is that most familiar to the anaesthetist except that those methods which rely on ventilation with volatile agents as a major component may be impossible to combine with reliable spinal cord monitoring. Tubocurarine is still a satisfactory relaxant and, whilst others are not absolutely contraindicated, it seems unnecessary to use agents which maintain or increase systolic blood pressure prior to attempting to reduce it. Ganglion or α-adrenergic blockade may cause tachycardia as a side-effect, though this may be modified by beta blockade. The combined alpha and beta blocking effects of labetalol make for an effective agent. Sodium nitroprusside is, again, a successful hypotensive agent, but its use has revealed tachyphylaxis and resistance to the drug in some patients. Increasing dosage to high levels should be avoided because fatal cyanide intoxication has occurred (Davies, 1975). Provided that maximum dosage and rate of administration have been restricted, this agent has proved satisfactory in use in adults and in children (Bennett and Abbott, 1977). Glyceryl trinitrate infusions may similarly be used.

Rapid blood loss occurs at particular stages of posterior spinal surgery. A moderate loss occurs during incision and stripping of the muscles from the vertebrae, but is rarely great and is easily seen by the anaesthetist. Greater losses occur during decortication of the laminae and removal of donor bone from the iliac crest. These may not be fully revealed initially, as the operative site is packed for a period before the swabs are available for display. Anticipation of this loss avoids under transfusion at the time of distraction when consequent hypotension is undesirable.

The level of systemic blood pressure during most of the surgery is not critical to the patient, but during distraction of the spine reversible changes in transmission in the cord may occur (Hall *et al.*, 1978). The short time course of the impaired conduction indicates a vascular origin (Sudhir *et al.*, 1976), and case reports and animal studies suggest it is sensible to permit the blood pressure to approach normal levels at the time of distraction in patients where a wake-up test or cord function monitoring is indicated (Grundy *et al.*, 1981). Changes in cord function have been clearly demonstrated following clamping of anterior spinal arteries (Apel *et al.*, 1991).

Apart from blood loss and interference with anaesthetic and monitoring connections to the patient, the other rare but significant problem is a pneumothorax. This is more likely if costotransversectomy is undertaken.

Postoperative management

It is the intention of all anaesthetic techniques to result in a smooth transition from anaesthesia to consciousness with the patient being as comfortable as possible on awakening. In some spinal surgery there are other considerations which require rapid return to alertness, but most patients can be allowed to wake up more slowly if it facilitates adequate analgesia. Even when spinal cord monitoring has limited the anaesthetic technique, it is possible to introduce longer acting analgesic agents before surgery is complete.

Some spinal surgery, especially when an anterior approach has been used, is very amenable to epidural analgesic techniques and to postoperative local anaesthetic or narcotic infusions provided suitable care facilities are available. Non-narcotic analgesic can be very effective and should be used when appropriate. Prophylactic use of anti-emetics should be considered especially if the patient is to be nursed supine. Postoperative ileus should be anticipated after correction of spinal deformity.

In appropriate cases, a chest radiograph should be taken soon after recovery from anaesthesia to exclude pneumothorax and to check the position of the spine and its internal fixation.

Fluid and blood replacement should continue especially as both overt and covert blood loss can be significant.

General nursing care and physiotherapy (Sawyer, 1983; Brosnan, 1991; Brown and Seltzer, 1991; Dartyka, 1991) has to be of a high standard as major thoracic interventions commonly result in areas of pulmonary atelectasis or collapse and respiratory infections are fairly frequent. Urinary infections may also be a problem as may the consequences of prolonged nursing in a supine position. These include pressure area damage, deep vein thrombosis and occasionally pulmonary embolism (Dickson and Harrington, 1973).

The lumbosacral spine

The lumbar spine is involved in many of the processes which affect the thoracic region and frequently surgical intervention encompasses both. It is rather more prone to intervertebral disc lesions than other spinal areas and spondylolysthesis at the lumbosacral junction is a relatively frequent problem.

The anaesthetic considerations are in the main general ones except where the thorax is also involved or there are distant associations of the disease process.

Anterior approach to lumbo-sacral spine

The lumbar spine is usually approached from the front as part of major thoracolumbar corrective surgery (see Thoracic spine) though some surgery isolated to the lumbar spine is undertaken. Access to the lumbosacral region is occasionally needed when posterior fixation of spondylolysthesis has failed.

The anaesthetist will be familiar with abdominal surgery for other purposes and standard techniques are appropriate. Internal organs have to be displaced during surgery and are vulnerable to damage, though circulatory changes from handling the aorta and particularly the inferior vena cava are likely to be more common. Blood loss is again a potential hazard but is usually apparent.

Monitoring requirements are standard and access to the patient is not unusually restricted. Where surgery involved both the thoracic and lumbar spine, intravascular monitoring and preparations for major haemorrhage should be considered (see Thoracic spine). Most operations are performed in the supine position and are transperitoneal though a lateral approach which may be retroperitoneal is occasionally possible.

Posterior approach to lumbo-sacral spine

Most anaesthetists will be familiar with some cases where this approach is used, especially for decompression and fusion. Routine premedication may be given except for some patients whose primary problem also involves thoracic deformity. The prone position is usually used, though some operations can be performed satisfactorily in a lateral position with the spine flexed. For operation on the lower spine, variations on the knee-chest position (Lipton, 1950) supporting the patient on the pelvis, chest and elbows may be used. Many centres have developed supporting frames of various designs to facilitate positioning of the patient (Relton and Hall, 1967; Martin, 1978; Wayne, 1984).

The object of all these is to support the patient adequately whilst allowing free movement of the abdomen during respiration and, preferably, to avoid obstruction of the inferior vena cava and accentuated lordosis during surgery of the lumbar spine. The legs may also be arranged to be partly dependent to further reduce venous engorgement. In the knee-chest position, care should be taken to prevent the patient sitting on his calves and kinking his popliteal arteries (Martin, 1978).

The anaesthetic technique may vary, both with the usual practice of the surgical unit and with the patient's position. Some centres employ regional anaesthesia in conscious patients and large series of lumbar laminectomies disc protrusion performed under spinal anaesthesia have been reported (Silver *et al.*, 1976). An isobaric mixture of local anaesthetics is administered by the lumbar route, together with supplementary skin infiltration. Some patients are reluctant to accept this technique and general anaesthesia is used, as it is when a block in cerebrospiral fluid (CSF) circulation has been demonstrated myelographically.

In most centres general anaesthesia is preferred for lumbar spine surgery. Spontaneous respiration is practicable in the lateral position and in the well positioned prone patient, but few spinal procedures are completed in under an hour and many are considerably longer, so a technique involving controlled ventilation is favoured. If surgery for fixation of a spinal fracture is being performed, a wake-up test may be needed and again a relaxant/IPPV technique is indicated (see Spinal cord monitoring). Somatosensory evoked potentials may also be used for monitoring purposes during surgery for lumbar spinal stenosis (Herron *et al.*, 1987).

Usually any anaesthetic combination may be used, though recent injuries to the head or impaired spinal cord function may impose limitations. The degree of patient monitoring and number of intravascular lines depends very much on the magnitude of the proposed surgery. Blood loss is not usually excessive in lumbar spinal surgery, except in major infected lesions, provided the patient is positioned satisfactorily. In most cases, a venous cannula, electrocardiograph monitoring and a means of measuring blood pressure and peripheral oxygen saturation, with end tidal carbon dioxide monitoring used if the patient is ventilated or prone, are adequate. If sudden or prolonged haemorrhage is likely, then intra-arterial pressure monitoring and a central venous catheter or additional peripheral cannula should be considered. In extreme cases where satisfactory positioning of the patient is unlikely to be possible because of obesity or when head and other injuries are present, arterial cannulation for blood gas sampling may be considered. These may help in adjusting ventilation pressures to a minimum in the obese patient, allowing least impairment of surgical conditions by venous congestion. Negative end-expiratory pressure (NEEP) is no longer favoured in these cases as it may accentuate pulmonary atelectasis. Where extensive soft tissue stripping and cancellous bone exposure are necessary, a degree of systemic hypotension may also be of value in reducing blood loss.

Postoperative management

Patients recovering from anterior lumbar surgery may have all the problems associated with intraabdominal surgery as well as those related to their spinal intervention. The usual methods for control of pain, including epidural analgesia, and for suppression of emesis are applicable. The possibility of ileus must not be overlooked. Fluid sequestration in the abdomen can confuse the assessment of postoperative losses especially when some continued haemorrhage is anticipated. Early mobilization may be restricted in these patients and also in some after major posterior lumbar surgery, and care by experienced nurses and physiotherapists is essential. Other patients may be mobilized very rapidly after limited posterior surgery.

In all patients the combination of specific therapies and good general care are essential for rapid, effective and acceptable recovery.

References

Abott, T. R. and Bentley, G. (1980). Intra-operative awakening during scoliosis surgery. *Anaesthesia*, **35**, 298–302.

Akinglini, O. O. (1979). Complications of guided blind endotracheal intubation. *Anaesthesia*, **34**, 590–2.

Apel, D. M., Marrero, G., King, J., Tolo, J. P. and Bassett, G. S. (1991). Avoiding paraplegia during anterior spinal surgery: the role of somatosensory evoked potential monitoring with temporary occlusion of segmental spinal arteries. *Spine*, **16**, S365–70.

Bedbrook, G. M. and Hardcastle, P. H. (1991). Spinal injuries. In G. Bentley and R. B. Greer (eds), *Rob and Smith's Operative Surgery, Orthopaedics Part 1*. Butterworth-Heinemann, London, pp. 624–9.

Ben David, B. (1988). Spinal cord monitoring. *Orthopaedic Clinics of North America*, **19**, 427–8.

Bennett, N. R. and Abbott, T. R. (1977). The use of sodium nitroprusside in children. *Anaesthesia*, **32**, 456–63.

Bergofsky, E. H. (1979). Respiratory failure in disorders of the thoracic cage. *American Review of Respiratory Disease*, **119**, 643–69.

Bjure, J. and Nachemson, A. (1973). Non-treated scoliosis. *Clinical Orthopaedics and Related Research*, **93**, 44–52.

Boltshauser, E., Steinmann, B., Meyer, A. and Jerusalem, F. (1980). Anaesthesia induced rhabdomyolysis in Duchenne muscular dystrophy. *British Journal of Anaesthesia*, **52**, 559.

Brosnan, H. (1991). Nursing management of the adolescent with idiopathic scoliosis. *Nursing Clinics of North America*, **26**, 17–31.

Brown, M. D. and Seltzer, D. G. (1991). Perio-operative care in lumbar spine surgery. *Orthopaedic Clinics of North America*, **22**, 353–8.

Brownell, A. K. W., Daasuke, R. T., Elash, A., Fowlow, S. B., Seagram, C. G. F., Diewold, R. J. and Friesen, C. (1983). Malignant hyperthermia in Duchenne muscular dystrophy. *Anaesthesiology*, **58**, 180–2.

Calancie, B., Klose, K. J., Baier, S. and Green, B. A. (1991). Isoflurane-induced attenuation of motor evoked potentials caused by electrical motor cortex stimulation during surgery. *Journal of Neurosurgery*, **74**, 897–904.

Calder, I. (1987). Anaesthesia for transoral and craniocervical surgery. *Balliere's Clinics in Anaesthesia*, **2**, 441–57.

Carstens, C., Paul, K., Niethand, F. U. and Pfeil, J. (1991). Effect of scoliosis surgery on pulmonary function in patients with meningomyelocoele. *Journal of Paediatric Orthopaedics*, **11**, 459–64.

Crockard, H. A. and Ransford, A. O. (1991). Transoral approach to the cervical spine. In G. Bentley and R. B. Greer (eds), *Rob and Smith's Operative Surgery, Orthopaedics Part 1*. Butterworth-Heinemann, London, pp. 453–62.

Dartyka, M. B. (1991). Practical points in the care of the post-lumbar spine surgery patient. *Journal of Post-Anaesthetic Nursing*, **6**, 185–7.

Davies, J. A. H. (1968). Blind nasal intubation using doxapram hydrochloride. *British Journal of Anaesthesia*, **40**, 361–3.

Davies, D. W., Greiss, L., Kadar, D. and Steward, D. J. (1975). Sodium nitroprusside in children. *Canadian Anaesthetic Society Journal*, **22**, 553–60.

Dawson, E. G., Sherman, J. E., Kanim, L. E. A. and Nuwer, M. R. (1991). Spinal cord monitoring. Results of the Scoliosis Research Society and the European Spinal Deformity Society survey. *Spine*, **16**, S361–4.

Dickson, J. H. and Harrington, P. R. (1973). Evolution of the Harrington instrumentation technique in scoliosis. *Journal of Bone and Joint Surgery*, **55A**, 993–1002.

Dvorak, J., Herdmann, J., Janssen, B., Thailer, R. and Grob, D. (1990). Motor evoked potentials in patients with cervical spine disorders. *Spine*, **15**, 1013–16.

Dwyer, A. F. (1973). Experience of anterior correction of scoliosis. *Clinical Orthopaedics and Related Research*, **93**, 191–206.

Eichhorn, J. H., Cooper, J. B., Cullen, D. J., Maier, W. R., Philip, J. H. and Seeman, R. G. (1986). Standards for patient monitoring during anaesthesia at Harvard Medical School. *Journal of the American Medical Association*, **256**, 1017–20.

Emery, S. E., Smith, M. D. and Bohlman, H. H. (1991). Upper-airway obstruction after multilevel cervical corpectomy for myelopathy. *Journal of Bone and Joint Surgery of America*, **73**, 544–51.

Flynn, J. C., Price, C. T. and Zink, W. P. (1991). The third step of total autogous blood transfusion in scoliosis surgery. Harvesting blood from the postoperative wound. *Spine*, **16**, S328–9.

Flynn, J. C., Metzger, C. R. and Csencsitz, T. A. (1982). Intra-operative autotransfusion (IAT) in spine surgery. *Spine*, **7**, 423–35.

Friedman, W. A. and Grundy, B. L. (1987). Monitoring of sensory evoked potentials is highly reliable and helpful in the operating room. *Journal of Clinical Monitoring*, **3**, 38–44.

Gardner, R. C. (1970). Blood loss after spinal instrumentation and fusion in scoliosis (Harrington procedure). *Clinical Orthopaedics and Related Research*, **71**, 182–5.

Gokel, E., Arkan, A., Sagiroglu, E., Karci, A. and Maltape, F. (1991). Continuous infusions of fentanyl-propofol and alfentanyl-propofol as anaesthetic methods in spinal surgery and the 'wake-up' test. In C. Prys-Roberts (ed.), *Focus on Infusions – Intravenous Anaesthesia*. Current Medical Literature, London, pp. 180–3.

Grundy, B. L., Nash, C. L. and Brown, R. H. (1981). Arterial pressure manipulation alters spinal cord function during correction of scoliosis. *Anaesthesiology*, **54**, 249–53.

Hall, J. E., Levine, C. R. and Sudhir, K. G. (1978). Intra-operative awakening to monitor spinal cord function during Harrington instrumentation and spinal fusion. *Journal of Bone and Joint Surgery*, **60A**, 533–6.

Hamblen, D. L. (1991). Anterior fusion of the cerival spine. In G. Bentley and R. B. Greer (eds), *Rob and Smith's Operative Surgery, Orthopaedics Part 1*. Butterworth-Heinemann, London, pp. 463–70.

Hamblen, D. L. (1991). Posterior fusion of the cervical spine. In G. Bentley and R. B. Greer (eds), *Rob and Smith's Operative Surgery, Orthopaedics Part 1*. Butterworth-Heinemann, London, pp. 471–81.

Herron, L. D., Tripps, A. C. and Gonyeau, M. (1987). Intra-operative use of dermatomal somatosensory-evoked potentials in lumbar stenosis surgery. *Spine*, **12**, 379–83.

Hoppenfield, S., Gross, A. and Andrews, C. (1991). The ankle clonus test: an alternative to the Stagnara wake-up test and somatosensory evoked potentials in the treatment of scoliosis. *Journal of Bone and Joint Surgery*, **73B**, suppl. 1, 31–2.

Husum, B. and Berthelsen, P. (1981). Allen's test and systolic arterial pressure in the thumb. *British Journal of Anaesthesia*, **53**, 635–7.

Jones, R. S., Kennedy, J. D., Owen, R. and Taylor, J. F. (1981). Mechanical inefficiency of the thoracic cage in scoliosis. *Thorax*, **36**, 456–61.

Kalkman, C. J., Traast, H., Zuurmand, W. W. and Bovill, J. G. (1990). Substitution of nitrous oxide by propofol improves posterior tibial nerve somatosensory evoked potentials. *British Journal of Anaesthesia*, **64**, 387P.

Kalkman, C. J., Ten Brink, S. A., Been, H. D. and Bovill, J. G. (1991a). Variability of somatosensory cortical evoked potentials during spinal surgery. *Spine*, **16**, 924–9.

Kalkman, C. J., Traast, H., Zuurmand, W. W. and Bovill, J. G. (1991b). Differential effects of propofol and nitrous oxide on posterior tibial nerve somatosensory cortical evoked potentials during alfentanyl anaesthesia. *British Journal of Anaesthesia*, **66**, 483–9.

Kelly, M. F., Spiegel, J., Rizzo, K. A. and Zwillenborg, D. (1991). Delayed pharyngoesophageal perforation: a complication of anterior spine surgery. *Annals of Otorhinolaryngology*, **100**, 201–5.

Lamalre, A., Hall, J. E., Weng, T. R., Aspin, N. and Levison, H. (1971). Pulmonary function in scoliosis one year after spinal correction. *Journal of Bone and Joint Surgery*, **53A**, 195.

Leatherman, K. D. and Dickson, A. R. (1988). *The Management of Spinal Deformities*. Butterworth, London.

Lindh, M. and Bjure, J. (1975). Lung volumes in scoliosis before and after correction by the Harrington instrumentation method. *Acta Orthopaedica Scandinavica*, **46**, 934–48.

Lipton, S. (1950). Mohammedan prayer position. *Anaesthesia*, **5**, 208–12.

Loughnan, B. A., Murdoch, L. J., Hetreed, M. A., Howard, L. A. and Hall, G. M. (1990). Effects of 2% lignocaine on somatosensory evoked potentials recorded in the extradural space. *British Journal of Anaesthesia*, **65**, 643–7.

MacLennan, F. M. and Robertson, G. S. (1981). Ketamine for induction and intubation in Treacher–Collins syndrome. *Anaesthesia*, **36**, 196–8.

Magnaes, B. and Hauge, T. (1980). Surgery for myelopathy in cervical spondylosis: safety measures and preoperative factors relating to outcome. *Spine*, **5**, 211–14.

Martin, J. T. (1978). *Positioning in Anaesthesia and Surgery*. W. B. Saunders, Philadelphia, PA.

Merwin, G. E., Post, J. C. and Sypert, G. W. (1991). Transval approach to the upper cervical spine. *Laryngoscope*, **101**, 780–4.

Miller, E. D., Sanders, D. B., Rawlingson, J. C., Berry, F. A., Scussman, M. D. and Epstein, R. M. (1978). Anaesthesia induced rhabdomyolysis in a patient with Duchenne's muscular dystrophy. *Anaesthesiology*, **48**, 146–8.

Moe, J. H., Winter, R. B., Bradford, D. S. and Lonstein, J. E. (1978). *Scoliosis and Other Spinal Deformities*. W. B. Saunders, Philadelphia, PA.

Nash, C. L. and Braun, R. H. (1989). Current concepts review: spinal cord monitoring. *Journal of Bone and Joint Surgery*, **71A**, 627–30.

Owen, J. H., Bridnell, K. H., Grubb, R., Jenny, A., Allen, B., Padberg, A. M. and Shimon, S. M. (1991). The clinical application of neurogenic motor evoked potentials to monitor spinal cord function during surgery. *Spine*, **16**, S385–90.

Prime, F. J. (1977). A review of lung function in scoliotic subjects. In P. A. Zorab (ed.), *Scoliosis*. Academic Press, London, pp. 329–38.

Recommendations for Standards of Monitoring During Anaesthesia and Recovery (1988). The Association of Anaesthetists of Great Britain and Ireland, London.

Relton, J. E. S. and Hall, J. E. (1967). An operation frame for spinal fusion: a new apparatus designed to reduce haemorrhage during operation. *Journal of Bone and Joint Surgery*, **49B**, 327–32.

Riseborough, E. J. (1973). The effects of scoliotic deformities on pulmonary function. *Israeli Journal of Medical Science*, **9**, 787–90.

Sawyer, M. W. (1983). The role of the physical therapist before and after lumbar spine surgery. *Orthopaedic Clinics of North America*, **14**, 649–59.

Secher-Walker, R. H., Ho, J. E. and Gill, I. S. (1979). Observations on regional ventilation and perfusion in kyphoscoliosis. *Respiration*, **38**, 194–203.

Shannon, D. C., Riseborough, E. J., Valenca, L. M. and Kazemi, H. (1970). The distribution of abnormal lung function in kyphoscoliosis. *Journal of Bone and Joint Surgery*, **52A**, 131–144.

Silver, D. J., Dunsmore, R. H. and Dickson, C. M. (1976). Spinal anaesthesia for lumbar disc surgery. Review of 576 operations. *Anesthesia and Analgesia, Current Researches*, **55**, 550–4.

Sneerson, J. M. (1977). The determination of pulmonary

artery pressure in thoracic scolisis. In P. A. Zorab (ed.), *Scoliosis*. Academic Press, London, pp. 193–201.

Stein, S. M., Kirchner, S. G., Horer, G. and Hernanz-Schulman, M. (1991). Atlanto-occipital subluxation in Down syndrome. *Paediatric Radiology*, **21**, 121–4.

Sudhir, K. G., Smith, R. M., Hall, J. E. and Hansen, D. D. (1976). Intra-operative awakening for early recognition of possible neurologic sequelae during Harrington-rod spinal fusion. *Anesthesia and Analgesia, Current Researches*, **55**, 526–8.

Taylor, P. A. and Towey, R. M. (1972). The bronchofibroscope as an aid to endotracheal intubation. *British Journal of Anaesthesia*, **44**, 611–12.

Trammel, T. R., Benedict, F. and Reed, D. (1991). Anterior spine fusion using Zielke instrumentation for adult thoracolumbar and lumbar scoliosis. *Spine*, **16**, 307–16.

Vauxelle, C., Stagnara, D. and Jouvinoux, P. (1973). Functional monitoring of spinal cord activity during spinal surgery. *Clinical Orthopaedics and Related Research*, **93**, 173–8.

Waldman, J., Kaufer, H., Hensinger, R. N., Callaghan, M. L. and Lieding, K. G. (1977). Wake-up technic to avoid neurological sequelae during Harrington rod procedure. A case report. *Anesthesia and Analgesia, Current Researches*, **56**, 733–5.

Wang, G. J., Whitehill, R., Stamp, W. G. and Rosenberger, R. (1979). The treatment of fracture dislocations of the thoracolumbar spine with halofemoral traction and Harrington rod instrumentation. *Clinical Orthopaedics and Related Research*, **142**, 168–75.

Waters, D. J. (1963). Guided blind endotracheal intubation. *Anaesthesia*, **18**, 158–62.

Wayne, S. J. (1984). A modification of the tuck position for lumbar spine surgery. A 15-year follow-up study. *Clinical Orthopaedics*, **184**, 212–16.

Westgate, H. D. and Johnson, B. E. (1971). Pre-operative pulmonary evaluation and postoperative respiratory management of patients with severe thoracic scoliosis. *Journal of Bone and Joint Surgery*, **53A**, 195.

Whitesides, T. E. and Shah, S. G. A. (1976). On the management of unstable fractures of the thoracolumbar spine. *Spine*, **1**, 99–107.

Wood, P. R. and Lawler, P. G. P. (1992). Managing the airway in cervical spine injury. A review of the Advanced Trauma Life Support protocol. *Anaesthesia*, **47**, 792–7.

Zorab, P. A. (1977). *Scoliosis*. Academic Press, London.

Zorab, P. A., Prime, F. J. and Harrison, A. (1979). Lung function in young persons after spinal fusion for scoliosis. *Spine*, **4**, 22–8.

Chapter 5

The management of postoperative pain

The problem

Postoperative pain is a complex subjective emotional experience of infinite range, its emotional aspect best demonstrated by dramatic responses to placebos. Between 5 and 10 per cent of patients appear to suffer no postoperative pain at all after minor procedures – an important finding for the interpretation of studies comparing means of pain relief. The intensity of pain may not be constant even in a given individual but will wax and wane in a cyclical pattern (Gjessing and Tomlin, 1979). There may be diurnal variations caused by superimposition of other diurnal rhythms (Lloyd, 1977), and women appear to have a lower requirement for analgesia than do men (Gjessing and Tomlin, 1979); McQuay *et al.*, 1980) perhaps because of a sex difference in the endogenous neuroendocrine mechanism of pain relief. It has been local experience that the greatest demands for analgesia have been made by fit, athletic young men! More neurotic patients suffer greater postoperative pain than do less neurotic patients (Parbrook *et al.*, 1973). Smokers metabolize analgesics considerably faster than non-smokers (Keeri-Szanto and Pomeroy, 1971) and need more as a result. Some authorities have claimed that limb surgery gives rise to little postoperative pain; however, Gjessing and Tomlin (1979) found that pain of visceral origin was easier to control than pain of musculo-skeletal origin. They ascribed this to the anatomical arrangement of afferent relays in the substantia gelatinosa of the spinal cord – visceral afferents are more superficial than musculo-skeletal afferents and therefore more accessible to drugs. Established work suggests, however, that both the outer layer and the sixth or innermost layer of cells of the dorsal horn are concerned with the relay of somatic pain, and conflicts with this suggestion.

Perhaps because of this variety of experience, postoperative pain is a neglected area of anaesthetic practice. From the viewpoint of patients, Freed (1975) found pain following surgery of the legs for trauma almost unbearable at night, and MacInnes (1976) was struck by 'the nonchalant attitude of the medical profession towards quite unnecessary suffering'.

Pain was seldom discussed in the literature prior to 1975 apart from papers comparing the qualities of analgesics; Utting and Smith, reviewing the subject in 1979, concluded that there had been little progress in 25 years and that the problem awaited a radical new approach. An Editorial (1976a) in the *British Medical Journal* pointed out that doctors and nurses were not assiduous in treating postoperative pain – possibly because it is self-limiting, possibly because of concern about the side-effects of controlled drugs. This approach was rightly condemned by the *Lancet* (Editorial, 1976b) as 'tight-fisted analgesia'.

The treatment of postoperative pain is not simply a question of the patient's comfort: it is possible that severe postoperative pain may have physiological consequences increasing the stress response to surgery and the time required for convalescence. Severe pain often causes patients to remain immobile, thus becoming vulnerable to deep vein thrombosis, pulmonary atelectasis, muscle wasting and urinary retention. Moreover, restlessness caused by severe pain may contribute to postoperative hypoxaemia.

At present a routine schedule of treatment is usually prescribed for postoperative pain because its changing nature allows insufficient time for adjustment of dosage to individual needs. This routine is most often an opiate given by intramuscular injection, 4-hourly as necessary. With this management there is abundant evidence that roughly half of all postoperative patients will suffer very severe pain (Smith and Utting, 1976). The treatment of postoperative pain is in the hands of the nursing staff, yet the study by Smith and Utting (1976) suggested that nurses were often unable to recognize when a patient had severe pain – a situation complicated by the North European ethic that demands that patients conceal their pain and keep a stiff upper lip.

The inadequacy of existing treatment is in part due to pharmacodynamic causes and in part to the logistic problems of administering controlled drugs. The logistic difficulties arise from the legal requirements for keeping and administering controlled drugs. At night, when pain tends to be magnified by fear and isolation, analgesic drugs are available virtually only when the night sister makes her round (Smith and Utting, 1976). The pharmacodynamic causes are due to the variable plasma concentrations of opiates which result from intramuscular injection; Austin *et al.* (1980) found that the minimum concentration required for analgesia was exceeded for only 35 per cent of the 4-hour interval between injections. Peak plasma concentrations may vary 5-fold between patients and 2-fold within patients following the same injection (Stapleton *et al.*, 1978). Absorption from the intramuscular site increases with the lipophilicity of the agent injected (Table 5.1) and the regional blood flow; this in turn may vary with body temperature, circulating blood volume and $PaCO_2$ in the immediate postoperative period. Final plasma concentrations, too, will depend upon the rate of elimination of the agent by the liver, also subject to immense variability at this time. Following accidental trauma, it is accepted practice not to give opiates intramuscularly because the effect is so unpredictable.

Postoperative pain reaches a peak at 3–6 hours after surgery and then declines to become minimal after 3–4 days. The drugs available for its treatment have been extensively reviewed by Bullingham (1981) and by Utting and Smith (1979), who comment that advances on this front have at best been marginal. Stapleton *et al.* (1978) considered that the drugs available were adequate and that further improvement in management could only come from improved means of administration. All the known analgesics are effective at suppressing steady background pain and poor at treating sharp incident pain which occurs when a wound is suddenly distracted or a fracture of bone moved. Side-effects are common: respiratory depression, sedation, dysphoria, hallucination, nausea and vomiting such that the treatment of postoperative pain can be positively disabling.

Orthopaedic patients who are not ill, who have no systemic disease and have undergone peripheral surgery may find the side-effects of conventional intramuscular analgesics disproportionate.

The deficiencies in the management of postoperative pain were recognized by the working party on Pain after Surgery, appointed by the Royal College of Surgeons of England and the College of Anaesthetists (1990). The working party report recommended fundamental changes in the way postoperative pain is managed: that an acute pain service should be established in each major surgical hospital and that a named member of staff should be responsible for a hospital policy which ensures satisfactory pain relief for all patients after surgery: that a high dependency unit and properly trained staff should be available to support the needs of the policy; that current methods of pain relief should be exploited to the full, and that new means should be devised by an active research programme. Finally, the report recommended that a patient's pain should be assessed and charted together with other observations such as blood pressure and heart rate.

Developments in assessment of pain and techniques of analgesia particularly suited to orthopaedic surgery are described in subsequent sections of this chapter.

Table 5.1 Lipophilicity of analgesics

Lipophilicity	Agent
High ↑	buprenorphine
	methadone
	fentanyl
	pethidine
	etorphine
	levorphanol
	morphine
Low	

Source: Bullingham (1981).

The assessment of postoperative pain

The difficulty in assessing postoperative pain remains an obstacle to further development in this field, and the construction of good clinical trials where like is compared with like and recognizable bias is excluded demands careful work at the design stage. Further difficulties arise from ethical requirements for patients in pain, the range or variability of the subject of investigation and the fact that, postoperatively, patients may be unsuitable for investigation or unable to cooperate.

The means available for assessing clinical pain are listed in Table 5.2. The most basic technique is a simple questionnaire but the number of possible grades of response is limited if the questionnaire is not to be overloaded. A more sensitive device is a scoring system or the visual analogue upon which the patient marks the severity of his or her pain at that time and without reference to previous records. Possible gradations now range from, say, 10 to infinity, but interpretation of the response poses problems; opinions differ over whether the measurement should be linear or logarithmic. A careful appraisal of pain questionnaires and their statistical evaluation has been given by Melzack (1975). An objective measurement such as vital capacity is superficially attractive, but in practice is limited and useful only after major thoracic or abdominal surgery.

Assessment of pain based on the patient's demand for analgesia provides answers to a different question; where the questionnaire assessments are based on the intensity of pain, the demand for analgesia involves a further subjective decision with the threshold differing in different patients. Commonly the two means of assessment are regarded as complementary and used together in a study. The patient's demand for analgesia creates objective data which may be interpreted relatively easily. This method is used in its most sophisticated form by McQuay *et al.* (1980), who recorded the timing and frequency with which patients demanded incremental doses of an intravenous analgesic from a demand analgesia apparatus (see pp. 68–71). The efficacy and duration of action of one intravenous agent may then be compared with another (standard) agent. By a further step, other analgesic techniques may be evaluated by the degree to which they fail to provide analgesia and thus cause the patient to make demands from the demand apparatus. With all studies of pain there is great need for a well-trained research assistant who is able to make clear to patients what is expected of them without creating a bias and to assist with questionnaires without colouring the replies.

Table 5.2 Techniques used for assessing clinical pain

Simple questionnaire:
'My pain is absent/mild/moderate/severe'

Scoring of pain intensity:
Patient assesses pain severity on a scale 1, 2, 3, 4, 5, 6, 7, 8, 9, 10

Visual analogue scale:
No pain at all ____________ Worst pain imaginable

Objective measurement
vital capacity

Demands for analgesia:
1. Time to first demand
2. Total dosage of analgesic required in a given time
3. Frequency of demand

At the Nuffield Orthopaedic Centre a full-time Sister is appointed as Pain Sister to oversee nursing management of pain and to train nurses to keep accurate observations of pain along with other nursing observations. The nursing staff of the high dependency unit are taught about new methods of pain control and feed back information about the success or failings of the methods chosen. Provision of adequate pain relief and monitoring of postoperation pain are rendered easier if patients are nursed postoperatively in a purpose designed postoperative ward (Fig. 5.1).

Intravenous analgesia

To achieve the best results from opiate analgesics in the immediate postoperative period, the drugs should be given by the intravenous route. This route has overwhelming advantages, compared with intramuscular administration, which may be summarized as:

1. a predictable, rapid onset of drug action, which produces prompt relief of pain;
2. an early attainment of peak plasma levels of drug, which makes assessment of need and titration of dose practicable;
3. a decline in plasma levels after initial peak concentrations, which limits the time in which toxic effects are likely to occur.

Because the action of the drug given intravenously is so short, it must be given either as a continuous infusion or as frequently repeated small incremental doses.

Stapleton *et al.* (1979) investigated a regimen of controlled intravenous infusion delivered from a

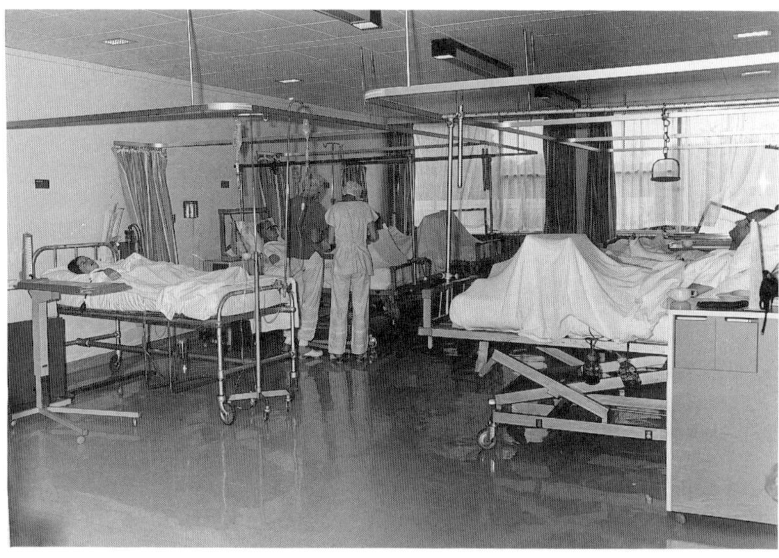

Fig 5.1 Postoperative ward, general view. Patients are admitted immediately following surgery and remain until the following day.

syringe pump in 10 female patients immediately following abdominal hysterectomy. Pethidine was infused at rates determined mathematically and designed to ensure that the minimum analgesic plasma concentrations (0.2 μ/ml) would be exceeded within half an hour of the start and that 80 per cent of the ultimate steady state concentration would be achieved by 6 hours (Table 5.3). The infusion was continued for 32 hours and good analgesia (assessed by questionnaire) was obtained in all the patients save during the first 3 hours when severe pain was felt by some.

Clearly, greater plasma concentrations than the minimal analgesic are required in the first few hours after surgery if pain is adequately to be controlled at this stage. The most suitable agent to choose for infusion is one of low lipophilicity since the chief determinant of plasma concentrations, given a steady infusion, is the rate of hepatic clearance of the drug from the plasma. This is higher for more lipophilic drugs (see Table 5.1), so the effect of variations in hepatic blood flow will be more obvious in plasma concentrations.

Table 5.3 Two regimens for continuous intravenous infusion of pethidine

1. Stapleton et al. (1978)	2. Church (1979)
(a) Loading dose of 1.0 mg per minute for 45 minutes	(a) Bolus dose of 0.3 mg/kg
(b) 0.53 mg per minute for 28 minutes	(b) Maintenance rate 0.3 mg/kg per hour
(c) Maintenance rate 0.4 mg per minute	
Duration of infusion: 32 hours	Duration of infusion: 'indefinite'

The Stapleton *et al.*, study (1979) was confined to a limited homogeneous group of patients. Wider experience of 300 general surgical patients who received narcotic infusions after major abdominal surgery was reported by Church (1979). His regimen was simpler than that of Stapleton (Table 5.3), consisting of a bolus dose followed by a constant infusion. The rate of infusion was adequate for 80 per cent of the patients and required adjustment for the remainder; 3 patients developed respiratory depression which needed reversal with naloxone. Assessment of results is confined to 41 patients who returned a postal questionnaire; unsatisfactory treatment was reported by 11 per cent of the trial group compared with unsatisfactory treatment in 44 per cent of a matched control group who received intramuscular opiates.

Demand analgesia systems

Constant intravenous infusion rates do not however cope with the problem of the range of variation of demand for analgesia. This is neatly overcome by patient activated demand systems preset to deliver a given bolus of a suitable agent intravenously when the patient requires it. In addition, some systems permit a constant background infusion to even out the peaks and troughs in plasma analgesic concentration. Patient controlled analgesia (PCA) is superior to intramuscular analgesia because patients have control of their own pain without the need for painful intramuscular injections; these are often given at inappropriately low dosage and long intervals, and suffer from the fact that drug absorption postoperatively from intramuscular sites is erratic and unreliable. The principle of PCA is popular with patients who like to have control and this reduces the anxiety component of pain, making it easier to treat.

The introduction of PCA in 1966 is described by Sechzer (1990) who, from the beginning, saw PCA as both a means of treating pain and a means of quantifying analgesic deficit. He set out criteria for safe, dependable function of the delivery system: it must be sterile and permit continuing delivery of sterile material; it must allow precise, consistent and replicable delivery of the dose set and it must be easy to standardize, maintain and calibrate. Sechzer also quickly noticed the enormous range of demands made and that some patients even appeared to have no postoperative pain and made no demands. The beginning of the report of the first 118 subjects (Sechzer, 1971) gave the name to the apparatus, 'A patient-controlled analgesic – demand. . . .'. Since this introduction PCA has been very slow in gaining acceptance. This may be because of the high cost of sophisticated demand analgesia pumps or the difficulty in training staff adequately in their use: now the introduction of a cheap disposable mechanical device (Rowbotham *et al.*, 1989) has given the technique added impetus (Fig. 5.2).

Notcutt and Morgan (1990) reported their experience introducing PCA in a district general hospital. They quickly achieved considerable success: only 29 per cent of patients complained of pain, of whom 8 per cent classified the pain as severe. However, the authors found that the pumps developed faults (one range of pumps was subsequently withdrawn) and that it was difficult to maintain the level of nursing vigilance. Untutored enthusiasts would fiddle with the machines, and security is a problem when dangerous drugs are left unattended. The authors abandoned background infusions which they believed increased the complication rate and reduced safety.

There is now a considerable body of literature confirming that PCA is effective in treating postoperative pain, without appreciable respiratory depression due to excessive demands by the patient. Wasylak *et al.*, 1990) demonstrated not only that PCA was better than conventional intramuscular analgesia in a group of women recovering from hysterectomy, but that postoperative morbidity was lower: minute ventilation recovered faster, ambulation was achieved more rapidly and patients were discharged home earlier. The additional cost of PCA can thus be justified economically.

Weller *et al.*, 1991) compared morphine PCA with epidural morphine for the relief of pain after hip or knee replacement in a prospective study in 30 patients. Pain was recorded by visual analogue scores and side-effects were charted. Marginally better analgesia was noted in the epidural group with fewer painful episodes but this group had more side-effects, principally pruritus and slow respiratory rates. However, had the PCA been set to deliver a larger bolus, (they used 1–1.5 mg) it is likely that these differences would disappear. Levels of analgesia are more likely to fluctuate during PCA since the stimulus to demand is more pain and if small boluses are chosen pain will return more frequently: patients will have longer pain-free intervals with epidural administration. In essence this is the argument for background intravenous infusions.

PCA is still in its infancy and much remains to be learned. There is wide variation in plasma opiate concentrations reported when patients are pain free. This might reflect the variation in severity of pain described by individuals but probably means that analgesia is not attained at a given plasma concentration: it is not simply a question of an ED_{50} for the opiate concerned.

Owen *et al.* (1990a) investigated the effect of bolus size on rate of demand. Surprisingly, they found that the number of demands made was independent of bolus size, casting doubt on the concept of plasma minimal effective analgesia concentration. Whatever the pain, patients would make a demand to seek its reduction, once they had learned that this was what happened: operant conditioning had occurred rather like the bar-pressing behaviour of rats fed on demand. Owen *et al.*, 1990b) also studied the use of brief infusions triggered by demand to provide rapid onset of analgesia while minimizing peak plasma concentrations to reduce euphoria and side-effects. They used alfentanil, a potent analgesic with a short latency. However, the latency was too great for alfentanil to be used in this manner and if the infusion rate was increased to reduce latency, peak plasma levels rose and respiratory depression became more prominent.

PCA equipment and its use

There are now a number of microprocessor-controlled electromechanical pumps available which cost about £2000 and a simple disposable device which costs about £20.

The disposable PCA device (the 2C1070 Travenol Infusor) is described in detail by Duthie *et al.* (1987). It is compact and completely portable, usually clipped to the patients clothes; it requires no external source of power; it is almost tamper proof since no adjustment can be made once it is loaded (Fig. 5.2). However, there are some patients who find it difficult to operate; a volume of schedule drug is left exposed and unlocked, and the system is inflexible since the size of the bolus is determined by the initial dilution.

The electromechanical pumps are very flexible, capable of giving a wide range of boluses and volumes, with or without a background infusion: they can be reprogrammed in use so that the setting can be 'fine-tuned' for a particular patient; the contained drug is locked away. But they are not suitable for ambulant patients because they are large and heavy, owing to the rechargeable battery, and are best clamped to a patient's bed. (Fig. 5.3) They are fickle, and anyone with access to the key can reprogramme them. The Graseby PCAS is described and evaluated by Jackson *et al.* (1991).

Any opiate can be used. At the Nuffield Orthopaedic Centre NHS Trust, we currently use morphine made up to give 1 mg/ml with a bolus of 1–2 mg and a lockout of 5–10 minutes. The Graseby performs poorly at volumes of less than 1 ml (Jackson *et al.*, 1991) and is subject to a variety of memory failures and electromechanical failures. The Travenol infusor delivers 0.5 ml only and therefore the opiate must be diluted to give 2 mg/ml or more. An anti-emetic such as droperidol 5 mg added to the solution markedly reduces nausea and vomiting.

Patient compliance is critical to the effectiveness of PCA and so patients should have the devices demonstrated preoperatively and have the chance to try them and familiarize themselves with the control. This also motivates patients to use the device afterwards and is generally a morale booster.

It is important that the nursing staff involved in PCA support the patients and make regular observations of pain score, respiratory frequency and the amount of drug consumed in order to detect side-effects or malfunction of the apparatus. Constant supervision remains necessary: Wakelin and Larsen reported a case of spouse controlled analgesia (?SCA) in which a well-intentioned husband triggered a bolus dose for his wife whenever he felt she might need it – even if she were already asleep.

PCA is particularly useful for those patients who undergo extensive or very painful surgery and for those patients who have been taking opiates in whom drug requirement is difficult to predict. It is also useful for haemophiliacs in whom intramuscular injections are contraindicated. PCA reduces the risk

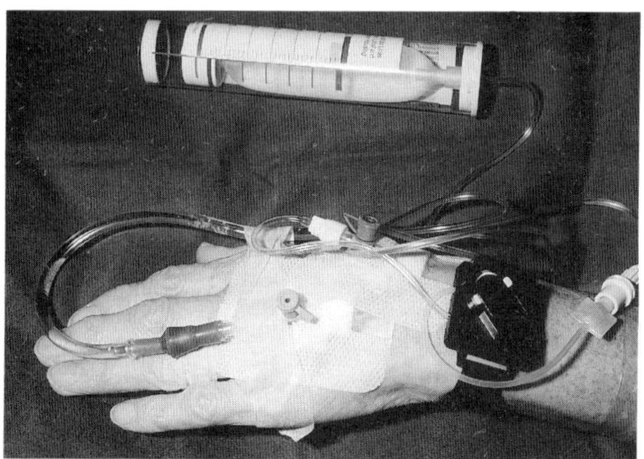

Fig 5.2 Disposable PCA device (2C1070 Travenol Infusor). Top is the graduated reservoir holding up to 60 ml of solution: a pushbutton is mounted on the dorsum of the wrist and 0.5 ml aliquots of solution are fed into a cannula separate from the intravenous infusion.

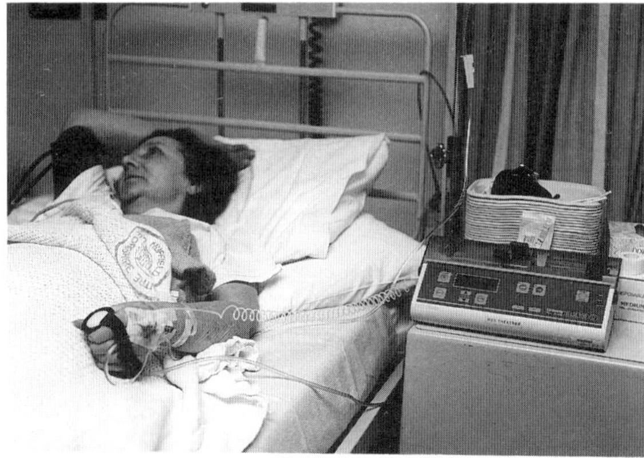

Fig 5.3 Electromechanical PCA equipment. The pump mechanism containing a locked reservoir of solution rests on the patient's bedside locker whilst the patient holds the hand control containing the pushbutton (white). The analgesic is fed into a separate cannula.

of contamination or needlestick injury to staff when patients are hepatitis B or HIV positive because it is a closed system with no requirement for injections.

Although at first sight a very simple system of analgesia, PCA demands considerable experience in its use and great attention to detail for good results: it is not a 'set and forget' system. Serious accidents are being reported and there is as yet no full Department of Health evaluation programme for PCA equipment.

Epidural and spinal analgesia

Bolus dosage

Epidural opiate analgesia has enjoyed widespread popularity since its introduction in 1979 because of its effectiveness, relative freedom from side-effects and long duration of action. More recent work has been directed towards refining the technique with new agents and adjuvants. Epidural opiates are particularly effective in elderly patients and require no patient compliance. Moore *et al.* (1990) studied differences in epidural morphine requirements between elderly and young patients. The elderly group was 65 years or older and the younger group was 50 years or younger. All patients received morphine (0.05 mg/kg) in 10 ml of solution. The elderly group derived significantly better and prolonged analgesia; most elderly patients did not require any further analgesia until towards the end of the first postoperative day and 2 required no further analgesia at all. There was no difference between the groups in plasma morphine concentration which was well below the 50 mg/ml level associated with intramuscular analgesia, confirming a focal spinal effect. Stuart-Taylor *et al.* (1992) used epidural bolus doses of diamorphine 2.5 mg diluted in 10 ml of saline administered 2–3 hourly as required by nursing staff. Eight hundred postoperative patients were studied and satisfactory analgesia was obtained in 94.6 per cent. Respiratory depression occurred in 7 patients in the early postoperative period and was readily reversed with naloxone 0.4 mg. They concluded that diamorphine was safe used in this way provided that other peri-operative opioids were avoided, that the dose of 2.5 mg was not exceeded and that the technique was not used after dural puncture.

Local anaesthetic agents may potentiate the epidural opioid. Bisgaard *et al.* (1990) compared regular boluses of morphine (4 mg) every 8 hours with a mixture of bupivacaine 2.5 mg/ml and morphine 0.06 mg/ml given as an epidural infusion of 9 ml/hour after major abdominal surgery. The combination proved significantly more successful than morphine alone.

Given epidurally, clonidine has analgesic properties. Clonidine is an a_2 adrenoceptor agonist used in the treatment of hypertension which was found to produce analgesia when given intrathecally to patients with chronic pain syndromes. This action is ill understood, although it is known that noradrenergic neuronal systems are involved in the modulation of pain at both spinal and supraspinal levels, mediated by a_2 receptors. Van Essen *et al.* (1990) found epidural clonidine inferior to epidural morphine: the average reduction in pain score with clonidine was only 37 per cent compared with 57 per cent for morphine. In combination however clonidine looks more promising. Vercauteren *et al.* (1990) compared epidural clonidine (1 μg/kg) and sufentanil (25 μg) with sufentanil (50 μg) alone. The mixture gave better analgesia and the smaller dose of opioid led to fewer side-effects.

Sufentanil may have particular promise as an epidural analgesic: it is a short-acting opioid with a high lipid solubility and high receptor affinity. It should therefore rapidly induce analgesia with a low incidence of unwanted effects. Leicht *et al.* (1990) found that epidural sufentanil was very effective in providing analgesia in parturients after caesarian section. This is a group of patients in whom epidural analgesia with opioids is particularly difficult, possibly because of the dynamic epidural circulation at delivery which quickly redistributes any drug. However sufentanil provided more than 90 per cent pain relief in all patients. In addition, if adrenaline (300 μg) was added to the sufentanil, the duration of analgesia was extended from a mean of 266 minutes to a mean of 348 minutes. The adrenaline here may either be acting as a vasoconstrictor conserving sufentanil or it may be modulating activity in the spinal neurones concerned with nociception, potentiating the effects of sufentanil.

Management of top-up doses during the period of blood loss and circulatory instability which follows major surgery is not simple, and severe hypotension due to hypovolaemia and autonomic blockade is easily provoked by an injudicious dose of local anaesthetic or by allowing blood replacement to fall behind cumulative loss. Hypotension impairs cerebral perfusion and produces marked drowsiness, nausea and vomiting, thus losing many of the advantages of epidural analgesia. There remains the possibility that the epidural catheter might erode through into the subarachnoid space so that a subsequent top-up may inadvertently result in a high spinal block.

Resistance to epidural analgesia amongst orthopaedic patients was reported by Sprotte (1979), who noted failure of the block amongst patients who were taking antirheumatic drugs, especially indomethacin. Other failures occurred in patients who were taking anticonvulsants, antidepressants and alcohol in excess of 80 g/day (Ross *et al.*, 1980).

Epidural infusion

Epidural infusions are gaining in popularity because of their simplicity once systems are set up. The need for 'topping-up', which is so often a stumbling block when bolus doses are used is removed because doctors are unavailable or nurses are not trained.

Alexander *et al.* (1990) compared epidural infusion and intravenous infusion of the same drug, diamorphine. Fourteen patients were studied who had undergone major abdominal surgery. Half were given diamorphine 3 mg epidurally followed by an infusion of 20 mg over 48 hours, and half received the same dose intravenously. Additional analgesia was provided as required. The epidural group needed fewer supplementary doses and needed the first dose later than the intravenous group.

The pain after knee operations can be particularly severe, especially if continuous passive movement (CPM) devices are used to increase the range of movement at the joint postoperatively. Pettine *et al.* (1989) used an epidural infusion of bupivacaine after total knee replacement in patients who went on to receive CPM and compared analgesia with that obtained from intramuscular opiates in a second group which underwent the same procedures. Analgesia was markedly better in the epidural group, until the infusion was discontinued when such severe pain followed in one patient that CPM was interrupted. In the group which received intramuscular analgesia, 3 patients had totally ineffective analgesia which required continuous amendments to the prescription by the medical staff. Whilst the epidural group had a slightly better range of movement at discharge, by 3 months there was no difference. Plasma concentration of bupivacaine during continuous infusion was measured at 6 and 24 hours and all levels were well within the toxic levels of 4 μg/ml (1.6 + 0.72 μg/ml and 0.97 + 0.54 μg/ml respectively). In general, knee operations are extremely painful and analgesia after bilateral procedures (knee replacement for example) will be inadequate unless regional analgesia is used.

Although effective analgesia can be obtained with intravenous opioids, respiratory function is better preserved with an epidural infusion of local anaesthetic, (Clyburn *et al.* 1990). There is increasing evidence that changes in ventilatory rhythm and apnoeic episodes are common in patients receiving opioids for postoperative analgesia. Clyburn *et al.* found a significantly lower incidence of both obstructive and central apnoea if analgesia after upper abdominal surgery was provided with epidural infusion of bupivacaine 0.25 per cent delivered at up to 6 ml/hour rather than intravenous morphine at up to 4 mg/hour. Further, there was a lower incidence of tachyarrhythmias and ventricular ectopic beats in the epidural group, possibly because there was less hypoxia.

The difficulty with epidural infusions is that there is no end-point between ineffective analgesia at too low an infusion rate and systemic toxicity at too high an infusion rate. Complications are relatively uncommon with slow infusions and are easily treated by turning off the infusion or reducing the rate: precipitate falls in blood pressure such as might follow a top-up do not occur. However, if slow infusions are used 'breakthrough pain' is a problem and is best treated with an additional epidural bolus dose. Ross *et al.* (1980) secured good analgesia in 9 patients after abdominal surgery using an infusion of 20 ml/hour of 0.125 per cent bupivacaine. There were no complications but plasma concentration of bupivacaine rose steadily throughout the period of the study. Epidural infusions are unwise in patients with established organ failure. At present, the best results are obtained with an infusion of a mixture of fentanyl or diamorphine with bupivacaine 0.25 per cent and the infusion run at 3–7 ml/hour.

Epidural catheter techniques always give rise to worry about bacterial contamination of the catheter and subsequent epidural infection. Hunt *et al.* (1977) found an overall incidence of 22 per cent bacterial contamination of catheters removed from patients and one instance of deep seated infection: only with the greatest caution should continuous epidural analgesia be used in patients whose immunocompetence is reduced by disease or drugs (e.g. in rheumatoid arthritis).

Intrathecal opioids

Whilst intrathecal blocks can be used for surgery of the hip and thigh, they are particularly useful for surgery of the ankle and foot where epidural anaesthesia becomes unpredictable. Intrathecal opiates and intrathecal catheters and top-ups are the only means available to extend the action of subarachnoid blocks.

Wang *et al.* published a controlled study of intrathecal morphine in cancer patients in 1979 and demonstrated its remarkable analgesic properties and prolonged duration of action. Since the original research, there has been a plethora of papers: not only are spinal opioids effective in producing pain relief, but analgesia is achieved without any demonstrable motor, sensory or autonomic deficit. In addition, cephalad flow in the CSF occurs only slowly so that intracranial side-effects of spinal application – sedation, nausea and vomiting and respiratory depression – are few.

The choice of drug for subarachnoid administration has been largely empirical, with the majority of workers choosing morphine. In an attempt to obtain the same potency with fewer side-effects, others have used different opioids but in the same proportion of the systemic dose (i.e. about 10 per cent) as for morphine. However drugs differ in their ability to cross the blood-brain barrier and extrapolation from systemic potency in this way is not valid. Using a rat model, McQuay *et al.* (1989) compared the relative potency of 4 opioids all μ-receptor agonists and found that intrathecal potency of opioids was inversely related to lipid solubility (Table 5.1). Thus morphine and normorphine were more potent than pethidine, in turn more potent than methadone. For the present, therefore, morphine should remain the drug of choice for intrathecal analgesia. The effect of a range of different doses of intrathecal morphine was investigated by Yamaguchi *et al.* (1990) who attempted to find the optimum dose for minimum side-effects. Vomiting was commonest after spinal block alone with no morphine and also occurred with the largest doses, 0.15 and 0.2 mg. Respiratory depression with elevation of $PaCO_2$ was seen again with the largest doses. Itching, however, appears to be unrelated to dose and occurred both with and without effective pain relief. The dose of morphine which made additional analgesics unnecessary in 60 per cent of patients during the first 24 hours was 0.06–0.12 mg mixed with hyperbaric tetracaine. Yamaguchi and colleagues argue that it is preferable to use a small dose of morphine with few side-effects and add supplementary analgesia as necessary. Nursing procedures such as bathing or lifting onto a bedpan are particularly likely to increase the rate at which subarachnoid opioids reach the brain by creating turbulence in the cerebrospinal fluid. Similarly nursing patients head-down will cause increased central effects most noticeably vomiting.

Urinary retention requiring catheterization is common after opioids given either by the epidural or the spinal route. This may be because of loss of bladder sensation but Samii *et al.* (1981) have suggested that high concentrations of opioids in the cerebrospinal fluid might lead to inappropriate secretion of antidiuretic hormone and oliguria. Orthopaedic surgeons are often concerned at the risk of bacteraemia during catheterization and infection of a prosthetic joint; however, despite extensive use over many years of spinal and epidural opioids with a 40 per cent rate of catheterization, there has been no change in the incidence of joint infection. Many men with prostatic symptoms will require postoperative catheterization if immobilized in bed and the nursing of elderly patients may be simplified if a urinary catheter is passed: incontinence and a wet bed also promote infection and pressure sores, whilst repeated lifting on to bedpans predisposes to dislocation of prostheses. Suprapubic catheterization is associated less frequently with bacteraemia and should be performed soon after surgery under antibiotic cover.

The most threatening complication remains respiratory depression. In an extensive review of the problem Etches *et al.* (1989) emphasized the need for long-term (that is 24 hours) intensive observation in a high dependency unit if spinal or epidural opioids were to be used safely. They stress that somnolence should be monitored in addition to respiratory frequency and that apnoea alarms will not detect obstructive apnoea. They suggest that continuous monitoring with a pulse oximeter will provide an added measure of safety, and conclude that there is still inadequate evidence to decide whether equianalgesic doses of spinal or parenteral opioids differ in the degree of respiratory depression they cause. Much work remains to be done.

Regional blocks

Although underestimated by reviewers, local anaesthesia has a great deal to offer in orthopaedic surgery. Edmonds-Seal *et al.* (1980) examined the postoperative analgesia derived from simple limb blocks performed as part of the anaesthetic technique. Postoperatively, they found that no analgesic was required by 80 per cent of patients within 4 hours of surgery and by 41 per cent of patients within 8 hours of surgery (when blocks are beginning to fade). This interval is sufficient for patients to be fully recovered from light general anaesthesia and able to take non-opioid analgesics orally. This study was not controlled and the onset of pain was assessed solely by the patient's request for analgesia.

Even simple measures can have a profound effect upon the patient's well-being: the pain after arthroscopy can be treated very effectively by the injection of 20 ml of bupivacaine 0.5 per cent on completion of the procedure (Chirwa *et al.*, 1989) although analgesia is relatively brief. Longer-lasting analgesia was obtained by Joshi *et al.* (1992) who injected 5 mg morphine in saline 25 ml into the knee at the end of surgery and achieved good pain relief for 18 hours without side-effects. In this study, plasma morphine concentrations were measured and found to be minimal so that analgesia must have been mediated locally. This is surprising since opioid receptors have not yet been reported in synovium, but Stein *et al.* (1990) have shown that opioid agonists are effective at peripheral opioid receptors in inflamed tissue. Dinley and Dickson, orthopaedic surgeons, reported good pain relief after Keller's operation for hallux valgus from instillation of bupivacaine into the wound at the end of surgery.

Continuous nerve blocks

Continuous techniques of local nerve blockade have been reported where top-up doses of local anaesthetic agents may be given through an indwelling catheter, thus prolonging effective analgesia for many days (Table 5.4). In each case brachial blocks were established and fine catheters threaded through the needle before the needle was withdrawn and the catheter taped in position (see Chapter 9). Hempel *et al.* (1981) suggested a modification of the supraclavicular approach to the brachial plexus – a transverse supraclavicular approach – which both reduces the risk of a pneumothorax and renders fixation of the indwelling catheter easier. Continuous lumbar plexus analgesia after total knee replacement was reported by Serpell *et al.* (1991). An 18 swg cannula was positioned in the femoral sheath using the paravascular approach of Winnie and guided by a nerve stimulator. Bupivacaine 0.3 ml/kg as 0.5 per cent solution was injected and topped up with the same dose at 6–8 hour intervals and residual pain was assessed using a PCA device. A control group used the PCA alone which in some patients needed supplementation with intramuscular morphine. The study group had significantly better analgesia which Serpell and colleagues attributed chiefly to abolition of quadriceps muscle spasm.

Other analgesics

Non-steroidal anti-inflammatory drugs (NSAIDs) are a profitable field for pharmaceutical companies and the drugs are usually promoted beyond their abilities. Nevertheless, they have a place, particularly in orthopaedic pain and in day case surgery where potent opioids are undesirable. NSAIDs block prostaglandin synthesis. They all have analgesic properties whilst being devoid of central effects and in addition

Table 5.4 Continuous nerve blockade

	Cases	Nerve block	Initial dose	Top-up	Duration
Manriquez and Pallares (1978)	3 – trauma and vascular lesions	Interscalene	Bupivacaine 0.5% 30 ml	0.25% 20 ml 6-hourly	3 days
Rosenblatt et al. (1979)	1 – vascular	Axillary	Bupivacaine 0.75% 20 ml* 2-chloroprocaine	*	3 days
Vataschky and Aronson (1980)	1 – vascular	Interscalene	Bupivacaine 0.5% 40 ml	0.5% 15 ml 8-hourly	3 days
Hempel et al. (1981)	12 – not specified	Longitudinal	Prilocaine 2% 20 ml *or* lignocaine 2% 20–25 ml	The same as initial dose The same as initial dose	Not given

Note: *Continuous infusion.

have anti-inflammatory, anti-pyretic and anti-platelet activity. All are associated with gastrointestinal erosions and bleeding, reduction of renal and hepatic function, and a variety of hypersensitivity reactions. There are interactions with many drugs, especially oral anticoagulants and diuretics. Pain at the intramuscular injection site may be severe and for Diclofenac the site is specified (gluteus maximus) to avoid sterile abscesses and long-lasting complications.

Ketorolac was found to be almost as effective as morphine in a group of patients undergoing laparotomy (Powell *et al.*, 1990) but it was also associated with a similar incidence of vomiting. In elderly patients, Smallman *et al.* (1992) found Ketorolac was as effective as papaveretum when given intramuscularly and then orally for 8 days after orthopaedic surgery. However, neither form of treatment in this study could be said to be adequate, since in both the papaveretum group and the ketorolac group, almost 60 per cent of patients had moderate to severe pain 1 hour after treatment. Simple intramuscular analgesia is no longer good enough after major surgery whatever drug is chosen. This study also illustrated the wide range of response commonly obtained with NSAIDs: whilst some patients had clearly inadequate analgesia, others needed no further analgesia until the following day.

Perhaps a better way to view NSAIDs is demonstrated by Gillies *et al.* (1987), who assessed an infusion of Ketorolac as a morphine-sparing agent. In this study patients received either Ketorolac 1.5, or 3 mg/hour or saline by intramuscular infusion and used a morphine containing PCA as indicator. Patients who received Ketorolac required one-third less morphine than the control group and at the same time had lower pain scores. Further, there was significantly less respiratory depression in the trial group with the higher infusion rate, than in the control group. Because the trial groups had lower pain scores than the control group Gillies and colleagues argue that control patients modify their demand for morphine from the PCA because of unwelcome side-effects, such as drowsiness or nausea. Segstro *et al.* (1991) investigated indomethacin suppositories in combination with morphine PCA to provide analgesia after total hip arthroplasty. Lower pain scores were found in the group which had combination therapy with a significantly lower consumption of morphine and no increase in bleeding occurred. Combining indomethacin with a narcotic enhanced the quality of analgesia.

The rectal route has never been popular in the United Kingdom yet it has many advantages for NSAID administration; unpleasant intramuscular injections are avoided and sustained release of the drug provides steady plasma concentrations with a lower incidence of side-effects than is associated with oral administration.

Agonist-antagonist drugs

The agonist-antagonist drugs have been developed in the hope that the link between analgesia and respiratory depression can be broken. This class of drugs includes buprenorphine, meptazinol, nalbuphine and pentazocine. However, side-effects remain as prominent as with pure agonist drugs and they therefore offer few advantages. Buprenorphine is particularly suited to the sublingual route of administration. It is highly lipophilic (Table 5.1) and crosses the buccal mucosa rapidly, whilst its high receptor affinity allows pharmacologogically effective occupancy of receptors at the low plasma concentrations achieved by this means of administration. In postoperative patients buprenorphine is as effective as NSAIDs and provides long-lasting analgesia although long-lasting nausea can be a problem. Sublingual absorption of buprenorphine is poor immediately postoperatively because many patients have a dry mouth and initial doses of analgesic should be administered parenterally, but thereafter sublingual dosage may suit some patients. Because the drug is not a schedule drug, a small supply may be left with patients for self-administration.

Conclusion

The problem of how best to relieve postoperative pain has remained unresolved because of the difficulty in achieving analgesia for all patients without unacceptable side-effects. The variables include: differing degrees of pain following different operations; differing perception of pain for the same operation; differing degrees of effectiveness of the same drug in different patients, and, finally, the variety of analgesic drugs and treatments available. The journals are awash with papers showing how the majority of patients can be relieved of their pain using a given regimen but no papers showing how *all* patients can be helped.

If postoperative pain relief is effective, developing surgical complications – too tight a plaster or dressing, or a dislocation – may be more difficult to detect. It is important, therefore, that wounds, fingers and toes should be examined regularly even though the patient is comfortable.

In an important review, McQuay and Dickenson (1990) examined current concepts of the mechanism of pain and their implications for management. The nervous system is no longer considered a hard-wired line-labelled system like a telephone exchange: it is capable of plasticity, and may change in function with injury or experience. Thus, the phenomenon of phantom limb pain after the excision of its neural pathways is an example of moulding of the system. There is a suggestion that the development of phantom limb symptoms might be blocked if central neural blockade is used for anaesthesia (Jacobsen *et al.*, 1989) and central blocks have been used successfully in treatment (Jacobsen and Chabal, 1989). More acutely, multiple pain impulses arriving at the dorsal horn, e.g. after surgery or injury, might augment the effect of subsequent pain impulses, inducing a hyperexcitable state termed *wind-up*. Thus the prevention of pain or the reduction of its impact may make subsequent management easier. The imperative for effective early postoperative pain relief is not just humanitarian, but also physiological in terms of improved recovery.

References

Alexander, J. I., Kong, K. L., Black, A. M. S. (1990). Epidural and intravenous infusions of diamorphine. *European Journal of Anaesthesiology,* **7**, 309–15.

Austin, K. L., Stapleton, J. V., Mahter, L. E. (1980). Multiple intramuscular injections: a major source of variability in analgesic response to meperidine. *Pain,* **8**, 47.

Bisgaard, C., Mouridsen, P., Dahl, J. B. (1990). Continuous lumbar epidural bupivacaine plus morphine versus epidural morphine after major surgery. *European Journal of Anaesthesiology,* **7**, 219–25.

Bullingham, R. E. S. (1981). Synthetic opiate analgesics. *British Journal of Hospital Medicine,* **25**, 59.

Chirwa, S. S., MacLeod, B. A. and Day, B. (1989). Intra-articular bupivacaine (marcaine) after arthroscopic meniscectomy. *Arthroscopy,* **5**, 33–5.

Church, J. (1979). Continuous narcotic infusions for relief of postoperative pain. *British Medical Journal,* **1**, 977.

Clyburn, P. A., Rosen, M., Vickers, M. D. (1990). Comparison of the respiratory effects of i.v. infusions of morphine and regional analgesia by extradural block. *British Journal of Anaesthesia,* **65**, 596–7.

Commission on the provision of surgical services: report of the working party on pain after surgery (1990). Royal College of Surgeons of England, The Royal College of Anaesthetists, London.

Dinley, R. J., Dickson, R. A. (1976). The control of pain after Keller's operation by the instillation of local anaesthetic before closure. *Journal of Bone and Joint Surgery,* **58B**, 356.

Duthie, D., Davies, S. J., Nimmo, W. (1987). The Travenol Infusor. *Care of the Critically Ill,* **3**, 2.

Edmonds-Seal, J., Paterson, G. M. C. and Loach, A. B. (1980). Local nerve blocks for postoperative analgesia. *Journal of the Royal Society of Medicine,* **73**, 111.

Etches, R. C., Sandler, A. N. and Daley, M. D. (1989). Respiratory depression and spinal opioids. *Canadian Journal of Anaesthesia,* **36**, 165–85.

Editorial (1976a). Postoperative pain. *British Medical Journal,* **2**, 664.

Editorial (1976b). Tight-fisted analgesia. *Lancet,* **1**, 1338.

Freed, D. L. J. (1975). Inadequate analgesia at night. *Lancet,* **1**, 519.

Gillies, G. W. A., Kenny, G. N. C., Bullingham, R. E. S. and McArdle, C. S. (1987). The morphine sparing effect of ketorolac tromethamine. *Anaesthesia,* **42**, 727–31.

Gjessing, J. and Tomlin, P. J. (1979). Patterns of postoperative pain. A study of the use of continuous epidural analgesia in the postoperative period. *Anaesthesia,* **34**, 624.

Hempel, V., Van Finck, M. and Baumgartner, E. (1981). A longitudinal supraclavicular approach to the brachial plexus for the insertion of plastic cannulas. *Anesthesia and Analgesia,* **60**, 352.

Hunt, J. R., Rigor, B. M., Collins, J. R. (1977). The potential for contamination of continuous epidural catheters. *Anesthesia and Analgesia,* **56**, 222.

Jackson, I. J. B., Semple, P. and Stevens, J. D. (1991). Evaluation of the Graseby PCAS. *Anaesthesia,* **46**, 482–6.

Jacobsen, L. and Chabal, C. (1989). Prolonged relief of acute postoperative phantom limb pain with intrathecal fentanyl and epidural morphine. *Anesthesiology,* **71**, 984–5.

Jacobsen, L., Chabal, C. and Brody, M. C. (1989). Relief of persistent postamputation stump and phantom limb pain with intrathecal fentanyl. *Pain,* **37**, 317–22.

Joshi, G. P., McCarroll, S. M., Cooney, C. M., Blunnie, W. P., O'Brien, T. M. and Lawrence, A. J. (1992). Intra-articular morphine for pain relief after knee arthroscopy. *Journal of Bone and Joint Surgery,* **74B**, 749–51.

Keeri-Szanto, M. and Pomeroy, J. R. (1971). Pentazocine metabolism and atmospheric pollution. *Lancet,* **i**, 947–9.

Keeri-Szanto, M. and Heaman, S. (1972). Postoperative demand analgesia. *Surgery Gynaecology and Obstetrics,* **134**, 647.

Leicht, C. H., Kelleher, A. J., Robinson, D. E. and Dickerson, S. (1990). Prolongation of postoperative sufentanil analgesia with epinephrine. *Anesthesia and Analgesia,* **70,** 323–5.

Lloyd, J. W. (1977). Experiences in a pain relief unit. In A. Harcus, R. Smith and B. Whittle (eds), *Pain: New Perspectives in Measurement and Management.* Churchill Livingstone, Edinburgh and London, p. 122.

MacInnes, C. (1976). Cancer ward. *New Society,* **36,** 232.

McQuay, H. J., Bullingham, R. E. S., Paterson, G. M. C. and Moore, R. A. (1980). Clinical effects of buprenorphine during and after operation. *British Journal of Anaesthesia,* **52,** 1013.

McQuay, H. J. and Dickenson, A. H. (1990). Implications of nervous system plasticity for pain management (Editorial). *Anaesthesia,* **45,** 101–2.

McQuay, H. J., Sullivan, A. F., Smallman, K. and Dickenson, A. H. (1989). Intrathecal opioids, potency and lipophilicity. *Pain,* **36,** 111–15.

Manriquez, R. G. and Pallares, V. (1978). Continuous brachial plexus block for prolonged sympathectomy and control of pain. *Anaesthesia and Analgesia,* **57,** 128.

Melzack, R. (1975). The McGill pain questionnaire: major properties and scoring methods. *Pain,* **1,** 277.

Moore, A. K., Vilderman, S., Lubenski, W., McCann, J, Fox, G. S. (1990). Differences in epidural morphine requirements between elderly and young patints after abdominal surgery. *Anesthesia and Analgesia,* **70,** 316–20.

Notcutt, W. G. and Morgan, R. J. M. (1990). Introducing patient controlled analgesia for postoperative pain control in a district general hospital. *Anaesthesia,* **45,** 401–6.

Owen, H., Kluger, M. T. and Plummer, J. L. (1990a). Variables of patient controlled analgesia 4: the relevance of bolus size to supplement a background infusion. *Anaesthesia,* **45,** 619–22.

Owen, H., Brose, W. G., Plummer, J. L. and Mather, L. E. (1990b). Variables of patient controlled analgesia 3: test of an infusion demand system using alfentanil. *Anaesthesia,* **45,** 452–5.

Parbrook, G. D., Steel, D. F., Dalrymple, D. G. (1973). Factors predisposing to postoperative pain and pulmonary complications. *British Journal of Anaesthesia,* **45,** 21.

Pettine, K. A., Wedel, D. J., Cabanela, M. E. and Weeks, J. L. (1989). The use of epidural bupivacaine following total knee arthroplasty. *Orthopaedic Review,* **XVIII,** 894–901.

Powell, H., Smallman, J. M. B. and Morgan, M. (1990). Comparison of intramuscular ketorolac and morphine in pain control after laparotomy. *Anaesthesia,* **45,** 538–42.

Rosenblatt, R., Pepitone-Rockwell, F., McKillop, M. J. (1979). Continuous axillary analgesia for traumatic hand injury. *Anesthesiology,* **51,** 565.

Ross, R. A., Clarke, J. E. and Armitage, E. N. (1980). Postoperative pain prevention by continuous epidural infusion. *Anaesthesia,* **35,** 663.

Rowbotham, D. J., Wyld, R. and Nimmo, W. S. (1989). A disposable device for patient controlled analgesia with fentanyl. *Anaesthesia,* **44,** 922–4.

Samii, K., Chauvin, M. and Viars, P. (1981). Postoperative spinal analgesia with morphine. *British Journal of Anaesthesia,* **53,** 817.

Sechzer, P. H. (1971). Studies in pain with the analgesic-demand system. *Anesthesia and Analgesia,* **50,** 1–10.

Sechzer, P. H. (1990). Patient controlled analgesia (PCA) a retrospective. *Anesthesiology,* **72,** 735–6.

Segstro, R., Motley-Forster, I. K., Lu, C. (1991). Indomethacin as a postoperative analgesic for total hip arthroplasty. *Canadian Journal of Anaesthesia,* **38,** 578–81.

Serpell, M. G., Millar, F. A., Thomson, M. F. (1991). Comparison of lumbar plexus block versus conventional opioid analgesia after total knee replacement. *Anaesthesia,* **46,** 275–8.

Smallman, J. M. B., Powell, H., Ewart, M. C. and Morgan, M. (1992). Ketorolac for postoperative analgesia in elderly patients. *Anaesthesia,* **47,** 149–53.

Smith, J. M. and Utting, J. E. (1976). Postoperative pain. *British Medical Journal,* **2,** 875.

Sprotte, G. (1979). Some reasons for failure of regional analgesia. *Anaesthesia,* **34,** 395.

Stapleton, J. V., Austin, K. L. and Mather, L. E. (1978). Postoperative pain. *British Medical Journal,* **2,** 1499.

Stapleton, J. V., Austin, K. L. and Mather, L. E. (1979). A pharmacokinetic approach to postoperative pain: continuous infusion of pethidine. *Anaesthesia and Intensive Care,* **7,** 25.

Stein, C., Millan, M. J., Yassouridis, A. and Hertz, A. (1990). Intrinsic mechanisms of antinociception in inflammation: local opioid receptors and beta-endorphin. *Journal of Neurosciences,* **10,** 1292–8.

Stuart-Taylor, M. E., Billingham, I. S., Barrett, R. F. and Church, J. J. (1992). Extradural diamorphine for post-operative analgesia: audit of a nurse-administered service to 800 patients in a district general hospital. *British Journal of Anaesthesia,* **68,** 429–32.

Utting, J. E., and Smith, J. M. (1979). Postoperative analgesia. *Anaesthesia,* **34,** 320.

Van Essen, E. J., Bovill, J. G. Ploeger, E. J. and Schout, B. C. (1990). A comparison of epidural clonidine and morphine for postoperative analgesia. *European Journal of Anaesthesiology,* **7,** 211–18.

Vataschky, E. and Aronson, H. B. (1980). Continuous interscalene brachial plexus block for surgical operations on the hand. *Anesthesiology,* **53,** 356.

Vercauteren, M., Lauwers, E., Meert, T., De Heert, S. and Adriaensen, H. (1990). Comparison of epidural sufentanil plus clonidine with sufentanil alone for post-operative pain relief. *Anaesthesia,* **45,** 531–4.

Wakelin, G. and Larson, C. P. (1990). Spouse controlled analgesia. *Anesthesia and Analgesia,* **70,** 119.

Wang, J. K. (1979). Analgesic effect of intrathecally administered morphine. *Regional Anaesthesia,* **2,** 8.

Wasylak, T. J., Abbott, F. V., English, M. J. M. and Jeans, M. E. (1990). Reduction of postoperative morbidity following patient-controlled morphine. *Canadian Journal of Anaesthesiology*, **37**, 726–31.

Weller, R., Rosenblum, M., Conrad, P. and Gross, J. B. (1991). Comparison of epidural and patient-controlled intravenous morphine following joint replacement surgery. *Canadian Journal of Anaesthesia*, **38**, 582–6.

Yamaguchi, H., Watanabe, S., Motokawa, K. and Ishizawa, Y. (1990). Intrathecal morphine dose-response data for pain relief after cholecystectomy. *Anesthesia and Analgesia*, **70**, 168–71.

Chapter 6

Orthopaedic surgery for particular diseases

In this chapter diseases of special interest to the orthopaedic anaesthetist are discussed. Rheumatoid arthritis is a common condition which may pose considerable problems; haemophilia, sickle cell anaemia and malignant hyperpyrexia are rare but require special knowledge, whilst the problem of anaesthetizing patients in chronic renal failure is one that is likely to become more common.

Rheumatoid arthritis

Rheumatoid arthritis (RA) affects 1–2 per cent of the population, women three times as commonly as men. Whilst predominantly a polyarthritis, many other tissues of the body are affected, either as a complication of the disease or an unwanted effect of treatment, and the result is a crippling disease attacking young men and women in the prime of life and then progressing steadily.

The aetiology of RA remains unknown although there is abundant evidence of an immunological mechanism and a suggestion of an infective origin. The immunological mechanism gives rise to the high incidence of a specific rheumatoid factor, an IgM globulin; circulating and localized immune complexes; and an association with other immune complex diseases. Indeed, systemic lupus erythematosus (SLE) and RA may be regarded as intravascular and extravascular immune complex diseases respectively. RA is geographically ubiquitous and urban populations are more at risk than rural ones.

Suspicion remains that RA is caused primarily by viral disease in genetically susceptible people. Parvovirus infection is known to result in an acute inflammatory polyarthritis indistinguishable from RA (Naides *et al.*, 1990) but there is little epidemiological support for an infectious cause: there are no epidemics and the onset of disease in siblings occurs at random times. However, Lyme disease, which was considered to be an epidemic form of juvenile RA, has been shown to be caused by the spirochaete, *Borrelia burgdorferi* (Steere *et al.*, 1983).

There is now evidence to reinforce the clinical impression that both the incidence and the severity of RA are declining. Successive generations of patients with RA are less likely to be seropositive or to suffer erosive disease and subcutaneous nodules. As yet there is no explanation for these changes.

The principal manifestations of RA are seen in joint disorders, although systemic complications are common.

Joint disease in rheumatoid arthritis

Patients with rheumatoid arthritis frequently tolerate a surprising degree of dysfunction and deformity because the disease progresses at a rate that allows accommodation to disability. The disease advances as an insidious progressive polyarthritis favouring the smaller joints of the fingers and toes, the wrists and the neck. The joints themselves become bulky and the muscles acting across them suffer disuse atrophy and become wasted. Within the joints, cartilage and bone are eroded as a pannus of profuse granulation tissue, fibroblasts and chronic inflammatory cells spreads across the articular surfaces, whilst the synovial fluid becomes less viscous and contains an inflammatory exudate. The fluid also frequently contains cryoprecipitates with DNA and IgG/anti-IgG complexes.

The most prominent signs are seen in the hands where the joints become swollen, hot and tender. The hands become disfigured by the development of rheumatoid nodules beneath the skin and synovial swellings arising in relation to the synovial linings of joints, tendons and bursae. Synovitis of tendon sheaths and displacement of tendons lead to weakening of tendons, further muscle atrophy and occasionally to tendon rupture. Muscle power in the hands may be further reduced by motor nerve compression caused by synovitis in adjacent joints or tendon sheaths. Commonly, this involves the ulnar nerve at the elbow and the median nerve in the carpal tunnel at the wrist. It is rare to find muscle abnormality in RA but this can occur as a result of vasculitis of vessels of supply.

Although the joints of the spine are not usually involved in the rheumatoid process, radiographical studies show that 40–80 per cent of inpatients with RA have involvement of the cervical spine. This involvement may occur at an early stage when there are few other signs of disease and later, gross, radiological damage may be present without obvious neck symptoms. The significant lesions occur in the upper cervical vertebrae; erosion of the odontoid peg and increasing laxity of the transverse ligaments of the atlas lead to critical instability and eventual subluxation of the atlanto-axial joint in 25 per cent of patients. Despite this common occurrence the incidence of cervical cord compression is surprisingly low (Matthews, 1974), possibly because the spinal canal is widest at the atlanto-axial level. Progressive neurological deterioration is an indication for cervical fusion.

Involvement of the synovium of the temporomandibular joint leads to stiffening of the joint and eventually loss of much of its range of movement. The synovial joints of the cricoarytenoid articulation of the larynx are also subject to RA, giving rise to a feeling of fullness in the throat, pain and dysphagia during an acute phase. Eventually ankylosis may occur, with severe restriction of vocal cord movement and limitation of the airway.

Systemic complications of rheumatoid arthritis

Sjogren's syndrome

Keratoconjunctivitis sicca occurs in some form in up to 60 per cent, of patients, and in many cases – almost all female – forms part of a true Sjogren's syndrome (connective tissue disease, keratoconjunctivitis sicca and xerostomia). Of importance in this syndrome is the lymphocytic infiltration and secondary atrophy of the mucous glands of the bronchial mucosa, leading to atelectasis and frequent lung infection.

Blood

There is wasting of the formed elements of blood, with failure of incorporation of iron into erythrocytes, leucopenia and thrombocytopenia. Bone marrow depression or gastrointestinal haemorrhage caused by drug treatment may, however, complicate these changes.

Renal function

Amyloidosis occurs in 3–5 per cent of RA patients and may progressively impair renal function, producing a persistent proteinuria. Direct renal damage caused by vasculitis is rare. Analgesic nephropathy is becoming less common with improvements in management.

Rare syndromes

Felty's syndrome

This is an aggressive form of RA, with splenomegaly and neutropenia in addition to arthritis. The main problem is reduced resistance to infection, which is compounded if steroids or antimetabolites are used in treatment. Sjogren's syndrome is also sometimes present, when the overall disease carries a poor prognosis.

Systemic vasculitis

This, is progressive and widespread and clinically borders on polyarteritis nodosa. The presence of a vasculitis is suggested by finding small brown paronychial infarcts in the skin.

Pleural effusions

These are found occasionally: the fluid characteristically contains high titres of immune complexes and rheumatoid factor. Less commonly, other lesions occur in the lungs; rheumatoid nodules may form, cysts develop with honeycombing of the lung and there may be diffuse interstitial fibrosis. Rheumatoid lung involvement in combination with miner's pneumoconiosis is known as Caplan's syndrome.

Hyper-viscosity syndrome

This condition develops when the serum becomes laden with macromolecules, especially the IgM rheumatoid factor, and becomes increasingly viscous and treacly. This increases the work load of the heart and in time leads to dyspnoea and heart failure. Hyperviscosity syndrome may be treated by plasma exchange.

Treatment of rheumatoid arthritis

The growth of rheumatology as a specialty has led to the development of specialized centres where complementary forms of treatment are concentrated – maintenance of drug regimes, physiotherapy, rehabilitation, psychological support and orthopaedic surgery.

Drugs

A wide variety of drugs is available, which is summarised in Table 6.1. Individual patient tolerances and preferences seem to matter at least as much as differences between the drugs; comparative trials of efficacy are sparse and of limited value. To have appreciable analgesic effect in RA the drug must have an anti-inflammatory action: pethidine has little effect, and clinical trials of pentazocine and paracetamol have shown no superiority over placebo. The importance of these drugs for the anaesthetist lies in the wide range of adverse reactions which is associated with them.

Table 6.1 Drugs used in the treatment of rheumatoid arthritis

Salicylates	
Non-steroidal anti-inflammatory drugs (NSAIDs)	
Propionic acid derivatives	Ibuprofen, fenoprofen, naproxen
Fenemates	Ketoprofen, mefenamic acid
Pyrazolone derivatives	Flufenamic acid, phenylbutazone, oxyphenbutazone
Alclofenac, fenclofenac, diclofenac	
Indomethacin	
Sulindac	
Disease-modifying second-line drugs	
Gold salts	
Penicillamine	
Corticosteroids	
Immunosuppressive drugs	
Azathioprine	
Cyclophosphamide	

Many of the anti-inflammatory drugs cause gastrointestinal bleeding and bone marrow depression, with anaemia, leucopenia and reduced platelet counts. The pyrazolone derivatives are potent inducers of hepatic microsomal enzymes and may speed up metabolism of other drugs administered concurrently. They are also avidly protein bound and will displace other drugs (e.g. anticoagulants) from binding sites. Nephropathy is reported in association with gold salts, and may take the form either of a protein-losing nephrotic syndrome or acute tubular necrosis due to a membranous glomerulonephritis. Prolonged use of steroids leads to obesity, reduced resistance to infection and suppression of the pituitary-adrenal response to stress. Skin atrophy occurs due to thinning and fragmentation of connective tissue elements, so trivial injury often results in major skin damage requiring grafting (David, 1972). There is generalized osteoporosis which weakens bone, and its severity correlates with the degree of skin atrophy (McConkey *et al.*, 1963).

Surgical treatment

Experience is accumulating of the use of orthopaedic surgical procedures in patients with RA so that decisions about timing and type of intervention are becoming refined; it has been found, for example, that Austin Moore protheses are unsuitable for patients with RA because the bone is too soft and the metal head migrates into the pelvis. The overall aims of surgical treatment can be expressed as:

1. to stop disease progression,
2. to restore motion and relieve pain.

Progression of disease at a joint is slowed down by synovectomy, and this procedure can be used in young patients to buy time. Total joint replacement is better and will, in many cases, prevent further advance at that joint since the implant is not eroded by pannus. Finally, joint fusion with excision of articular surfaces stops progress; it is especially successful at the wrist where pain can be reduced, grip strength improved and the usefulness of the hand increased.

Joint replacement to restore motion and reduce pain is considered when progression of the disease has produced a joint with limited motion or one which is unstable. The staging of surgery is of vital importance: joints are considered in turn and a patient is not allowed to progress until 3 or 4 joints need replacing;

weight-bearing joints are given priority so that a patient can be mobile and at home: hip replacement precedes knee replacement because results are so much better in RA.

Anaesthesia

Preoperative assessment and premedication

Anaesthesia for the vast majority of patients with RA is perfectly straightforward but careful preoperative assessment is necessary to identify those in whom difficulties are present or in whom complications are likely to arise. At the preoperative visit, note should be taken of the patient's disabilities and the speed of progress of the disease; the anaesthetist should familiarize himself with the details of present and past drug therapy. When the patient is examined, body weight should be correlated with body habitus and the degree of obesity, and an assessment should be made of skin atrophy and overall frailty. The mobility of the head and cervical spine should be tested and the patient asked to open and close his mouth. If a local block is being considered, a check should be made that the patient's mobility is adequate for him to be positioned suitably. Investigations which should be available include a recent blood picture, serum electrolyte, urea and creatinine estimations, and *X*-rays of the chest and upper cervical spine. Consideration should be given to correcting severe anaemia preoperatively.

Chest *X*-ray is required to exclude pleural effusions, lung infection and pulmonary tuberculosis, particularly in patients receiving steroids. A solitary nodule seen on the film is more likely to be a carcinoma than a rheumatoid nodule (Hughes, 1979). A lateral *X*-ray of the neck in flexion is required to demonstrate upper cervical instability.

Suitable premedication should omit drying agents for those patients with possible Sjogren's syndrome and add a steroid supplement to cover surgery for those patients who have received steroids for more than 1 week in the last 6 months. For minor procedures a single intramuscular dose of hydrocortisone hemisuccinate 100 mg will suffice, whilst for more major procedures, cover should be maintained 6-hourly for 3 days.

Induction of anaesthesia

When patients are prepared for theatre, tender areas should be padded and a foam rubber collar should be fitted to support the neck and remind the anaesthetist of its instability. During surgery the general frailty of patients is a major problem; inadvertent injury may be caused by positioning without care, by the operating table and even by adhesive tape applied to the skin under tension. If pain is severe and the airway poses no problems, it may be kindest to induce anaesthesia in the bed before moving the patient to the transfer trolley. Establishing an intravenous line is usually easy because of the dilated veins over the dorsum of the hand, although occasionally peripheral vascular disturbances can lead to cold blue hands with no obvious infusion sites. Intubation of the trachea should not be taken lightly because, even in patients who have previously been intubated, progress of disease may have rendered it more difficult. Even if no difficulty is encountered, intubation should be carried out slowly and gently without rough or rapid movement of the head and neck.

The difficult intubation

Latto and Rosen (1985) offer advice to help with the difficult intubation, but actual practical experience is never more valuable. Difficulty with intubation must be expected in any patient with RA and an anaesthetic technique chosen which avoids intubation if possible. In many cases use of a laryngeal mask airway will suffice provided that the patient can open his or her mouth far enough to admit the mask. Insertion of the laryngeal mask is usually straightforward but it may be a little easier if a new mask is chosen – old ones more easily bend double and obstruct: it is important to pass the mask upwards in order to encourage it to follow the curve of the palate and it is less hard edged if a little air is left in the cuff.

If endotracheal intubation is essential, possible methods include awake intubation under local anaesthesia; blind nasal intubation with the patient awake or asleep; fibreoptic laryngoscopy; and intubation over a wire passed from below. When the patient has an unstable neck, support throughout intubation is necessary which may be provided by an assistant holding the neck manually or, as Birkinshaw (1975) has suggested, by the application of a plaster cast as a preliminary.

For intubation under local anaesthesia a suitable technique is as follows: the mouth is first anaesthetized by asking the patient to suck an amethocaine lozenge (60 mg), and to spit it out when he can no longer feel it; bilateral superior laryngeal nerve block is then carried out by advancing a pledget of wool soaked in cocaine solution 5 per cent held in Krause's forceps into each pyriform fossa and applying external pressure on the neck to hold the wool closely against the mucosa. Finally, an injection of cocaine solution 5 per cent is made through the cricothyroid membrane to anaesthetize the trachea itself. This is done by identifying the triangular cricothyroid membrane and advancing a fine needle in the midline directly through it until air can be aspirated into the syringe. The patient is then asked to breathe right out, and at the end of expiration, 2 ml of cocaine solution 5 per cent is injected into the trachea; during the immediate inspiration the needle can be withdrawn before coughing begins. The patient is allowed to breathe oxygen, and a syringe of thiopentone is attached to an indwelling intravenous needle. Laryngoscopy is then carried out with the blade of the laryngoscope well lubricated with lignocaine ointment and intubation completed. Despite the preparation, there is usually some coughing when the trachea is entered and this can be stopped by injecting a little thiopentone. The manoeuvre may not be successful, particularly if the anaesthetist is not practised – the technique is more popular in the USA than in the UK – but it will at least allow an assessment of the anatomical difficulties to be overcome without in any way hazarding the patient.

Blind nasal intubation can be attempted after local anaesthesia of the nose and upper airway or after induction of general anaesthesia; this technique may be used when movement of the jaw is limited, and has the advantage that spontaneous respiration is preserved throughout. Again, practice is necessary before reasonable success can be expected. Finally, the intubating laryngoscope can be used as mentioned in Chapter 2. This is a difficult technique; however, Bernstein (1980) has noted that in patients with RA it was not successful when most needed and that the most likely cause for failure was severe distortion of the larynx which came to face posteriorly so that it was impossible for the laryngoscope to negotiate the right-angle bend.

Finally, intubation may be carried out by introducing the endotracheal tube over a Seldinger wire passed upwards through the larynx from a needle passed through the cricothyroid membrane (as described for topical anaesthesia). The chief difficulty encountered is that, when passing the endotracheal tube, it tends to become hooked up on the margins of the larynx.

A technique of awake intubation using a laryngeal mask has been suggested by McCrirrick and Pracilio (1991). The mask was positioned over the glottis after topical anaesthesia of the oropharynx and a gum elastic bougie was passed into the trachea before the mask was withdrawn and an endotracheal tube passed over the bougie. The patient tolerated this with only light sedation from midazolam 2 mg intravenously. A similar technique in anaesthetized patients was reported by Chadd *et al.* (1989).

Maintenance of anaesthesia

Maintenance of anaesthesia is unremarkable except that patients with RA, particularly if under treatment with steroids, are less tolerant of depressive drugs, land doses of induction agents and opiate supplements should be conservative. If doses are calculated on a basis of body weight, due allowance should be made for the reduced muscle bulk due to wasting and the greater proportion of fat.

Meticulous cleanliness throughout is required, as many patients with RA have reduced resistance to infection because of bone marrow depression or because of treatment with steroids or antimetabolites.

Regional anaesthesia has much to commend it for surgery of the arm, hand or lower limb. However, nerve blocks about the wrist and elbow are contraindicated because nerve compression may result from the injected volume of local anaesthetic. Spinal and epidural blocks are usually possible because, in contrast to ankylosing spondylitis, the rheumatoid process spares the spine. There may, however, be difficulty in positioning patients comfortably for the blocks to be carried out.

Haemophilia

The incidence of haemophilia in the UK is small – 6 per 100 000, giving a total population of haemophiliacs of about 3000 – but over half of all elective surgery undergone by haemophiliacs is orthopaedic, to correct the musculoskeletal complications of previous bleeds. Patients with bleeding disorders are registered with their local haemophilia centre and carry a card giving details of the factor deficiency; no elective surgical treatment should be begun without the active cooperation and help of the haemophilia centre.

Haemophilia is a recessively inherited, sex-linked bleeding disorder of which two distinct types exist: haemophilia A due to a congenital absence of factor

VIII activity, and haemophilia B due to absence of factor IX (Christmas) activity. Haemophiliacs appear to synthesize the protein factors but these then lack clotting activity. The types of haemophilia are clinically indistinguishable but haemophilia A is about ten times more common than haemophilia B.

The first manifestations of haemophilia appear in early childhood, usually about 6–9 months of age, when the child develops extensive bruising and painful swellings caused by deep tissue haematomas. Younger children have an at present unexplained temporary immunity.

The most characteristic bleeding in haemophilia is into the joints, and 3 phases of joint involvement are described:

1. *The acute phase.* The joint is hot, swollen and tender (Fig. 6.1) and very painful. The joints most commonly affected are the knees, elbows, ankles, hips and shoulders. The pain and swelling of an acute haemarthrosis resolves rapidly with infusion of the appropriate factor.
2. *The subacute phase.* This is less well defined; the joint remains swollen and boggy after a second or third bleed, with persisting restriction of movement, and there is marked synovial thickening (likened to that of rheumatoid arthritis). There is seldom any pain.
3. *The chronic phase.* Finally, the joint is totally destroyed and surrounded by fibrotic contracted tissues. This usually follows 6 months or more of the subacute phase.

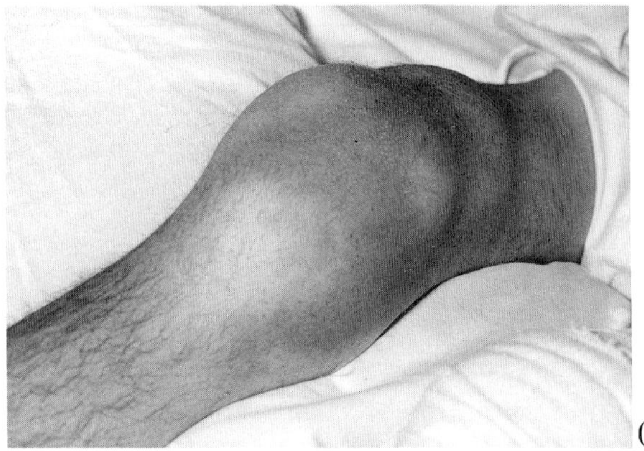

(a)

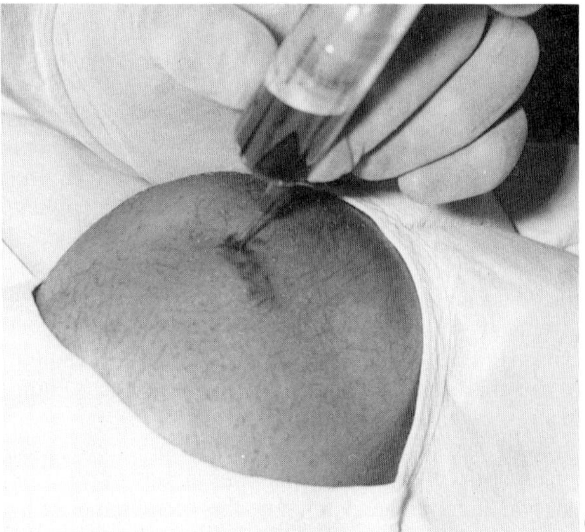

(b)

Fig 6.1(a) Haemophilia; acute haemarthrosis of the knee. The joint is hot swollen and tender. (b) Haemophilia; aspiration of blood from the joint.

Tissue haematomas may compress muscles, nerves or blood vessels and cause ischaemia and paralysis with patches of anaesthesia peripherally, and in fact lead to more disability than the haemarthrosis (Fig. 6.2). Bruising is extensive because the haematoma remains fluid and tracks through tissue planes; it remains interstitial and cannot be evacuated surgically. In the tongue and throat, haemorrhage can be immediately dangerous, putting the airway in jeopardy. Not all haemophiliacs are equally deficient in factor activity and the manifestations of bleeding will vary according to the percentage activity present (Table 6.2). Only severe haemophiliacs suffer spontaneous haemarthrosis; that is, those who have less than 5 per cent factor activity.

Inwood and Meltzer (1978) have reported 3 cases of female patients with a bleeding diathesis, and warn that, rarely, female carriers of haemophilia may have reduced levels of factor activity. This occurs due to the process of lyonization in sex chromatin formation when × chromosomes, some carrying normal factor genes and some carrying defective factor genes, are randomly inactivated, leading to a variability in ability to produce normal factor VIII or IX. These patients are at risk precisely because bleeding is seldom suspected in a female; Inwood and Meltzer (1978) suggest that if a female patient with a family history of haemophilia presents for surgery, investigations should be carried out to measure factor levels and to exclude von Willebrand's disease. In discussing the diagnosis and managements of abnormal bleeding peri-operatively, Ellison (1977) has stressed the importance preoperatively of routinely obtaining a history of the haemostatic response to previous surgery or trauma. Almost every patient has undergone

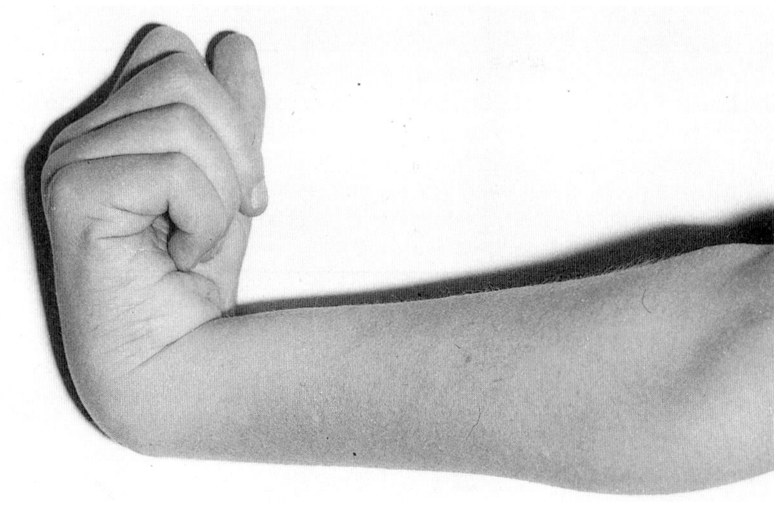

Fig 6.2 Haemophilia; forearm contracture resulting from a compartment syndrome caused by a tissue haematoma.

Table 6.2 The relation of observed blood levels of factor VIII to the severity of the clinical manifestations of defective haemostasis

Blood level of factor VIII (% normal)	Level of haemostatic efficiency
50–100	Normal
5–25	Severe bleeding after minor trauma or surgical operations
1–5	Gross bleeding after minor injuries. Some haemarthroses and spontaneous bleeding
0	Haemarthroses and crippling. Deep tissue haemorhages

dental extractions or tonsillectomy, both procedures carried out on vascular tissue which test adequately the haemostatic response; abnormal bleeding suggests the need for laboratory investigation.

Von Willebrand's disease

Von Willebrand's disease shares abnormal factor VIII function in common with haemophilia A but was the first bleeding disorder reported in women (by Von Willebrand in 1926). It is inherited as an autosomal dominant, unlike the sex-linked recessive pattern of classic haemophilia, and produces a spectrum of bleeding disorders depending on whether the patient is homozygous or heterozygous. Mild disease in a heterozygous patient occurs in 2–3 per cent of the general population and accounts for one-fifth of the 15 per cent of the population found to have an abnormality of haemostasis (Kobrinsky, 1988). The incidence of severe disease in homozygous patients is very much lower and similar to that of haemophilia A.

The presentation of Von Willebrand's disease is usually with cutaneous or mucosal bleeding and deep or muscle bleeding only occurs in severe disease. Most commonly therefore, the diagnosis follows investigation of epistaxis or menorrhagia or bleeding after dental extractions.

Bleeding in Von Willebrand's disease occurs because of a mild reduction in factor VIII activity and the absence of a co-factor which facilitates normal platelet activity. Factor VIII is now believed to be a bimolecular complex of haemophilia factor (VIIIC) and Von Willebrand factor (VWF) both of which must be present for coagulation: reduction in VWF will diminish the activity of the factor as a whole (Fulcher and Zimmerman, 1982). Thus infusion of purified factor VIII fails to correct the bleeding time in Von Willebrand's disease and should not be used.

Traditionally the abnormal bleeding in Von Willebrand's disease has been ascribed to abnormal platelets, but evidence suggests that it is the absence of a co-factor which is decisive. Thus, the infusion of normal platelets does not correct the bleeding time and bleeding in patients with aplastic anaemia may be stopped by infusing platelets from patients with Von Willebrand's disease.

Surgery should not be undertaken without help from a haemophilia unit. The basis of management is the replacement of VWF factor which is present in cryoprecipitate and in fresh frozen plasma (Table 6.3). Cryoprecipitate is much richer in VWF and so smaller volumes can be given avoiding the risk of overtransfusion. Usually 20 ml/kg FFP every 8 hours will control the bleeding (Cameron and Kobrinsky, 1990). Haemarthrosis and haematomas are rarely seen in Von Willebrand's disease and so orthopaedic surgery is rarely required.

Table 6.3 Therapeutic materials for use in bleeding disorders

1. *Dried Factor VIII fraction BP* is a freeze dried human factor VIII concentrate prepared from large pool plasma. Widely used in the UK.
2. *Porcine Factor VIII* is of value in management of patients with antibodies to human factor VIII.
3. *Cryoprecipitate* is a frozen concentrate from the cryoprotein fraction of human plasma. It is often reserved for the treatment of patients with mild factor VIII deficiency.
4. *Dried Factor IX fraction BP* is freeze dried factor IX concentrate and contains in addition factors II and X.
5. *High potency, high purity Factor VIII.* Recently introduced and extremely expensive, may be of value in patients who are HIV positive.

Source: Adapted from Rizza (1984) with permission.

Medical treatment of haemophilia

The dramatic development of the last decade has been the provision in adequate quantity of purified factor concentrates for intravenous infusion. With early infusion of factor following a bleed, rapid resolution of the haematoma is obtained and lasting damage to joints or tissues prevented.

The face of the disease is thus changing: young haemophiliacs less than 10 years old show none of the recognizable stigmata; mild or moderate joint damage is seen in patients 10–20 years old; and the severe crippling associated with haemophilia is now only seen in older patients. Consequently, the need for surgical intervention should dwindle as the newer generations grow up. Factor concentrates are prepared from fresh-frozen plasma such that the factor activity of 1 unit of blood is concentrated in 10 ml, therefore only small-volume infusions are required which can be administered to children without risk of overloading the circulation. Freeze-dried preparations are also available which are easier to store, and many parents have been taught how to give intravenous injections to their affected children at home so that treatment can begin promptly after a bleed without waiting for hospital admission. The consequences of bleeds are thus minimized, time spent in hospital is less and the impact of the disease on schooling and family life is reduced. In children, trauma requiring factor infusions occurs on average every 3 weeks and in the past children have spent the majority of their lives in hospital. A full account of management, drawn from extensive experience, is given by Biggs (1978). A list of preparations is given in Table 6.3.

Factor activity is measured in international units (i.u.): 1 i.u. is the amount of activity in 1ml of normal pooled plasma and is equivalent to 100 per cent activity. One i.u. per kilogram infused will raise activity by 2 per cent for factor VIII and 1.5 per cent for factor IX. The half-life of factor VIII is 6–12 hours and of factor IX 8–18 hours in the circulation, and injections of factor must thus be repeated every 12 hours if levels are to be maintained. The activity of factor concentrates varies between samples and each must be assayed. In addition, studies of factor survival in the patient's circulation are necessary to determine dosage. A rough guide to factor levels required for treatment is given in Table 6.4.

Many drugs interfere with platelet function and are best avoided in haemophiliacs: aspirin compounds; antihistamines; clofibrate; sulfamoxole; and anti-inflammatory agents, ibuprofen, indomethacin and phenylbutazone (Eipe, 1972). Propoxyphene, co-

Table 6.4 Factor levels required for surgical procedures

%	Surgical procedure
20	Necessary for haemostasis, postoperative physiotherapy
20–30	To control muscle haematomas (those of gastrocnemius and soleus are treated more vigorously to avoid contracture of the calf)
40	Necessary for suture removal
40–50	To control haemarthroses
100	To allow surgery, to control CNS bleeds and bleeds into the retroperitoneal space

Source: Data from Arnold and Hilgartner (1977).

deine, pethidine and methadone are suitable analgesics. Although trials appeared to show a reduction in frequency of bleeding episodes with e-aminocaproic acid (Strauss *et al.*, 1965) and tranexamic acid (Rainford *et al.*, 1973), they interfere with resolution of haematomas and may increase fibrosis and joint damage. In practice, they are little used in long-term management. During the postoperative period, however, antifibrinolytic agents reduce the need for factor replacement and currently tranexamic acid (Cyklokapron) 250–500 mg four times daily beginning with the premedication is favoured by the Oxford Haemophilia Centre.

Complications of treatment

Hepatitis and HIV

Transfusion of blood products carries with it the risk of infusion of undetected virus particles; both of hepatitis and Human Immuno-deficiency Virus (HIV). Haemophiliac patients receive many such transfusions and it is estimated that more than half are infused with hepatitis infected material each year (Biggs, 1978). Anti-haemophilic factors are extracted from large pool plasma and much of the material is still imported due to delay in establishing an up-to-date facility in Britain capable of supplying the needs of the haemophiliacs in this country. In the early 1980s many haemophiliac patients were infected with HIV contaminated factor transfusions (knowingly, in France!). The risk of infection has diminished with heat treatment of factor concentrates and as a consequence the number of HIV positive haemophiliacs should begin to fall. High potency purified high cost factor VIII concentrates have been marketed but initial claims that these concentrates had an important sparing effect on the immune system of patients with haemophilia have not been justified. There is also no evidence that high potency factors are of special benefit in patients who are HIV positive but they may be of some value in patients who have developed antibodies to intermediate factor VIII concentrates.

Some haemophiliac patients become drug abusers, partly from regular exposure to opiates and partly from despair, and this opens up a further avenue for infection with both HIV and hepatitis. Although the hepatitis and HIV status of haemophiliac patients is generally known prior to surgery, it is our practice to assume that all are positive and all precautions are taken to avoid exposing staff to risk of infection. General guidelines for the management of HIV-infected patients were published by the Association of Anaesthetists in 1988.

Antibodies to factors

Management of factor replacement may be complicated in a small number of patients by the development of antibodies directed specifically against clotting factors and which destroy infused factor. Replacement therapy is reserved for more serious bleeds and larger doses of factor are needed. After 5 days of treatment, antibody can be expected to rise to dangerously high titres; therefore, if surgery is required, it should be carried out immediately after the first dose of factor. A greater problem is presented by the patient with an already high antibody titre: for these patients only life-saving surgery should be contemplated.

Surgical treatment of haemophilia

The aims of surgical treatment are:

1. to reduce bleeding episodes by removal of bleeding sites.
2. to correct joint deformity by reconstruction or replacement.

Bleeding sites may be reduced by joint debridement when bony spurs or osteophytes are removed – these occur particularly at the medial and lateral margins of the knee – and by synovectomy. Overgrowth of the head of the radius at the elbow may be treated by its removal. Reduction of disability is effected through: osteotomy to realign bones; arthrodesis of joints which are destroyed to restore function of a limb (e.g. of the ankle, shoulder or subtalar joint); and surface or replacement arthroplasty at the hip and knee joint. There is controversy about when knee replacement should be carried out; continuing pain is a strong indication. If there are contractures around the knee, it is unlikely that joint replacement will increase the range of movement.

Anaesthetic management

Safe management of anaesthesia and surgery depends upon the controlled infusion of calculated quantities of factor concentrate, and this must be supervised by the haemophilia centre. The first infusion is given within the hour before surgery and followed by further infusions 12-hourly until the wound is healed. Thus the amount of factor and the duration of infusion therapy depend on the severity of the operation, the time taken for the wound to heal, the extent to which the operation site can be immobilized postoperatively and the half-life of infused factor in the patient. Postoperatively, progressively lower levels can be accepted as healing proceeds, but if it is necessary to remove sutures or to manipulate a joint then higher levels must be restored for these procedures. Initial doses of 50 i.u./kg preoperatively and 25 i.u./kg on the evening of operation are suggested by Biggs (1978); pre- and postinfusion factor activity must be assayed, and a safe objective is to keep the postinfusion factor activity near 100 per cent and the preinfusion factor near 50 per cent for the first postoperative week (Fig. 6.3).

Oral premedication using a benzodiazepine is effective, avoids intramuscular injection and is preferable, although Sampson and Hamstra (1979) found that, provided that factor was given within the hour, no

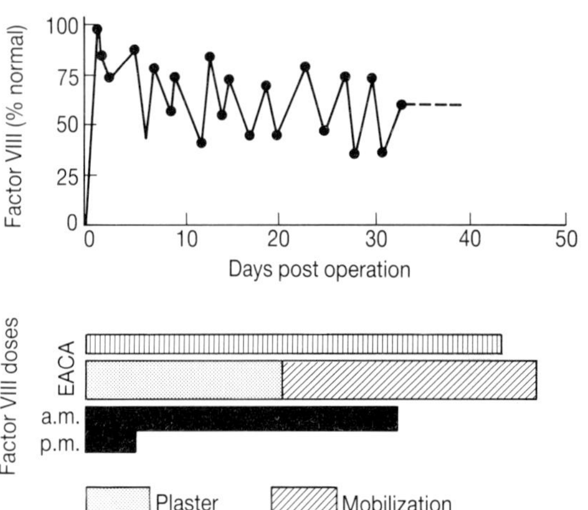

Fig 6.3 Haemophilia; management after hip replacement. e-aminocaproic acid (EACA) was given throughout and the joint immobilized in a plaster-of-paris hip spica for 3 weeks. The fluctuation of factor levels is shown.

haematomas followed an intramuscular premedication. An intravenous infusion should be established with care to avoid multiple punctures and patients should be handled gently throughout to prevent any unnecessary trauma. Endotracheal intubation should be carried out under ideal conditions with the patient fully relaxed so that the larynx is not traumatized; in the series reported by Sampson and Hamstra (1979) no complications followed intubation in 11 patients. Although haemophilia is a contraindication to local anaesthesia, the same series included 2 patients who successfully had an axillary block; no objection could be raised to the use of an intravenous regional technique. Spinal and epidural blocks, however, could be followed by permanent cord damage if an extradural haematoma were to form, and should not be used. At the end of surgery most patients will have a plaster cast applied to ensure immobilization of the wound, and this may add considerably to the duration of anaesthesia. Traction is not usually used since the presence of pins requires the maintenance of higher factor levels postoperatively.

Haemophiliac patients should be scheduled for the end of the list and their operations performed in the Charnley enclosure, which limits spread of contamination. The anaesthetist should wear gloves and eye protection and should use disposable breathing systems, masks and equipment wherever possible. If a ventilator is used it should be taken out of service afterwards and sterilized – hepatitis and HIV are susceptible to heat, ethylene oxide and proprietary bleach solutions. Disposable gowns and drapes should be used and placed in containers clearly marked 'contaminated' afterwards and any pathology specimens should also be clearly marked.

Needles should never be resheathed or passed to an assistant but dropped into an open tray placed nearby for the purpose and then disposed of in a rigid, clearly marked container. It is preferable that surgeons use hand tools. Power tools used on bone throw up a very fine aerosol of infectious material which could be inhaled around a face mask. This gives cause for concern, even though there is at present no evidence for airborne spread of either HIV or hepatitis viruses. Surgeons should use closed systems of drainage of large collections of blood or serum in haematomas before opening the cavity in order to minimize spill of infectious material. The number of health workers known to have been infected with HIV from patients has reached 60 (Royal College of Pathologists, 1992) and the risk of infection from a needlestick wound contaminated by an HIV carrier is 0.37 per cent (Jeffries, 1992).

During anaesthesia, high inspired concentrations of oxygen may be required to maintain oxygenation since significant impairment of gas exchange can result from infection of the lungs with *Pneumocystis Carinii*.

Postoperatively, patients should be nursed in a separate room by a dedicated nurse with disposable equipment available for cardiopulmonary resuscitation: mouth-to-mouth resuscitation should be avoided by early intubation of the trachea. Postoperative analgesia is best provided with a demand analgesia system using a programmable pump. This obviates the need for repeated intravenous injections and is a closed system which limits contamination. Careful adjustment of dose and lockout are necessary to cope with the likely habituation of patients to opiate analgesics. The postoperative pain of patients who are drug abusers is extremely difficult to manage and the best approach seems to be to use a combination of opioid, NSAID and sedative.

Although the situation with respect to hepatitis has improved recently due to the safety and efficacy of recombinant hepatitis B vaccine there is still no vaccine for hepatitis C or HIV. Thus although 86 per cent of British anaesthetists are now immunized against hepatitis B (O'Donnell and Asbury, 1992) it is still important to take all possible measures to reduce the possibility of infection with these latter agents. Reassuringly, there is no evidence that routine ward care or orthopaedic surgery has yet led to the infection of staff (Jeffries, 1992). If inoculation with HIV positive material does occur, a course of zidovudine could begin immediately, although there is no evidence that this will prevent seroconversion and a number of failures have been reported (Lange *et al.*, 1990).

Malignant hyperpyrexia

Malignant hyperpyrexia (MH) is widely recognized as the only iatrogenic disease of anaesthesia. Its reported frequency varies but, in the UK, Ellis and Halsall (1980) found 1 case per 200 000 general anaesthetics administered – that is, a given anaesthetist might expect to see a case once every 150 working years! MH is a condition characterized by thermal runaway, such that the patient's core temperature rises by at least 1°C per hour, leading to exhaustion of the tissue oxygen supply, breakdown of membrane function and death. The syndrome occurs only when a susceptible individual is exposed to certain rigger substances; halothane, enflurane and isoflurane and possibly depolarizing muscle relaxants. A similar syndrome clearly related to severe environmental stress occurs in swine (upon which most of the experimental work has been carried out) and in wild animals during pursuit and capture. Therefore it has been suggested that MH in man represents an abnormally developed stress response (Wingard, 1974). A similar syndrome of metabolic over-stimulation and muscle necrosis has been reported after poisoning with the amphetamine derivative 'ecstasy' (Campkin and Davies, 1992). The first case of malignant hyperthermia was reported in 1960 – coinciding with the growing use of halothane – and despite the development of effective treatment, the overall mortality of unrecognized cases continues to be high.

Susceptible cases are thought to suffer from an inherited myopathy (Ellis and Harriman, 1973) and consequently present for minor orthopaedic surgery or at the accident and emergency department with trauma. Almost half of the cases collected by Ellis and Halsall (1980) arose in this way. MH is seldom reported in connection with surgery of body cavities. MH myopathy is inherited as an autosomal dominant, with a range of expression. Evidence is accumulating that the culprit is the gene on chromosome 19 which codes the ryanodine receptor, which controls one of the calcium ion channels in the sarcoplasmic reticulum (MacLennan *et al.*, 1990). The observed increase in skeletal muscle metabolism is then thought to be caused by abnormal free calcium ion movement following breakdown in intracellular calcium control. Free calcium ion affects the permeability and control of both excitable and non-excitable tissue, which may account for the subtle evidence of widespread biochemical abnormality in MH-susceptible patients; differing exercise thermogenesis, altered glucose/insulin ratios and changes in lactate and pyruvate levels with feeding, and abnormal glucose tolerance.

Because MH is familial, cases tend to be grouped in geographical localities and the occurrence of one case should alert anaesthetists in the region to the possibility of others.

Clinical picture

Reported cases are usually discovered when the anaesthetist notices that the patient or the anaesthetic hoses are hot. In practice this appears to be a late sign preceded by others and indicating established MH. The temperature increase may be explosive with core temperature rising 1 degree every 5 minutes, and temperatures greater than 43°C may be achieved. The vastly increased metabolic rate results in tachypnoea, tachycardia, with extra systoles and cyanosis, despite an adequate inspired oxygen concentration. Muscle rigidity (particularly masseter spasm) following succinylcholine correlates well with the subsequent development of MH and occurs in 70 per cent of cases. Rarely, MH has occurred without significant fever (Schmitt *et al.*, 1975); the cases have been either young children, in whom heat loss is proportionately greater, or have taken place when excessive heat loss might mask the pyrexia such as could occur in a Charnley enclosure.

As intracellular metabolism runs out of control, there is breakdown of membrane function and loss of cell contents from striated muscle cells – myoglobin, creatinine phosphokinase, potassium and lactate ions – and there is a growing metabolic acidosis. Venous blood from muscle is desaturated and has a high $PVCO_2$. Myocardial function is depressed and arrhythmias become more likely. Whilst specific abnormality of myocardial cells has been postulated (Huckell *et al.*, 1978) analogous to that of striated muscle cells, it is more likely that cardiac function is altered secondary to the electrolyte abnormalities and increased sympathetic nervous system activity. Lucke *et al.* (1976) found a dramatic rise in plasma catecholamine during MH, and some authorities would have argued that sympathetic activation was not simply secondary to the enormous increase in muscle metabolism but was a partial trigger in itself (Wingard 1974; Lister *et al.*, 1975; Williams *et al.*, 1978). In the laboratory, α and β-adrenergic agonists have been found to trigger MH (Hall *et al.*, 1977; Gronert *et al.*, 1980) whilst sympathetic antagonists have been thought to offer modest protection (Lister *et al.*, 1976).

Acute cerebral oedema with coma, areflexia and fixed dilated pupils results from hypoxia, pyrexia, acidosis and hyperkalaemia; the quality of the recovery depends chiefly upon the speed with which MH is diagnosed and effective measures are instituted.

Respiratory changes include tachypnoea, hyperventilation, Va/Q abnormalities with raised $PaCO_2$ and a reduced PaO_2, and ultimately pulmonary oedema. Effluent venous blood from muscle beds shows marked desaturation and an enormous increase in CO_2 production; these changes are reflected in the mixed venous blood gases.

Renal function may diminish to eventual anuria as a result of shock, ischaemia and myoglobinaemia.

Assessment of patients

Assessment of patients depends first upon their history of previous anaesthetic experience and that of their immediate relatives. Unfortunately, MH may occur after uneventful previous anaesthesia in which either trigger agents were not used or the exposure was too brief to pass the point of no return (Halsall *et al.*, 1979). Physical examination may reveal, typically a patient in early adulthood, well-muscled but with marginal skeletal weakness. Ellis and Halsall (1980) have noted that thigh muscle development may be prominent. The majority of MH-susceptible individuals have an elevated resting serum creatinine phosphokinase, and this has been used as a screening test. Ellis *et al.* (1975) warn, however, that this test will fail to identify all those at risk when used without a muscle biopsy. Definitive diagnosis can only be achieved by the *in vitro* testing of a muscle biopsy specimen from the left vastus internus. A histological examination should be carried out for evidence of MH myopathy and tissue bath experiments should be conducted to measure the muscle threshold to contracture in the presence of caffeine, and halothane, according to the protocol of the European Malignant Hyperpyrexia Group (1984). Patients are classified as; susceptible to MH when abnormal responses are obtained to both halothane and caffeine challenges (MHS); or not susceptible (MHN) when responses are normal. Since 1984 an intermediate category (MHE) has been created for those patients in whom one response is abnormal but not both: such patients are best managed as for those who are MHS.

Treatment

There are many causes of pyrexia occurring during anaesthesia (Table 6.5) but anaesthetists should always remember the possibility of MH: early treatment is almost always successful but delay in diagnosis will compound the problem. Fulminant MH, indicated by an explosive rise in temperature of 1° per 15 minutes and rapid onset of cyanosis, is a clinical emergency and immediate treatment is required if the patient is to survive. In children and in conditions of substantial heat loss, the metabolic changes may be more dramatic than the rise in body temperature. The

Table 6.5 Causes of pyrexia during anaesthesia

Cerebrovascular accident	
Osteogenesis imperfecta	
Thyroid crisis	
Lymphoma	
Epileptic seizure	
Reaction to blood transfusion	
Drugs:	monoamine oxidase inhibitors
	tricyclic antidepressants
	ketamine
	atropine overdosage, especially in children
	phencyclidine

following scheme of treatment is based upon that of Ellis and Halsall (1980).

1. Discontinue all triggering anaesthetic agents and if possible switch to a clean machine; continue with oxygen alone. Non-depolarizing muscle relaxants may be given but the response may be poor since contracture is not a motor end-plate phenomenon.
2. Body temperature should be measured with pharyngeal and skin probes and an arterial line inserted for direct measurement of arterial pressure and for blood gas estimation. Blood should be taken for serum potassium estimation.
3. Begin cooling and terminate surgery as soon as possible. Surface cooling can be carried out using towels soaked in ice-cold water and ice-packs placed in the groins and axillae; its effectiveness can be increased by giving a vasodilator. In addition, gastric lavage with chilled solutions can be used and, if readily available, peritoneal dialysis using cold dialysis solution.
4. Give potassium free intravenous fluids liberally, running them through a blood warmer filled with ice-cold water. Use mannitol to protect the kidneys against deposition of myoglobin.
5. Give glucocoritcoids such as methylprednisolone 14 mg/kg (i.e. 1 g to an adult).
6. Give dantrolene 1 mg/kg intravenously and repeat up to 10 mg/kg by rapid infusion. Dantrolene has been shown to be effective in preventing MH if given prophylacticly to susceptible pigs (Harrison, 1975) and in inhibiting contracture in MH susceptible muscle *in vitro* (Austin and Denborough, 1977). Dantrolene is presented in vials containing dantrolene 20 mg, mannitol 300 mg and sodium hydroxide to pH 7.5 when made up with 60 ml of sterile water. The unreconstituted vials have a shelf life of 2 years and are expensive. At present the policy in Oxford is to have a limited supply of dantrolene available in each theatre suite with a single full course of treatment stored centrally. It may be necessary to continue treatment with 1–2 mg/kg 4 times daily for 1–3 days.
7. Immediate symptomatic treatment is required to control hyperkalaemia, metabolic acidosis and hypoglycaemia, whilst β-adrenergic-blocking agents may be required to treat extrasystoles.
8. Beware of late complications; disseminated intravascular coagulation may occur and clotting should be checked twice in the first 12 hours or immediately if there is abnormal bleeding from surgical wounds; renal failure may occur early, if renal protection has been inadequate, or later due to myoglobinaemia. The nephrotoxicity of myoglobin is reduced if urine is alkaline.

Anaesthesia for known or suspected susceptible patients

Patients may be anaesthetized successfully provided certain precautions are observed.

1. Known triggering agents are avoided and a machine is obtained from which vaporizers have been removed. The machine should be equipped with fresh disposable tubing and face mask which will not contain dissolved inhalational agents.
2. Adequate monitoring is employed: skin and core temperature, ECG and facilities for blood gas estimation.
3. Drugs which may be required, including dantrolene, should be immediately available and arrangements made for admission to the intensive therapy unit for postoperative observation.
4. A safe technique of anaesthesia should be used:
   a) premedication with diazepam;

b) induction of anaesthesia; thiopentone or propofol (Harrison, 1991);
c) maintenance; oxygen and nitrous oxide (no longer considered a trigger) with fentanyl supplements;
d) non-depolarizing muscle relaxants may be used but their action should be allowed to wear off unreversed;
e) local anaesthesia appears safe although opinion is divided about amide-linked local anaesthetic agents.

The fulminant classic case of MH is now thankfully rare because anaesthetists are more aware of the possibility and comprehensive monitoring is available. However, there has been an increase in the number of aborted or inconclusive cases, which need further investigation to define the risk. These cases should have a muscle biopsy performed for examination at a specialist centre such as that at Leeds (Leeds MH Investigation Unit, University Department of Anaesthesia, St James University Hospital, Leeds LS9 7TF).

Renal disease

A steadily increasing population of patients in the community is surviving with end-stage renal failure due to the success of the dialysis and renal transplant programmes. These patients present for orthopaedic surgery to manage complications both of long-term dialysis and of renal transplantation. In addition, pathological fractures may occur as a result of osteoporosis caused by hyperparathyroidism secondary to advanced renal failure.

A specific syndrome associated with long-term renal dialysis-haemodialysis amyloidosis is now recognized. Beta2 microglobulin accumulates in patients on long-term dialysis because the dialysis membrane is impermeable to proteins of this size. The microglobulin is converted into amyloid and laid down chiefly in the connective tissues of the musculoskeletal system; joint capsules, synovia, articular cartilage and soft tissues adjacent to joints and bones (Noel *et al.*, 1987). This causes severe joint pain with restriction of movement and little relief is obtained from analgesics or anti-inflammatory drugs.

Surgical treatment is required for carpal tunnel syndrome caused by accumulation of amyloid in the carpal tunnel, trigger finger due to accumulation in tendon sheaths and spontaneous rupture of tendons weakened by amyloid deposition.

Bone cysts may occur where amyloid accumulates in bone, typically in the bones of the hand first but later in the long bones and vertebrae. This leads to pathological fracture and vertebral collapse. Initially, fractures of the neck of the femur were treated with internal fixation but this commonly led to non-union, possible because of the inhibitory effects of beta2 microglobulin on calcification of osteoblasts, and total hip arthroplasty is now preferred (Kurer *et al.*, 1992). Cyst formation in cervical vertebrae may lead to vertebral collapse and instability of the cervical spine, so that preoperative *X*-rays of the cervical spine should be taken of any patient on long-term dialysis and great care taken during anaesthesia.

Successful renal transplantation is at present the only treatment available for dialysis amyloidosis.

Secondary hyperparathyroidism with parathyroid hypertrophy occurs in all patients with chronic renal failure; there is increased mobilization of calcium from bone, leading to weakness of long bones. The cause of these changes is not clear but may be related to resistance to vitamin D and reduced absorption of dietary calcium. Rarely, the parathyroids may become autonomous (tertiary hyperparathyroidism), when serum calcium concentrations are usually increased. This is associated with decreased neuromuscular excitability and muscle weakness, bone pain and a general feeling of malaise.

Successful renal transplantation is not uncommonly followed by erosion of the acetabulum and avascular necrosis of the head of the femur, possibly caused by the high doses of steroids employed postoperatively for immunosuppression (Chan *et al.*, 1980).

The consequence of chronic renal disease thus include a variety of orthopaedic problems but especially the need for internal fixation of pathological fractures and early hip replacement.

Anaesthesia for patients on dialysis

Preoperative preparation

Preoperative assessment of patients on chronic haemodialysis should focus on the patient's dialysis regimen. From the notes, pre- and postdialysis measurements of body weight, serum potassium and haemoglobin concentrations should be obtained together with readings of blood pressure. The period between dialyses is marked by increase in body weight and haemodilution due to retention of fluid, often associated with a rise in blood pressure. There is also a rise in serum potassiumn and patients feel progressively more 'off-colour'.

Hypertension is common amongst these patients and often only becomes controllable after nephrectomy. The majority of hypertensives have a 'fluid overload hypertension' where the blood pressure is closely related to the fluid load; as this increases, blood pressure rises and is treatable by dialysis. A small proportion of patients have severe hypertension which is controlled only with the greatest difficulty. Associated with hypertension there may be left ventricular hypertrophy and myocardial ischaemia.

Severe anaemia is the rule amongst patients on dialysis, with haemoglobin concentrations ranging between 4 and 8 g/dl. This degree of anaemia is usually surprisingly well tolerated, and if the patient is active without dyspnoea, then anaesthesia is uneventful. Attempts to correct the anaemia by transfusion are only briefly successful and run the risk of sensitizing the patient to infused antigens, prejudicing future renal transplantation. If a tourniquet is to be used for surgery, it is possible that blood replacement may be avoided. Low platelet counts may occur after dialysis and, if severe, cause bleeding difficulties postoperatively; this may be exacerbated by any residual heparin activity.

Physical examination, electrocardiogram and chest *X*-ray should exclude pleural and pericardial effusions. Any complaint by the patient that he does not feel well, or as well as he should, must be taken seriously and surgery postponed until patient and anaesthetist are reassured or the underlying cause is found.

Technique of Anaesthesia

The chief problems for anaesthesia in these patients are the anaemia, the delicate fluid balance and the impaired excretion of drugs administered. Local anaesthesia may be used where a suitable block is available and avoids some of the difficulties, but spinal or epidural block should be used only with the greatest caution. The patients tend to behave as though hypovolaemic, so the vasodilatation associated with central neural blockade easily leads to severe hypotension and impaired coronary perfusion. Further, corrective autonomic reflexes may be impaired by antihypertensive medication or uraemic autonomic neuropathy (Kersh *et al.*, 1974). There remains also the risk of creating an epidural haematoma if clotting function is reduced.

Before coming to the anaesthetic room, the patient's arm which contains his fistula should be wrapped in Gamgee, both to protect it and to serve as a marker (Fig. 6.4). The arm should not be used for intravenous infusions – the venous pressure is increased by the fistula – but kept straight by the patient's side. When choosing a site for an intravenous infusion, alternative fistula sites in the forearm must be avoided and preserved for use later. For any surgical procedure where appreciable blood loss is likely, it is best to weigh the swabs and keep a running total of loss. For major surgery, a central venous line inserted through the internal jugular vein or the subclavian vein and measurement of central venous pressure should be used to guide fluid replacement. During general anaesthesia, episodes of hypoxia should be prevented as far as possible by preoxygenation, careful technique and administration of oxygen postoperatively even for the smallest cases because of the reduced oxygen-carrying capacity due to anaemia.

Drug dosage should be conservative since the absence of the renal route of excretion of drugs and their metabolites means that smaller quantities are needed, and prolonged effects of both barbiturates (Dundee and Richards, 1954) and opiates (Don *et al.*, 1975) have been reported. Succinylcholine is best avoided because of the rise in serum potassium it produces, but non-depolarizing muscle relaxants may be used provided that the dose is cautious and that increments are given only when some movement of the patient makes clear the need. Atracurium is the drug of choice. Gallamine is excreted entirely by the kidney and prolonged neuromuscular blockade is likely to follow its use. Automatic ventilation should be such that PaC02 is little changed in order to prevent changes in pH with electrolyte

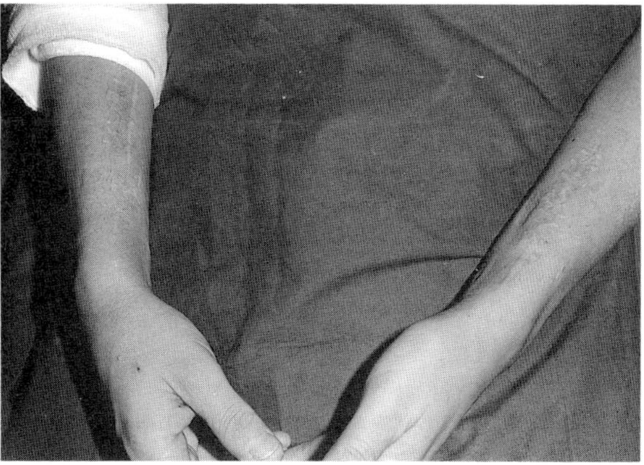

Fig 6.4 Haemophilia; scars of multiple shunts in both forearms of a patient after renal dialysis and renal transplantation.

shifts and reduction in oxygen availability due to shift of the haemoglobin dissociation curve.

Anaesthesia for renal transplant patients

For the patient with a renal homograft the problems are different. Following successful transplantation, renal function is restored, generally marked by an improvement in haemoglobin concentration to near normal levels; excretion of drugs and drug tolerance are improved; fluid loads can be excreted and patients are less sensitive over their fluid balance. However, it is of paramount importance that during the operative period immuno-suppression is continued, daily azathioprine and prednisolone being the standard therapy in most units. These drugs must be given on the day of surgery and continued without interruption postoperatively. As always, care must be taken over cleanliness of technique during anaesthesia so that infection is not introduced by the anaesthetist. During positioning of the patient, care must be taken not to compress the graft with a pelvic or other table support. Blood replacement during surgery remains a subject for debate; the risk of introducing further antigens must be set against that of reduced perfusion and graft hypoxia. Quite clearly, volume lost must be replaced assiduously and perfusion of organs maintained; systemic hypotension should be avoided. As with patients on dialysis, forearm veins which may be required in the future for fistulas should be preserved, and if the patient still has a patent fistula this too should be protected.

Improvements in the management of patients with renal failure will both diminish the frequency with which complications occur and increase the population of patients who survive their disease, so that, for the foreseeable future, patients with renal failure will continue to appear on orthopaedic operating lists.

Sickle cell disease

Sickle cells were first described in 1910 by Herrick, a Chicago physician, who noted the 'peculiar and elongated sickle shaped red corpuscles' in the blood of a West Indian medical student suffering from severe anaemia. The disease results from the presence of an abnormal haemoglobin (HBS): an inherited abnormality of the beta chain of haemoglobin such that at low oxygen tensions the haemoglobin forms spindle-shaped liquid crystals called tactoids which distort the red cell envelope and produce the recognizable sickle cells. When the oxygen tension rises, young red cells are able to resume their original shape but after repeated hypoxic episodes, they remain irreversibly sickled and are removed from the circulation in the reticuloendothelial system. The life of red cells is thus shortened and patients have a haemolytic anaemia with increased haematopoiesis and extension of active bone marrow. Patients who are homozygous for HBS are severely affected, with sickle cell anaemia (SCA), whilst patients who are heterozygous, have sickle cell trait and are relatively well. Other haemoglobinopathies, such as thalassaemia, may also be present.

When sickled, the deformability of red cells is reduced and blood viscosity is increased so that the microcirculation of tissues is impaired. Sickled cells tend to aggregate in larger capillaries, plugging them and causing distal hypoxia which in turn leads to further sickling. Many of the clinical consequences of sickle cell disease are due to these vaso-occlusive episodes which produce tissue infarcts. The distribution of tissue infarcts is capricious and any organ may be affected.

Intense pain results from infarcts in bone which subsequently can become infected often with unusual organisms leading to osteomyelitis. Repeated infarction in renal papillae causes reduced renal function and ultimately end-stage renal failure. Vaso-occlusion in the central nervous system can lead to convulsions and hemiplegia or multiple small episodes may lead to dementia. Widespread pulmonary vascular occlusion may cause pulmonary hypertension and interstitial fibrosis with consequent right ventricular hypertrophy and cor pulmonale by middle age.

Patients who are heterozygous are generally well and in this group anaesthetic disasters have only occurred when the risk went unrecognized. The HBS gene is present in approximately 10 per cent of the British black population with the main concentration of patients in London and Birmingham (Davis *et al.*, 1981). Travellers from Africa, the Mediterranean, and India constitute a further reservoir of cases. Screening tests should be used for any patient who might be at risk (see Chapter 2).

Musculoskeletal lesions (Table 6.6) occurred in the majority of cases of SCA reviewed by Bennett and Naminyak (1990): osteomyelitis was common principally due to infection with salmonella, to which these patients are particularly susceptible. Surgery was kept to a minimum but was needed for drainage of abscesses, sequestrectomy and late complications such a osteoarthritis of large joints.

Anaesthesia for patients with sickle cell anaemia

In vitro studies suggest that polymerization of HbS begins at an oxygen saturation less than 85 per cent and is complete at a saturation of 38 per cent (Bromberg and Jensen, 1967). Thus, patients with sickle cell disease are constantly sickling because mixed venous blood is at the critical point. Sickle trait cells (HbAS) do not begin to sickle until oxygen saturation is below 40 per cent and heterozygous patients are relatively little at risk. Techniques of anaesthesia should be chosen to avoid hypoxia, to avoid stasis of blood, body cooling, acidosis and preferrably any use of tourniquets. The actual technique chosen matters less than the skill with which it is applied.

Preoperative preparation

Any patient who is found to have HbS on routine screening should be referred to a haematologist for investigation and confirmation of the diagnosis. The assistance of a haematologist will be invaluable, particularly in centres which do not normally see many cases of sickle cell disease. In addition to haematology investigations, a chest X-ray and electrocardiogram should be performed to assess cardiomegaly and cor pulmonale. Preoperative transfusion is controversial (reviewed by Esseltine *et al.*, 1988) but is probably needed if the haemoglobin is less than 7 g/dl. This will dilute the haemoglobin S and depress haematopoiesis whilst also increasing oxygen transport. However, transfusion leads to alloimmunization, may transfer infection and causes accumulation of iron so that increasingly strict criteria for transfusion are being adopted (Davies and Wonke, 1992). Supplementary folic acid should be given to make good any deficiency and prophylactic antibiotics should be considered for all but the most minor procedures.

An intravenous fluid infusion should be started from the beginning of the period of preoperative starvation to ensure that there is no dehydration, hypovolaemia and increased viscosity due to hyperosmolality. Promethazine 1 mg/kg can be given as premedication because of its possible benefit inhibiting sickling of deoxygenated HbS (Kaufman and Sumner, 1979).

Table 6.6 Clinical details in 57 patients with sickle cell anaemia

Initial findings	Number of patients
Bone and joint pain	46
Osteomyelitis	35
Splenomegaly	19
Joint effusion	8
Deep soft tissue abscess	8
Cellulitis	7
Jaundice	5
Septic arthritis	4
Flexion contracture of hip	3
Haemarthroses	2

Source: Bennett and Namnyak (1990).

Technique of Anaesthesia

Added oxygen should be given from entry to the anaesthetic room to 24–48 hours postoperatively, preoxygenation is important to avoid hypoxia during induction or during any unexpectedly difficult intubation. Oxygen delivery and tissue saturation should be monitored throughout anaesthesia and regional or general anaesthesia may be chosen as appropriate. If epidural, spinal or caudal block is used, care must be taken to ensure that hypotension does not occur and the blood pressure maintained with adequate intravenous fluid therapy rather than by using sympathomimetic agents which might cause vasoconstriction. Epidural anaesthesia has also been used safely to treat pain during vaso-occlusive crises (Esseltine *et al.*, 1988).

Ventilation should be adjusted to normocapnia to avoid acidosis or shifts in the haemoglobin dissociation curve due to overventilation, and acid-base status should be measured from time to time from arterial blood gas samples.

Active warming of the patient should be undertaken using warmed air blankets, warmed infusion fluids and warmed, humidified inspired gases and both central and peripheral temperatures should be monitored. Warming should be continued in the recovery room. Skin cooling may be a crucial insult, stimulating vascular reflexes which divert blood from bone marrow and cause avascular necrosis (Serjeant and Chalmers, 1990). Cooling should be avoided at all costs.

Postoperative management

Recognition of peri-operative crises is likely to be difficult as the chief sign, pain, is likely to be masked by drugs given and organ infarction may be mistaken for operative complications. The most likely cause of major organ dysfunction, however, remains a vascular crisis and should be treated by exchange transfusion.

Postoperative analgesia is best provided by regional blocks and NSAIDS such as ketorolac (Goodman, 1991). Opioids cause respiratory acidosis and hypoxemia and may contribute to morbidity whilst pethidine appears to be toxic in the doses required, leading to fits caused by the metabolite Nor-pethidinic acid (Pryle *et al.*, 1992).

Hydroxyurea may be used in the future to raise the plasma levels of haemoglobin F in patients with SCA. There is experimental evidence that hydroxyurea increases production of haemoglobin F and reduces the incidence of painful crises in patients (Goldberg *et al.*, 1990). Thus, it may be that the need for surgical intervention will be reduced.

References

Arnold, W. D. and Hilgartner, M. W. (1977). Hemophiliac arthropathy. *Journal of Bone and Joint Surgery*, **54A**, 287.

Association of Anaesthetists (1988). *AIDS and Hepatitis B Guidelines for Anaesthetists*. Association of Anaesthetists, London.

Austin, K. L. and Denborough, M. A. (1977). Drug treatment of malignant hyperpyrexia. *Anaesthesia and Intensive Care*, **5**, 207.

Bennett, O. M. and Naminyak, S. S. (1990). Bone and joint manifestations of sickle cell anaemia. *Journal of Bone and Joint Surgery (Br)*, **72-B**, 494–9.

Bernstein, R. L. (1980). Anesthesia for total hip replacement. In M. L. Zauder (ed.), *Anesthesia for Orthopaedic Surgery*, F. A. Davies, Philadelphia, PA, p. 75.

Biggs, R. (1978). *The Treatment of Haemophilia A and B and Von Willebrand Disease*. Blackwell Scientific, Oxford.

Birkinshaw, K. (1975). Anaesthesia in a patient with an unstable neck. *Anaesthesia*, **30**, 46–9.

Bromberg, P. A. and Jensen, W. N. (1967). Blood oxygen dissociation curves in sickle cell disease. *Journal of Laboratory and Clinical Medicine*, **70**, 480–7.

Chadd, G. D., Ackers, J. W. L. and Bailey, P. M. (1989). Difficult intubation aided by the laryngeal mask airway. *Anaesthesia*, **44**, 1015.

Cameron, C. B. and Kobrinsky, N. (1990). Perioperative management of patients with Von Willebrand's disease. *Canadian Journal of Anaesthesia*, **37**, 341–7.

Campkin, N. T. A. and Davies, U. M. (1992). Another death from Ecstasy. *Journal of the Royal Society of Medicine*, **85**, 61.

Chan, L., French, M., Beare, J., Oliver, D. O., Morris, P. J. (1980). Prospective trial of high dose versus low dose prednisolone in renal transplant patients. *Transplantation Proceedings*, **12**, 323.

David, D. J. (1972). Skin trauma in patients receiving corticosteroid therapy. *British Medical Journal*, **12**, 614.

Davies, S. C. and Wonke, B. (1992). The management of haemoglobinopathies. *Bailliéres Clinical Haematology*, in press.

Davis, L. R., Huehns, E. R. and White, J. M. (1981). *British Medical Journal*, **283**, 1519.

Don, H. F., Dieppa, R. A. and Taylor, P. (1975). Narcotic analgesics in anuric patients. *Anesthesiology*, **42**, 745.

Dundee, J. W. and Richards, R. K. (1954). Effect of azotaemia upon the action of intravenous barbiturate anaesthesia. *Anesthesiology*, **15**, 333.

Eipe, J. (1972). Drugs affecting therapy with anticoagulants. *Medical Clinics of North America*, **56**, 255.

Ellis, F. R. and Halsall, P. J. (1980). Malignant hyperpyrexia. *British Journal of Hospital Medicine*, **24**, 318.

Ellis, F. R. and Harriman, D. G. F. (1973). A new screening test for susceptibility to malignant hyperpyrexia. *British Journal of Anaesthesia*, **45**, 638.

Ellis, F. R., Clarke, I. M. C., Modgill, M., Currie, S. and Harriman, D. G. F. (1975). Evaluation of creatinine phosphokinase in screening patients for malignant hyperpyrexia. *British Medical Journal*, **3**, 511.

Ellison, N. (1977). Diagnosis and management of bleeding disorders. *Anesthesiology*, **47**, 171.

Esseltine, J. W., Baxter, M. R. N. and Bevan, R. C. (1988). Sickle cell states and the anaesthetist. *Canadian Journal of Anaesthesia*, **35**, 385–403.

European Malignant Hyperpyrexia Group (1984). A protocol for the investigation of malignant hyperpyrexia (MH) susceptibility. *British Journal of Anaesthesia*, **56**, 395–423.

Fulcher, C. and Zimmerman, T. (1982). Characterization of the human factor VIII procoagulant protein with a heterologous precipitating antibody. *Proceedings of the National Academy of Science, USA*, **79**, 1648–52.

Goldberg, M. A., Brugnara, C., Dover, G. J., Schapira, L., Charache, S. and Bunn, H. F. (1990). Treatment of sickle cell anaemia with hydroxyurea and erythropoietin. *New England Journal of Medicine*, **323**, 366–72.

Goodman, E. (1991). Use of Ketorolac in sickle-cell disease and vaso-occlusive crisis. *Lancet*, **338**, 641–2.

Gronert, G. (1980). Malignant hyperthermia. *Anesthesiology*, **53**, 395.

Hall, G. M., Lucke, J. N. and Lister, D. (1977). Porcine malignant hyperthermia V. Fatal hyperthermia in the pietrain pig associated with the infusion of a-adrenergic agonists. *British Journal of Anaesthesia*, **49**, 855–63.

Gravallese, E. M., Baker, N., Lester, S., Kay, J. and Owen, W. F. Jr (1992). Musculoskeletal manifestations in beta 2-microglobulin amyloidosis. Case discussion (Clinical Conference). *Arthritis and Rheumatology*, **35** (5), 592–602.

Halsall, P. J., Cain, P. A. and Ellis, F. R. (1979). Retrospective analysis of anaesthetics received by patients before susceptibility to malignant hyperpyrexia was recognised. *British Journal of Anaesthesia*, **51**, 949–54.

Harrison, G. G. (1975). Control of the malignant hyperpyrexia syndrome in MHS swine by dantrolene sodium. *British Journal of Anaesthesia*, **47**, 62–5.

Harrison, G. (1991). Propofol anaesthesia in pharmacogenetic states. In C. Prys Roberts (ed.), *Focus on Infusion: Intravenous Anaesthesia*. Current Medical Literature, London, pp. 186–91.

Herrick, J. B. (1910). *Archives of Internal Medicine*, **6**, 676.

Huckell, V. F., Staniloff, H. M., Britt, B. A., Waxman, M. B., Morch, J. E. (1978). Cardiac manifestation of malignant hyperthermia susceptibility. *Circulation*, **58**, 916–22.

Hughes, G. R. V. (1979). Rheumatoid arthritis. *British Journal of Hospital Medicine*, **21**, 584.

Jeffries, D. J. (1992). Doctors, patients and HIV. *British Medical Journal*, **304**, 1258–9.

Inwood, M. J. and Meltzer, D. B. (1978). The female carrier of haemophilia – a problem for the anaesthetist. *Canadian Anaesthetists Society Journal*, **25**, 266.

Kaufman, L. and Sumner, E. (1979). *Medical Problems and the Anaesthetist.* Edward Arnold, London, pp. 139–51.

Kersh, E. S., Kronfield, S. J., Unger, A., Popper, R. W., Cantor, S, and Cohn, K. (1974). Autonomic insufficiency in anaemia as a cause of haemodialysis induced hypotension. *New England Journal of Medicine*, **290**, 650.

Kobrinsky, N. (1988). Bleeding problems in children. *Contemporary Pediatrics*, **4**, 9–20.

Lange, J. M. A., Boucher, C. A. B., Hollak, C. E. M., Wiltinu, E. H., Reiss, P., Van-Royen, E. A., Roos, M., Danner, S. A. and Goudsmit, J. (1990). Failure of Dizovudine prophylaxis after accidental exposure to HIV-1. *New England Journal of Medicine*, **322**, 1375–7.

Latto, I. P. and Rosen, M. (1985). *Difficulties in Tracheal Intubation.* Balliére Tindall, London.

Lister, D., Hall, G. M. and Lucke, J. N. (1975). Malignant hyperthermia: a human and a porcine stress syndrome. *Lancet*, **1**, 529.

Lister, D., Hall, G. M. and Lucke, J. N. (1976). Porcine malignant hyperthermia III: Adrenergic blockade. *British Journal of Anaesthesia*, **48**, 831.

Lucke, J. N., Hall, G. M. and Lister, D. (1976). Porcine malignant hyperthermia 1: Metabolic and physiological changes. *British Journal of Anaesthesia*, **48**, 297.

McConkey, B., Frazer, G. M., Bligh, A. S. and Whitely, H. Transparent skin and osteoporosis. *Lancet*, **1**, 693.

MacLennan, D. H., Duff, C., Zorato, F., Fujii, J., Phillips, M., Korneluk, R. G., Frodis, W., Britt, B. A. and Worton, R. G. (1990). Ryanodine receptor gene is a candidate for predisposition to malignant hyperthermia. *Nature*, **343**, 559–61.

McCrirrick, A. and Pracilio, J. A. (1991). Awake intubation: a new technique. *Anaesthesia*, **46**, 661–3.

Matthews, J. A. (1974). Atlanto-axial subluxation in rheumatoid arthritis: a 5 year follow-up study. *Annals of the Rheumatic Diseases*, **33**, 526.

Naides, S. J., Scharosch, L. L., Foto, F. and Howard, E. J. (1990). Rheumatologic manifestations of human parvovirus B19 infection in adults. *Arthritis and Rheumatology*, **33**, 1297–309.

Noel, L. H., Zingraff, J., Bardin, T.*et al.*(1987). Tissue distribution of dialysis amyloidosis. *Clinical Nephrology*, **27**, 175–8.

O'Donell, N. G. and Asbury, A. J. (1992). The occupational hazard of human immunodeficiency virus and hepatitis B virus infection. *Anaesthesia*, **47**, 923–8.

Pryle, B. J., Grech, H., Stoddart, **?.**, Carson, R., O'Mahoney, T. and Reynolds, F. (1992). Toxocity of nor-pethidine in sickle cell crisis. *British Medical Journal*, **304**, 1478–9.

Rainford, S. G., Jouhar, A. J. and Hall, A. (1973). Tranexamic acid in the control of spontaneous bleeding in severe haemophilia. *Thrombosis and Diathesis Haemorrhagica*, **30**, 272.

Rizza, C. R. (1984). Haemophilia A and B. *Prescriber's Journal*, **24**, 71–81.

Royal College of Pathologists (1992). *HIV Infection: Hazards of Transmission to Patients and Health Care Workers During Invasive Procedures.* Royal College of Pathologists, London.

Sampson, J. G. and Hamstra, R. (1979). Management of haemophiliac patients undergoing surgical procedures. *Anesthesia and Analgesia*, **58**, 133.

Schmitt, H. P., Simmendinger, H. J. and Wagner, H. (1975). Severe morphological changes in skeletal muscles of a five-month-old infant dying from an anaesthetic complication with general muscle rigidity. *Neuropadiatre*, **6**, 102–6.

Serjeant, G. R. and Chalmers, R. M. (1990). Is the painful crisis of sickle cell disease a 'steal' syndrome? *Journal of Clinical Pathology*, **43**, 789–91.

Steere, A. C., Grodzicki, R. L., Kornblatt, A. N., Craft, J. E., Barbour, A. G., Burgdorfer, W.*et al.*(1983). The spirochaetal etiology of Lyme disease. *New England Journal of Medicine*, **308**, 733–9.

Strauss, H. S., Kevy, S. V. and Diamond, L. K. (1965). Ineffectiveness of prophylactic epsilon aminocaproic acid in severe haemophilia. *New England Journal of Medicine*, **273**, 301.

Von Willebrand, E. A. (1926). Hereditor pseudohomople. *Finskia Laeksaellsk Handl.*, **68**, 87–122.

Williams, C. H., Howch, G. P. Jr and Roberts, J. T. (1978). Experimental malignant hyperthermia. *Anesthesiology*, **49**, 58.

Wingard, D. W. (1974). Malignant hyperthermia: a human stress syndrome? *Lancet*, **4**, 1450.

Chapter 7

Paediatric orthopaedic anaesthesia

John Stevens

Surgeons and Anaesthetists should not undertake occasional paediatric practice. The outcome of surgery and anaesthesia in children is related to the experience of the clinicians involved.
The report of the National Confidential Enquiry into Peri-operative Deaths (NCEPOD) 1989. (Campling *et al.*, 1989).

Introduction

The day of the anaesthetist and surgeon who, as true generalists, could tackle any case that came their way has passed, and this passing is enshrined in the recommendations of the NCEPOD report. Subspecialization in anaesthesia has reached the stage where occasional practice is no longer acceptable in many areas, and this particularly applies to paediatric anaesthesia.

The important role played by subspecialization in delivering high-quality care has been amply demonstrated by the findings of the report which showed that mortality and morbidity were extremely low when children were cared for by senior specialists and the recommendation that all hospitals should have anaesthetists and surgeons designated to care for paediatric patients was made. The British Paediatric Association has acknowledged these findings, and indeed goes further to recommend that if such specialists are not available then the patient should be transferred to a regional hospital where they are. The British Association of Paediatric Surgeons also now recommend that all children under 3 should be cared for in specialist units (Atwell and Spargo, 1992).

The report also recommends that 'consultants who take responsibility for the care of children must be kept up-to-date and competent in the management of children' and the specialist societies have responded positively to these words. Refresher courses, seminars and workshops have been designed to keep these designated specialists abreast of new developments. The Association of Paediatric Anaesthetists (APA) is reviewing its membership qualifications in an attempt to meet the needs of those anaesthetists who wish to keep in touch with paediatric practice but whose commitment in terms of regular working paediatric sessions is small.

Many orthopaedic hospitals such as the Nuffield Orthopaedic Centre, exist in isolation without resident anaesthetists and paediatricians, and accept and treat children of all ages and the wisdom of this must be questioned. The concept of self-contained children's hospitals or units has reappeared and now regularly features in discussions on the future of health care in Britain.

The establishment of specialist societies such as the APA of Great Britain and Northern Ireland has created a forum at which developments can be publicized, and a consensus reached in the most appropriate way of managing particularly vexing problems, thus providing a focus for change and a stimulus for research and development. Articles of interest to paediatric anaesthetists have hitherto been scattered through journals too numerous to follow in detail and the publication of the first editions of a specialist journal, *Paediatric Anaesthesia* should facilitate the assimilation of new information rapidly once it has found its place in the complex hierarchy of journals.

The aim of this chapter is to add to this specialist approach and to highlight the areas of development in paediatric anaesthetic practices that may be of reference to orthopaedic surgery.

Age distribution

Figure 7.1 shows the age distribution of children operated on for elective procedures at the Nuffield Orthopaedic Centre during the 12 month period April 1991–March 1992. Surgery under 1 year is rare and consists entirely in this series of clubfoot surgery and procedures for congenitally dislocated hips. The physiological and pharmacological variations in the infant are consequently of relatively less concern in paediatric orthopaedic anaesthesia for the vast majority of patients. Much elective surgery is timed to fit with growth patterns and social and educational needs and is spread fairly evenly through childhood with peaks in the preschool years and in early adolescence where orthopaedic procedures are the most common performed across the specialities. The relatively small numbers of children under 3 should indicate that anaesthetic problems per se in orthopaedic practice should hopefully be few and far between as it is this group that consistently appear to feature in morbidity reports (Tiret *et al.*, 1988), but the correspondingly high proportion of orthopaedic patients with multi-system diseases must also be included in the equation (Cohen *et al.*, 1990). These reports also reflect that the smaller the child the greater the likelihood of a major procedure being undertaken, thus increasing the incidence of complications.

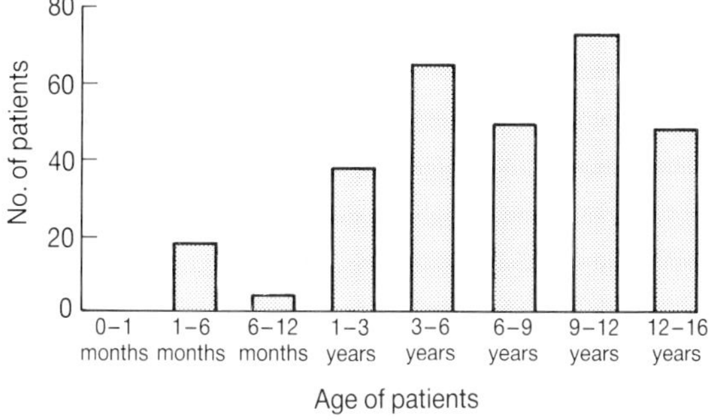

Fig 7.1 Age distribution of children operated on for elective procedures at the Nuffield Orthopaedic Centre.

Preoperative considerations

Premedication

A great deal of emphasis has been directed towards making the childs stay in hospital as pleasant as possible, and the National Association for the Welfare of the Child in Hospital (NAWCH) must take much of the credit for this. They have constantly fought against dogma enshrined and unquestioned over the years and have urged the health professions to review practices. Perhaps the most obvious areas of this public pressure has been the thorny question of whether parents should accompany the child to the anaesthetic room and the recovery area, and, to a lesser extent, the effect of the ever-present and often questioning parent on the frequency of use of intramuscular premedication. An anaesthetist's preference for injectable premeds tends to waver when he is questioned week in and week out as to whether it is really necessary or if a tablet or some other form of medicine would be just as effective. The introduction of alternative routes of drug administration may further relegate intramuscular injections in children to the annals of medical practices.

Rectal premedication with benzodiazepines, thiopentone and ketamine have proved popular on the continent but have never become established in the UK, and the worries surrounding the increased frequency of child abuse reports may lead to a further decrease in their use. Locally, the decision whether to allow school teachers and council carers to administer rectal diazepam to epileptic children has caused considerable worry in community care circles and the possible administration of rectal premedication to the unwilling and struggling child is clearly unacceptable.

Fentanyl lollipops have been produced, seem to be effective and have the added benefit of allowing sugar intake in the preoperative period thus decreasing the theoretical risk of hypoglycaemia, but they appear to be only of academic interest this far (Goldstein-Dresner *et al.*, 1991).

Much greater interest however, has been shown in the transdermal and intranasal routes of administration.

Trials have been undertaken on the applicability of transdermal fentanyl patches in paediatric practice in postoperative analgesia but a considerable degree of variability in absorption and effect have been demonstrated in this situation. On theoretical grounds it would seem likely that drug delivery would be more predictable in a preoperative situation in a physiologically stable child, whereas blood flow and body temperature changes might lead to variable absorption in the intra- and postoperative period (Gourlay *et al.*, 1990). If a pool of drug could accumulate in the dermis of the acutely hypovolaemic shut down patient and then be washed into the circulation when reestablishment of normal peripheral blood flow occurs, there would be a risk of respiratory depression or arrest. These difficulties also apply to the use of subcutaneous infusions in pain management, and may limit the usefulness of the transdermal route which is otherwise extremely attractive, to premedication and pre-emptive analgesia.

Intranasal administration of midazolam is effective, relatively easily undertaken and considerable quicker in action than oral or IM administration and only marginally slower than rectal administration (Rose *et al.*, 1990; Walbergh *et al.*,). There is in some patients an unpleasant burning sensation, and again the social implications of encouraging children to 'snort' drugs which induce a pleasurable sensation for medical purposes has been questioned. Sufentanil and ketamine can also be effectively administered by this route and further work on correct dosage and method of administration is being undertaken (Morrison *et al.*, 1992). Perhaps the major advantage of such a method is its rapidity, allowing a child to be quickly calmed for investigations, intravenous emplacement or when the running of a list descends to its customary bagatelle and the patient is called for whilst still fully dressed in the play room.

The advent of the eutectic mixture of local anaesthetics (EMLA cream, Astra) has revolutionized paediatric practice and is perhaps the single most important development of the last 10 years. It allows virtually pain free intravenous cannulation, and rapid smooth induction of anaesthesia and might be said to have rendered the whole question of premedication mostly irrelevant. It is, however, most important that time is allowed in list planning for EMLA to work, at least one hour (Maunuksela and Korpela, 1986).

Psychosocial considerations

In an ideal environment where the child is introduced to an area in the hospital, near the operating theatre, where only other healthy children are held, and helped into the acceptance of his new surroundings by trained staff and cooperative parents, EMLA may be the only premedication required. Children should be allowed to keep their own clothes or be dressed in colourful, comfortable and warm outfits, not the scratchy, voluminous shrouds of yesterday. If the change of setting can be accomplished without endless waits for lifts or half-mile journeys through cold, forbidding corridors, the pre- and postoperative experience can be made very tolerable and, if pain is adequately controlled, even pleasant. All these factors should have a bearing in hospital design but it is generally only in children's hospitals where much consideration to such elements is given.

The success of preparation of the child for anaesthesia and surgery depends on the age and demeanour of the child, the expectations of the parents, the attitude of the anaesthetist and to some extent on local practice and the experiences of the provision of a service. Steward (1989) has conveniently classified children into age ranges in which the considerations vary. From birth to 6 months the child is unaware of any threat to its well-being, whereas the parent feels most vulnerable and must be approached in a sympathetic fashion. From 6 months to around 4 years the child fears separation from the parent yet is unable to comprehend the need for this. At 4 to 6 years a meaningful dialogue can be undertaken and the child should be involved in decisions such as the route of premedication or choice of induction technique but too much detail may confuse and frighten. From 6 years to adolescence reliance of the child on the opinion of the parent is paramount and the concepts of pain, death, suffering are beginning to take root. Adolescence is a time of challenge, of decision-making and self-awareness and care must be taken to respect opinions, fears of loss of control and the maintenance of face and dignity. The judgement from the House of Lords in the Gillick case (*Gillick* v. *West Norfolk*, 1986) reinforces the rights of the older child to informed consent and to reasoned and reasonable discussion of various approaches to treatment (Pace, 1991).

Parental involvement

The role of the parent is central in the management and psychological preparation of the child. The NAWCH charter, which has been broadly accepted by all involved in paediatric care calls for the continued presence of the parent with the child throughout an admission, providing this is not obviously to the detriment of the child's care, or the sanity of the parent, and the argument against parents in the anaesthetic room has more or less abated. With sympathetic handling and confidence in one's own ability this should not present major problems and may serve to alter the anaesthetist's approach to premedication or induction. Time spent explaining to the parent, particularly if the child is in the 6 month to 4 years age group, that it may be necessary to restrain the child during induction if he or she becomes uncooperative or restless will prevent anger or resentment. Parents like to feel helpful and useful at a time of great stress, and allowing them to take part in some small way in the induction pays dividends. Those who for personal reasons find it too upsetting to accompany their child should not be disparaged.

Preoperative investigations

Preoperative investigations should be kept to a minimum and if blood tests are essential on the day of surgery, ward staff should be encouraged to employ indwelling cannulae which can be subsequently utilized for intravenous induction, saving precious veins and repeated venepuncture. The value of routine haemoglobin investigations in children has been questioned. Able and Howard (1992) in an audit of practice in a childrens hospital found that of 2468 Hb requests in children prior to surgery only 9 patients had surgery cancelled due to a low haemoglobin and all had a chronic compensated anaemia of nutritional origin. The acceptable level of haemoglobin seems to have fallen in recent years, most anaesthetists being happy with a level of 8 gms per cent or more. A high index of suspicion should be maintained in children with poor diets and those who have spent time in tropical climates, as evidenced by an Asian child presenting for minor surgery which proceeded uneventfully, but whose blood on venepuncture looked a little thin, and was consequently dispatched for analysis. The result came back at 3.4 gms per cent and the child, who had recently spent some months in Pakistan, was found to be heavily infested with threadworm.

Baseline electrolytes and creatinine should be recorded in children with spina bifida and cerebral palsy as renal problems are common in this group, and cross-match should be performed for major bony surgery, extensive soft-tissue surgery and spinal procedures.

Much orthopaedic surgery in children is for congenital anomalies many of which are associated with abnormalities in other systems, particularly the cardiovascular system. Echo cardiography has revolutionized the assessment of such problems and a skilled cardiologist will be able to clarify cardiac function and offer advice as to suitable management. Small children may need sedation in order to acquire good images.

Repeat anaesthesia is common in paediatric orthopaedic surgery whether it be for 2-stage procedures for scoliosis surgery or repeated plaster changes for hip or knee deformity correction or for knee surgery. Although rare, halothane hepatitis does seem to occur even in very young children (Whitburne and Summer, 1986), and access to the records of previous anaesthesia is essential. Wark (1983) estimated the incidence in children to be 1 in 82 000. Fulminant liver failure requiring transplantation may occur, so it seems prudent to avoid repeated exposure.

Malignant hyperpyrexia may also occur even in the very young (Wilhoit *et al.*, 1989), so a detailed family history of previous anaesthesia is extremely important.

Starvation

Preoperative starvation has undergone a major rethink in recent years (Goresty and Maltby, 1990). The timetable of the child usually means that the last oral intake is at around 7 pm at night. Thus the child for surgery at the end of the following morning may be without food or fluid for 12–16 hours if the traditional regimes are followed. This causes unnecessary suffering and may indeed be harmful. Clear non-particulate fluids exit the stomach in the child very quickly and it has been demonstrated that a drink of clear fluid such as apple juice taken up to 2 hours before surgery has little effect on gastric pH and actually decreases intragastric volumes (Sandhar *et al.*, 1989; Splinter *et al.*, 1989). However most parents are reluctant to wake their child in the middle of the night, and early admission, with a drink given by ward staff on arrival, seems to be the safest policy, particularly for day case surgery.

Coughs, colds and cancellations

One of the commonest and most vexing problems encountered in the preoperative stage is what to do with the child with a runny nose. Is this the beginning of an upper respiratory tract infection or is this allergic rhinitis? Is there a risk of complications if surgery and anaesthesia is allowed to proceed?

Published studies are at variance. Some have

shown no increased incidence of respiratory complications (Tait and Knight, 1987), and indeed seem to demonstrate a beneficial effect on the time course of symptoms of upper respiratory tract infections after short periods of anaesthesia (Tait *et al.*, 1988). Others do report increased complications particularly in children under one year, both during induction and in the postoperative period (Di Sito *et al.*, 1988; Williams *et al.*, 1992).

Many factors must be taken into account. If the parents feel the child is unwell, are apprehensive as to the safety of the procedure and the surgery is not urgent, then it would be sensible to postpone until the child is fit again and 4 weeks seems a suitable period for complete resolution of symptoms. If the child has no fever or lymphadenopathy and no cough then the implications of secretions in the airway leading to complications during induction should be made clear to the parents. Anticholinergic premedication may help to prevent problems and 50 μg/kg orally of glycopyrrolate at least 30 minutes before surgery is an effective drying agent and does not increase the viscosity of secretions (Berry, 1990). Inhalation induction may be more stormy in the presence of excessive secretion and marked desaturations may occur particularly with the more pungent vapours such as isoflurane (Crean *et al.*, 1991), and an intravenous technique may be preferable.

The urgency and type of the procedure must also be considered. If a child needs a plaster change without which the primary surgery may be compromised, then to cancel the case would be unwise. Likewise, major scoliosis surgery with its attendant respiratory complications should probably be cancelled even if rescheduling would be difficult.

Choice of technique

The choice of technique will depend on patient age, type and duration of surgery, position, ease of access, and of course individual preference. The trend has shifted away from inhalational induction to intravenous techniques due mainly to the introduction of EMLA cream but also to the difficulty in obtaining cyclopropane which was rightly much favoured in paediatric anaesthesia. Thiopentone is still the mainstay for IV use and the dose requirements have been well-described, ranging from 7 mg/kg in the infant to 4–5 mg/kg in adolescence. Ketamine still has its advocates but has been limited in its usefulness by psychic disturbance, and the need for quiet isolated recovery areas. It has also recently found popularity as a drug of social use, particularly at 'rave' parties where its dissociative properties are much sought after, and is likely to become a controlled drug, perhaps limiting its use further. Perhaps its main role is in the management of the asthmatic patient (Corssen, 1972). Propofol has recently been introduced and is gaining in popularity. Children require considerably more than adults, infants 3–5 mg/kg and older children 2.5–4 mg/kg (Westrin, 1991). Pain on injection may be a problem but with the addition of 40 mg Lignocaine to 200 mg of Propofol the incidence has been around 5 per cent in 100 patients receiving anaesthesia for MRI in our unit. Exaggerated myoclonic movements are common (Sneyd, 1992), and it is as well to mention this to accompanying parents as this may be misinterpreted as seizure activity or inadequate anaesthesia. Recovery with Propofol is rapid and appetite seems to return more quickly, making it a most appropriate agent for short cases such as changes of plaster or procedures where there is little painful stimulus. Its role is less clear in major cases when rapid recovery is likely to be compromised by the use of analgesia and it may be counter-productive to have a child awake and active too soon after a major procedure. Its use as a total intravenous technique combined with regional anaesthesia in children is currently being evaluated.

Halothane still remains most anaesthetists drug of choice for inhalational induction, particularly as the availability of cyclopropane has declined. Newer agents, such as desflurane, are not yet freely available but may have much to offer in paediatric practice, although use requires expensive complex vaporizers.

Nitrous oxide is associated with a higher incidence of postoperative nausea and vomiting. This may be due in part to changes in middle ear pressure (Casey and Drake-Lee, 1982), as nausea is much less common in children after myringotomy. Abdominal distension may compromise respiration particularly if the child is placed in a spica postoperatively and many anaesthetists are moving to the use of oxygen-air mixtures with correspondingly increased doses of volatiles. The non-depolarizing neuromuscular blocking agents and in particular the newer agents such as atracurium and vecuronium, have all been well-researched in paediatric practice and have proven safety records (Gondsouzian, 1991). Orthopaedic surgery tends to be performed in children at an age when the neuromuscular function shows less variability in its response to blockade and a high degree of predictability is found. The duration of action and sensitivity to atracurium is fairly similar in neonates, infants and children as its termination is independent of renal or hepatic function (Meakin *et al.*, 1988), whereas vecuronium has a prolonged duration of action in the first year of life (Meretoja, 1989). Hypothermia prolongs the action of all these agents and must be taken into consideration and it is unwise to attempt reversal and extubation if the core temperature has fallen below 35°C.

Succinyl choline has always had a special place in paediatric anaesthesia and has been widely employed, perhaps because myalgia 'scoline pains' did not seem to occur but is becoming less popular. Children of 4 years and over do, however, seem to experience myalgia. The possibility of hyperkalaemia in trauma cases must be born in mind as should the association between succinyl choline, malignant hyperthermia, acute rhabdomyolisis and muscular dystrophy. The use of succinyl choline has been reported to produce masseter spasm and difficulty with intubation. This may be due to the use of an inadequate dose, 2–3 mg/kg is currently recommended (Meakin, 1988), or a normal response to the drug which occurs at the end of the period of fasciculation, the time one is traditionally taught to attempt intubation (Leary and Ellis, 1990). If 30 seconds is allowed after fasciculation has ceased, jaw movements are usually relatively free. Isolated masseter spasm does not seem to be related to the development of malignant hyperpyrexia, as is generalized rigidity after succinyl choline (Hackl *et al.*, 1990). It seems reasonable to reserve the use of succinyl choline for patients in whom definite indications exist (Delphin *et al.*, 1987). All the available narcotics have been utilized in paediatric surgery and shown to be safe. The half-life of morphine is prolonged for at least the first 3 months of life (Lynn and Slattery, 1987) and may be as long as 12 hours whereas fentanyl has a half-life of around 2 to 3 hours, not greatly different in infants and larger children. Ventilatory depression appears to be greater with water-soluble opiates such as morphine in the neonate perhaps due to an immature blood brain barrier, but after three months, the degree of ventilatory depression is similar to that in the adult for any given plasma concentration (Hertzka *et al.*, 1989).

Regional techniques

The use of regional techniques such as epidurals has increased greatly in recent years partly as a result of the production of needles and catheters designed with the child in mind (Fig 7.2). Epidural cannulation is a relatively simple technique in the anaesthetized child and may be accomplished by the thoracic, lumbar, sacral or caudal approaches (Dalens and Chrysostome, 1991). The catheters used are of necessity fine gauge and problems may be encountered with kinking at the skin, and leakage or occlusion at the hub. These soft, fine catheters are somewhat unpredictable in the direction they take, but appear less likely to puncture the dura or epidural veins that the stiffer adult catheters. Ultra-fine catheters are becoming available but need a stylet for stiffening and this may render them more likely to puncture. Epidural cannulae and catheters can also be used for continuous brachial plexus blockade. Regional techniques have numerous advantages, improving blood flow and aiding healing, allowing the use of lower doses of other agents and hence a more balanced technique. The sympathectomy effect may be particularly beneficial in microvascular techniques such as fibula grafting and pollicization. The technique can safely be carried into the postoperative period to allow excellent analgesia by continuous infusion (Marat *et al.*, 1987), but if this is planned, full explanation must be undertaken as a waking child may find paralysed, insensate limbs extremely frightening.

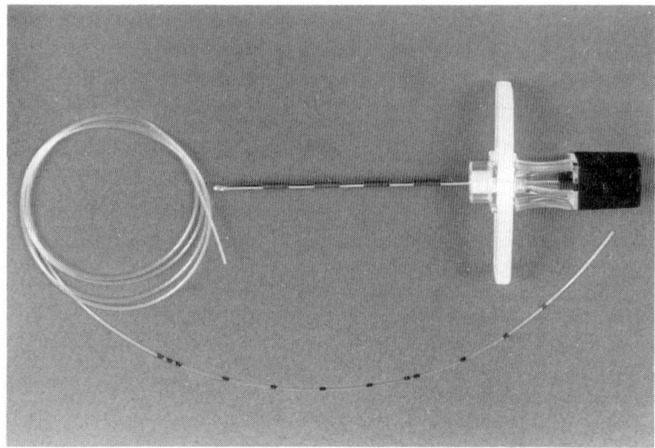

Fig 7.2 A Paediatric epidural needle (19 gauge) and catheter (23 gauge). The needle has detachable wings (Portex Ltd, UK).

Intraoperative monitoring

Monitoring policies are broadly similar to those adopted in adult practice. It is, however, not always possible or wise to attach monitoring to the child before anaesthesia begins as this may be frightening, particularly if the child associates wires and screens with seriously ill patients seen on television or on hospital visits. Movement usually dislodges the leads or gives rise to erroneous and worrying readings.

Temperature monitoring is particularly important in orthopaedic theatres as high airflow is often employed and the child can cool very quickly. Heating blankets should be used particularly in lengthy procedures, bearing in mind that it is always possible to overheat the patients. Hot-air cushions are particularly effective and also help to alleviate pressure areas. Fluid warming devices that heat the fluid line right up to the cannula are now becoming available and these should prove particularly useful in small children with small cannula where slow flow rates reduce the effectiveness of remote heating systems. As surgery has become more ambitious, it has also lengthened and urinary catheterization and output measurement is more often required and should be carried well into the postoperative period, particularly if the patient is heavily plastered.

Much surgery is accomplished under tourniquet and consequently intraoperative blood loss is minimal. The exception to this is scoliosis surgery in which a blood volume exchange is not uncommon. Central venous and intra-arterial pressure monitoring should be employed in such cases, and access to the central circulation may be achieved in 70 per cent of children over 3 years, using a Seldinger technique via the external jugular vein (Taylor *et al.*, 1991). In the younger child, cannulation of the internal jugular is more reliable.

Airway management

Prolonged surgery, and surgery in the prone position will require intubation and controlled ventilation, as does surgery where access is limited, and it is valuable in small children to apply a small amount of positive end-expiratory pressure in order to maintain FRC above closing volume. Ventilation using the Nuffield 200 ventilator with the Newton valve, driving a T-piece, is particularly suitable as the controlled leak through the Newton valve supplies 2–3 cms positive end-expiratory pressure (PEEP), and reversion to hand ventilation is simple. More sophisticated ventilators have PEEP valves included.

Shorter cases may be managed with face mask anaesthesia, but the advent of the laryngeal mask airway (LMA) has brought a new dimension to anaesthesia (Brain, 1991). The laryngeal mask can be easily inserted into the hypo-pharynx without laryngoscopy, where the cuff when inflated forms a seal which leaks at an airway pressure of approximately 20 cms H_2O. Although some protection is offered to the airway this should not be relied upon and an LMA should not be used if the patient has a full stomach. The recent introduction of intermediate sizes has increased the ease of use in children (Mason, 1990). Assisted ventilation is more easily accomplished with the LMA than with a face mask and capnography can be readily employed. The ability of propofol to obtund pharyngeal and laryngeal reflexes makes it a particularly suitable induction agent for use with the laryngeal mask, and the moist mucosa of unpremedicated patients makes insertion easier. The epiglottis may adopt a variety of positions inside the mask, as seen with fibreoptic instrumentation or MRI (Fig. 7.3) but this does not seem to compromise the airway. PEEP can readily be applied to the system by insertion of a fixed orifice at the end of the bag of the Jackson Rees modification. The laryngeal mask may also be used to facilitate fibreoptic-guided intubation of the difficult airway particularly in the young child who would not tolerate awake fibreoptic intubation (Brimacombe and Johns, 1991). An added benefit of the laryngeal mask is that it provides a safe, secure airway while the anaesthetist and assistant are gainfully occupied performing regional blocks or siting intravenous line.

The difficult intubation in the young child may also

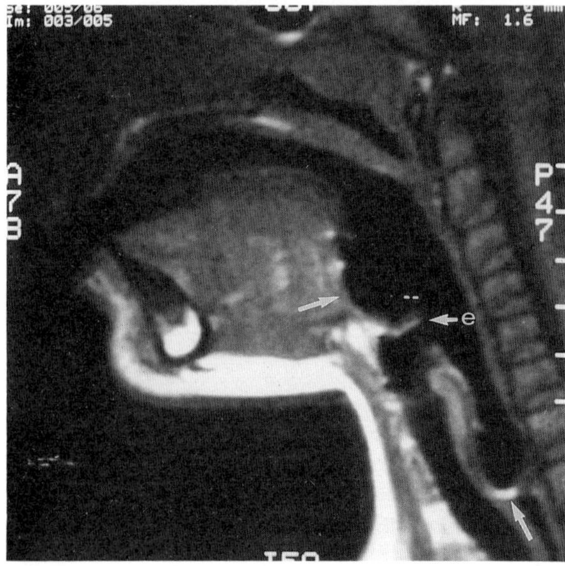

Fig 7.3 A magnetic resonance image of a 3 year old with a laryngeal mask airway inserted. The plain arrows indicate the upper and lower parts of the cuff. The epiglottis (e) appears to be pushed down over the laryngeal inlet by the upper cuff, but no airway obstruction was evident. The lower cuff is well down the oesophagus and slightly displaces and indents the trachea anteriorly.

be managed by insertion of a transtracheal cannula under sedation and local anaesthetic infiltration (Fig 7.4). The child can then be anaesthetized and ventilated via the transtracheal cannula with a venturi system, while fibreoptic intubation is accomplished in a controlled fashion. This technique should not be used if there is any evidence of laryngeal obstruction as high intra-thoracic pressures may be generated leading to barotrauma (Craft *et al.*, 1990).

In older children and adolescents, awake fibreoptic intubation can be employed and in particularly useful in patients with cervical trauma, in halo traction and with fixed cervical spines.

Fluids

Fluid replacement should be calculated taking into account the period of starvation, urine output if measured, environmental factors such as airflow and temperature, inspiratory gas humidification and concurrent medical problems. The extent of surgery and trauma must also be considered, so called 'third space' losses mainly due to oedema of traumatized tissues. A basic rate of 4 mls/kg/hr for the period of starvation and surgery with 2–4 mls/kg/hr added for thirdspace losses in extensive surgery is a good general rule but each anaesthetist and author has his own method of calculating requirements.

There has been much recent discussion as to the most appropriate crystalloid solutions. The use of solutions with a high glucose content has been questioned (Steward, 1992; Hongnat, 1991). Except in the very small infant, or those patients on beta-blockers, the risk of hypoglycaemia in the peri-operative period is small, and hyperglycaemia, as part of the stress response to surgery and anaesthesia, is more usual. This may be exacerbated by use of intravenous glucose, and as hyperglycaemia may increase the extent of brain damage should cardiac arrest or severe hypoxaemia occur, it seems prudent therefore to monitor blood glucose and only give glucose when indicated. The hyperglycaemic response is, however, blocked by regional anaesthesia and high-dose opiates and added glucose may be required if such techniques are employed. Hyponatraemia is a common complication of surgical and anaesthetic care, a result of inappropriate ADH secretion and water retention, and seizures may occur in the postoperative period particularly in children with a history of seizures, such as in cerebral palsy, and it is perhaps wise to refrain from the use of low sodium fluids. Dubois *et al.* (1992) suggest that lactated Ringer with 1 per cent Dextrose may be the ideal solution for peri-operative fluid therapy in the majority of children.

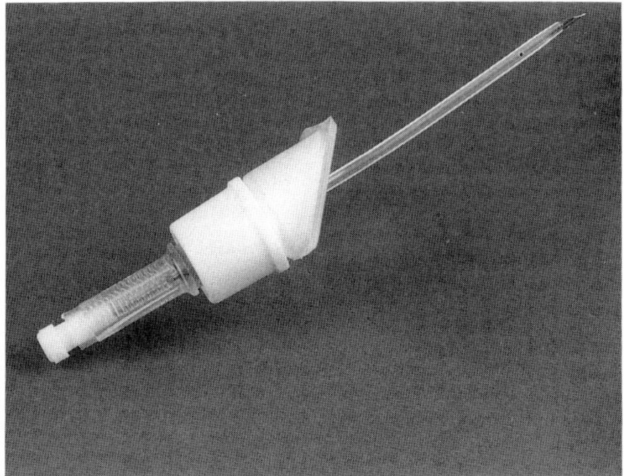

Fig 7.4 A trancricothyrotomy device. This 14-gauge cannula, for use in children, has two lateral eyes and a 15 mm connection for breathing circuits. There is also an internal luer-lok hub to which an injector can be connected (VBM Medizintechnik, Germany).

Blood replacement should be aimed at maintaining a haematocrit of 30–35 per cent. Fresh whole blood has an average haematocrit of about 35 per cent, but the plasma-reduced blood most commonly supplied has a haematocrit ranging from 60–70 per cent. In practice even 2 or 3 volume transfusion does not give rise to coagulation defects providing the child is not allowed to become shocked, acidotic or hypothermic, and reflex administration of fresh frozen plasma or platelets should be avoided. Blood products are rare and valuable commodities but potentially harmful and should be preserved for specific purposes. Guidelines for the use of blood products have recently been published (BCSH, 1992), and also provide a useful framework for dealing with coagulation problems.

Postoperative care

One of the primary considerations for the anaesthetist in the postoperative period is the provision of adequate analgesia and major changes have occurred in this area in recent years. In 1988 a survey of British paediatric anaesthetists revealed that although the majority considered that neonates could perceive pain and react to it, few were prepared to prescribe opiates for postoperative pain (Purcell-Jones, 1988). At around the same time, a major landmark was reached when the stress response to surgery was demonstrated to be essentially similar in neonates and adults (Anand *et al.*, 1987). Analgesia or the lack of it in infants and neonates became a hot topic and much debate ensued in the medical and national press (MPs attack . . . 1987; MP concerned by surgery on babies, 1987).

As a result of this, postoperative pain relief in all children, as in adults, has improved immensely, but there is still some way to go (McGrath, 1990).

The primary aim in children is to avoid repeated intramuscular injections.

Local techniques, such as blockade of lower limb nerves (McNicol, 1985; 1986), axillary plexus, and epidurals performed under anaesthesia are all valuable in specific circumstances and relatively free from complications (Dalens and Chrysostome, 1991). Bupivacaine is the usual agent of choice, but there may be a greater risk of toxicity in children under one year, as the drug-binding proteins albumin and alpha-I-glycoprotein are in lower concentration and the free fraction of the drug is thus greater. Epidural opiates also appear to be relatively safe, and effective in children of all ages (Shapiro *et al.*, 1984). (Fig. 7.5).

Continuous infusion of opiates are more effective than repeated intramuscular injections (Bray, 1983), but the constant worry of pump failure and overdose necessitates a high-level of nursing care and is not advised in younger patients outside the intensive care or high dependency environment. Titration of the required dose against effect and side-effect are also difficult and time-consuming and the concept of patient-controlled analgesia has devolved the responsibility for this from medical staff to the patient, nurse or even the parent. Patient-controlled analgesia (PCA) has been used effectively in children down to 5 years, and under this age the nurse or possibly a parent can take the part of the patient to good effect (Gillespie, 1992). Morphine is the most commonly employed agent. Whether or not to use bolus administration or bolus plus background infusion is a matter of personal preference but there is a greater risk of accumulative overdose and possibly the development of tolerance if a background infusion is used. PCA pumps are now supplied with an integrated apnoea monitor increasing the safety in the general ward environment. Disposable PCA units also appear to be safe and effective in children, but are somewhat less flexible in their potential uses (Irwin *et al.*, 1992).

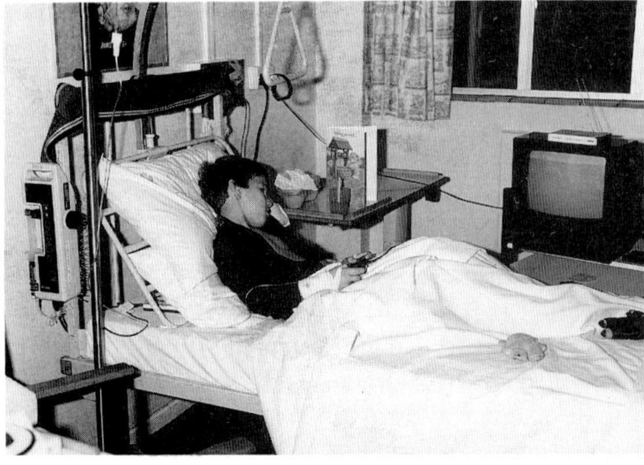

Fig 7.5 A 8 year-old boy 12 hours after bilateral femoral and tibial derotation osteotomies. Pain relief has been provided with a continuous infusion of a mixture of 0.25 per cent bupivacaine and fentanyl. The child is completely pain free, wide awake and able to complete a computer game.

Yet another approach is the siting of an indwelling intramuscular cannula through which analgesia may be administered for prolonged periods, again with good effectiveness and low side-effects (Underwood, 1991). Non-Steroidal anti-inflammatory compounds are useful agents in orthopaedic pain and can be given by a variety of routes, but may be contraindicated for procedures, such as leg lengthening, which depend on callus formation as osteoblastic activity may be impaired (Brimacombe, 1993).

Special conditions and considerations

Downs syndrome

Atlanto-axial instability is present in up to 20 per cent of children with Down's syndrome and if subluxation occurs, producing neurological signs, cervical fusion may be necessary (Lee *et al.*, 1991).[65]

Deceleration injury in road traffic accidents (RTA) may produce acute subluxation and all Down's syndrome children in a RTA should have neck *X*-ray. Anaesthesia and surgery may also give rise to acute neurological changes (Moore *et al.*, 1987), perhaps due to inappropriate positioning or over-vigorous manipulation of the neck during laryngoscopy in children who may be more difficult to intubate as a result of the large tongue. Congenital heart disease occurs in 25–50 per cent of Down's syndrome children and it is important to remember that a repaired heart is not a normal heart. Pulmonary hypertension may be present and conduction defects, particularly in repaired tetralogy of fallot and A-V canal defects, may also present problems (Kobel *et al.*, 1982). Postextubation stridor is more common in Downs children particularly if intubation has been problematical or if the tube is a tight fit. Dexamethasome 0.5–1.0 mg/kg may help to ameliorate this (Berry, 1990). Respiratory and wound infections are more common, and prophylactic antibiotics and physio should be routinely requested. Smaller endotracheal tubes than for a child of similar age and size may be required.

Cerebral palsy

The requirement for orthopaedic surgery in cerebral palsy seems to be increasing as parental expectations alter. Procedures may be for pain relief, to increase mobility, to allow easier positioning in a wheelchair or to improve toiletting. Cerebral palsy covers a wide spectrum but the severely afflicted patients create the greatest problems. Chronic malnutrition and dehydration are common, and mild renal impairment may result. Gastro-oesophageal reflux may lead to aspiration and chronic lung changes. Sympathetic hyperactivity may be part of the condition and poor peripheral circulation and hypertension may result (Korolenko and Klimenko, 1990). Seizures are common and may be a problem in the postoperative period particularly if hyponatraemia is allowed to occur.

Recently, baclofen has become increasingly popular to control spasticity (Dralle *et al.*, 1985), either alone or in combination with carbamazepine. Unfortunately baclofen, a GABA agonist, can only be given orally or intrathecally and withdrawal in the peri-operative period may lead to seizures, hallucinations or exaggeration of pre-existing movement disorders, such as choreoathetosis (Barker and Grant, 1982; Terrence and Fromm, 1981). Benzodiazepines may be substituted but the risk of regurgitation, aspiration and pneumonia is increased. Spasm in the muscles involved in surgery is also a particular problem, but can be controlled, either with heavy doses of benzodiazepines or alternatively by regional block. A continuous infusion of a mixture of 50 mls 0.25 per cent marcain plus 200 μg fentanyl at a rate of approximately 0.1 mls/kg/hour has proved effective for up to 4 days and without complication (personal data). Hypotension does not seem to occur with epidural blockade in cerebral palsy, possible due to the sympathetic hyperactivity previously mentioned. Urinary catheterization is advisable in these children. Sensitivity to muscle relaxants seems to be within normal limits.

Plaster casts and tourniquets

Body plasters such as hip spicas may restrict respiration particularly in the younger child who is a diaphragmatic breather, and have been associated with acute gastric dilation, paralytic ileus and in thin patients, aortic or mesenteric arterial compression and subsequent bowel ischaemia. Inexplicable pain and restlessness in the child, who cannot communicate, may be related to the plaster. Pressure sores may result and go unnoticed particularly if sensation is diminished by regional block. Blood loss into the plaster may go unnoticed and cases of hypovolaemic death have been reported. Any child in plaster in whom the surgery may give rise to bleeding should be closely observed particularly if the plaster has been applied whilst a tourniquet is in use. Tourniquets appear to be well-tolerated in children and release, even after prolonged inflation, is associated with fewer haemodynamic changes than in the adult (Lynn *et al.*, 1986).

Most theatre units have a separate area for plaster application and monitoring and temperature control may be problematical. Access to patient may be limited during the procedure and all lines and tubes are at risk.

Arthrogryposis

A wide range of presentations may occur and the aetiology appears to be intra-uterine contraction of muscles and tendons leading to dislocation and deformity. Other anomalies of concern to the anaesthetist may be manibular hypoplasia, laryngo-trachea nalacia, rib-cage softening and deformity which may alter lung mechanics (Fig. 7.6) and a 10 per cent association with congenital heart disease, particularly of the aorta. Multiple procedures may be necessary and venous access may be particularly difficult in deformed and scarred limbs.

Juvenile rheumatoid arthritis (Stills disease)

As in adults, this is a multi-system disease and a child may have cardiac involvement, chronic anaemia, renal damage and severe poly arthritis. Joint replacement may be performed in teenagers. The main problem for the anaesthetist is the possibility of

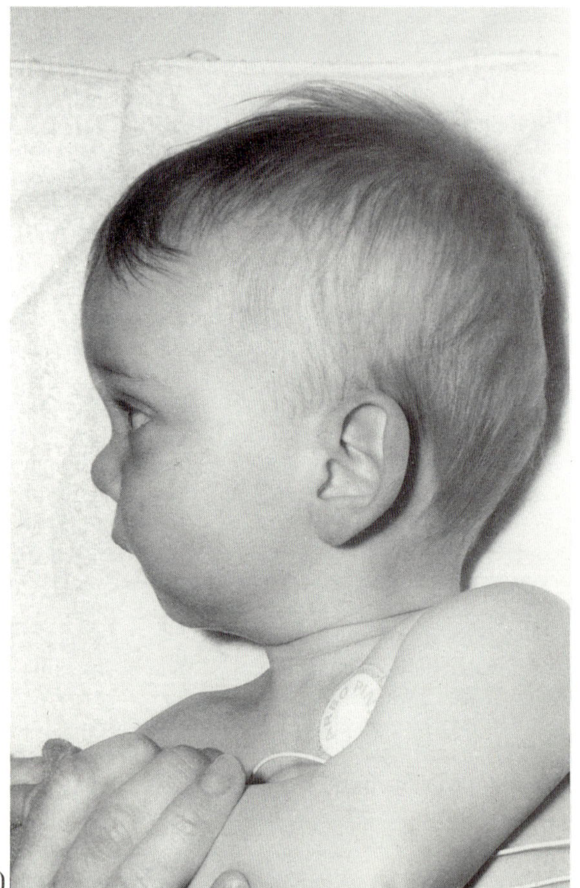

(a)

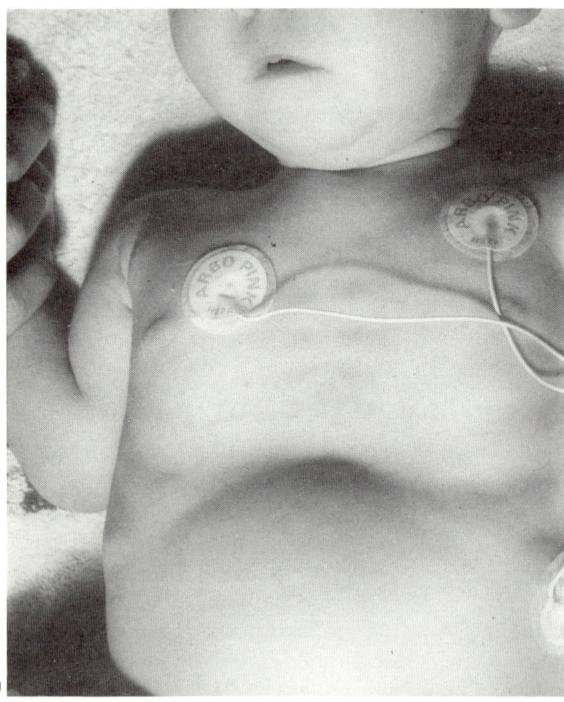

(b)

Fig 7.6 A 14 month-old child with arthrogryposis, exhibiting mild mandibular hypoplasia (a), and marked subcostal indrawing which worsened considerably on induction of anaesthesia (b). It was possible with only light pressure to displace the sternum posteriorly to touch the spinal column. There was also severe laryngo-tracheomalacia which has more or less resolved after 2 years further maturation.

intubation difficulty. Tempero-mandibular ankylosis, crico-arytenoid arthritis, atlanto-axial subluxation and cervical spinal amkylosis may all be found. Figure 7.7 shows a 15 year old boy presenting for bilateral hip replacement with fusion of vertebra and a very small gap between occiput and the spinous process of the first cervical vertebra, reducing extension of the head on the neck. Intubation was accomplished by fiberoptic endoscopy using cocaine for intranasal anaesthesia and 4 per cent lignocaine sprayed down the suction channel of the fiberscope as it was passed through the pharynx. Postoperative analgesia was provided with a continuous epidural infusion as his hands were too deformed by the disease to operate a patient-controlled analgesia (PCA) pump effectively.

Muscular dystrophies

Of the muscular dystrophies, Duchenne is the most common in childhood and cardiac abnormalities are the major anaesthetic problem. Cardiomyopathy develops with age and echocardiography should always be performed if possible. Resting sinus tachycardia is indicative of potential intraoperative dysrhythmias or cardiac arrest. Respiratory muscle weakness leads to retention of secretions and smooth muscle involvement to acute gastric dilatation and ileus. Patients are more sensitive to non-depolarizing relaxants and succinyl chlorine may trigger acute rhabdo myolysis, hyperkalaemia and malignant hyperthermia. The risk of volatile agents triggering a similar train of events is not as clear but it would seem wise to avoid them if possible (Warde, 1992). The most common orthopaedic procedure is scoliosis correction and respiratory complications are high and postoperative analgesia a difficult problem. Again, PCA seems to offer the best chance of avoiding too much respiratory depression.

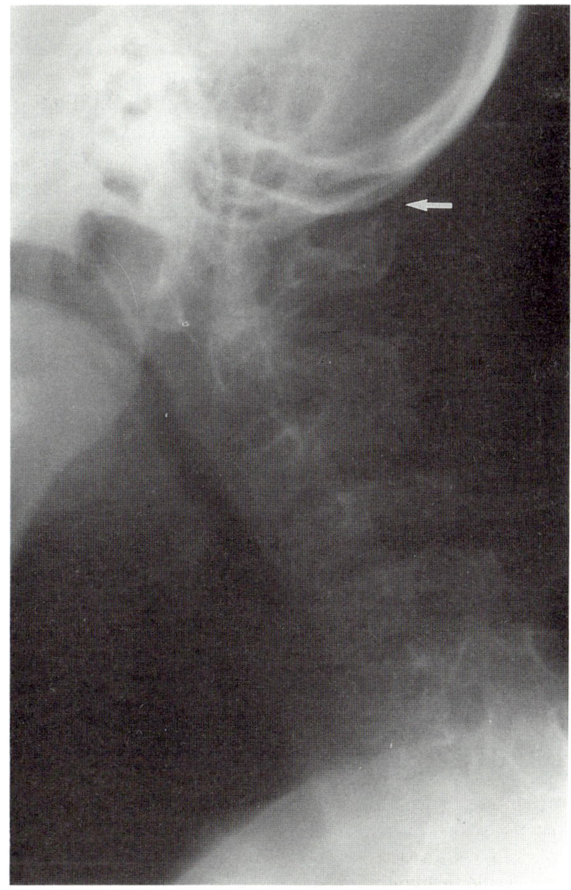

Fig 7.7 A 15 year-old boy with Stills disease (see text). The arrow indicates the reduced space between the occiput and CI spinous process.

Spina bifida

Scoliosis surgery, ankle arthodesis and hip relocation may be required. There may be renal impairment from chronic infection and reflux, and urinary diversion may have been performed. Pelvic surgery such as this may give rise to deep vein thrombosis particularly in wheelchair bound patients and pulmonary embolism may occur. Associated hydrocephalus may have required shunting and symptoms of shunt malfunction should be sought preoperatively. Delayed recovery and postoperative vomiting may be due to raised intracranial pressure. Mother and child will often request that venepuncture is performed in an anaesthetic area, usually in the feet but this can be extremely difficult and time consuming, and the use of EMLA cream may be a better option.

Limb discrepancy correction

Discrepancy, if unilateral, can be corrected either by arresting growth in the normal limb by epiphysiodesis or by lengthening the abnormal limb by slow distraction. Epiphysiodesis is usually performed at around 12–14 years of age and is not a particularly painful procedure, but may require numerous plaster changes. However, the concept of surgery to the normal limb may be more difficult for the parents and child to accept and lengthening of the abnormal limb may be more appropriate.

Lengthening of the abnormal limb can be achieved by a variety of techniques and up to 25–30 cms may be achieved. Small discrepancies up to 5–7 cms are usually treated at 12–15 years of age. Greater discrepancies are treated in 2 stages at around 9 years of age and then 13–15 years of age.

Bilateral limb lengthening may be performed on children with achondroplasia, Hurler's syndrome or hypothyroidism as well as for congenital dysplasias. This type of surgery is a major undertaking and may take 2–3 years to complete. In achondroplasia, the ideal age for commencement of surgery is 6–7 years.

Psychological and familial fortitude are a primary requirement for selection, and the management of postoperative pain of great importance in preventing a breakdown in the surgeon/patient relationship (Green, 1991). Epidural analgesia using again a combination of opiate and local anaesthesia (Saleh and Burton, 1991), or PCA have been employed successfully. Multiple anaesthetics may be required for pin-hole infection or angulation and distortion of the osteotomy site. Early movement is necessary to prevent contracture of stretched muscles, and again good analgesia facilitates this. Achondroplasia is associated with spinal stenosis but epidural cannulation does not appear to be problematical in this age group. Hypertension, perhaps due to stretching of the sciatic or sympathetic nerves, as in clubfoot surgery (Akbarnia *et al.*, 1990) has been reported in the postoperative period.

Osteogenesis imperfecta (OI)

OI is an inherited disease, characterized by brittle bones and frequent fracture such that a misdiagnosis of child abuse may occur. Surgery may be frequent and extensive (Fig. 7.8) and anaesthesia may be complicated (Hall *et al.*, 1992).

Hyperthermia may occur, due in part to thyroid overreactivity (Cropp and Myers, 1972), so it may be wise to avoid anticholinergic premedication.

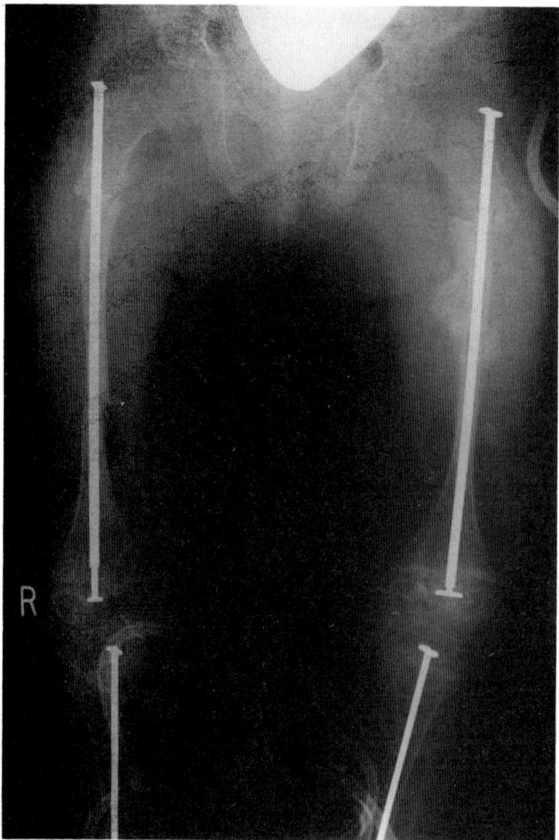

Fig 7.8 A 3 year old with osteogenesis imperfecta who has had bilateral tibial and femoral Sheffield expanding rods inserted. Considerable haemorrhage and 2°C temperature rise occurred during insertion of the femoral rods.

Platelet dysfunction may lead to excessive bleeding and teeth are also brittle (Hathaway and Solomons, 1970) and easily dislodged or broken during intubation. Great care must be taken during positioning, and suxamethonium fasciculation may induce fractures. Scoliosis may lead to severe respiratory impairment.

Fractures

Fractures in children rarely require internal fixation, the major exception being those of the elbow joint. Manipulation and plastering under anaesthesia may be required and the implications of the patient with a full stomach must be considered.

Traction, particularly for fractures of the femur may be complicated by severe and painful muscle spasm and PCA is particularly appropriate for management in the older child (Stevens, 1992). Surgery may be required if closed compartment syndrome develops and is urgent if ischaemic muscle damage is to be prevented (Willis and Rorabeck, 1990). Fat embolism seems to be rare perhaps because the marrow is more active and hence more vascular in this age group.

Magnetic resonance imaging (MRI)

MRI may soon become the imaging technique of choice in orthopaedics, both for bony abnormalities and soft-tissue delineation (Watt, 1991). Anaesthesia is required in many children as imaging sequences take some time, stillness is essential and the environment somewhat forbidding (Sury *et al.*, 1992). Poor access to the patient, interference of monitoring with image acquisition, malfunction of monitoring equipment in a high magnetic field and cooling in the high air-flow through the tunnel are all potential problems. The monitoring problem has hopefully been solved by the construction of specialized monitors built to function in this environment, such as the Maglife Monitor (Odam, Bruker), but these are as yet extremely expensive. A technique using continuous propofol infusion alone, a laryngeal mask and the Jackson–Rees modification of the T-piece allows respiration to be monitored visually, rapid recovery and has a zero incidence of postoperative nausea and vomiting (personal data).

References

Anand, K. J. S., Sippell, W. G. and Aynsley-Green, A. (1987). Randomised trial of Fentanyl anaesthesia in preterm babies undergoing surgery, effects on the stress response. *Lancet*, **i**, 243–8.

Able, A. and Howard, R. (1992). Preoperative haemoglobin estimations in a children's hospital. Presented at the APA March, London.

Akbarnia, B. A., Shapiro, J., Ziaee, M. and Akbarnia, N. (1990). Hypertension after operative correction of clubfoot deformity. *Journal of Bone and Joint Surgery*, **72A**, 1330–3.

Atwell, J. D. and Spargo, P. M. (1992). The provision of safe surgery for children. *Archives of Disease in Childhood*, **67**, 345–9.

Barker, I., Grant, I. S. (1982). Convulsions after abrupt withdrawal of baclofen. *Lancet*, **II**, 557.

Berry, F. A. (1990). Miscellaneous Potholes. In F. A. Berry (ed.), *Anesthetic Management of Difficult and*

Routine Pediatric Patients, 2nd edn. Churchill Livingstone, New York, p. 421.

Berry, F. A. (1990). The child with a runny nose. In F. A. Berry (ed.), *Anesthetic Management of Difficult and Routine Pediatric Patients*, 2nd edn. Churchill Livingstone, New York, p. 275.

Brain, A. I. J. (1991). The development of the laryngeal mask airway. *European Journal of Anesthesiology*, **4**, 5–18.

Bray, R. J. (1983). Postoperative analgesia provided by morphine infusion in children. *Anaesthesia*, **38**, 1075–8.

Brimacombe, J. and Johns, K. (1991). A modified Intavent laryngeal mask airway to assist fibreoptic endotracheal intubation. *Anaesthesia and Intensive Care*, **19**, 607.

Brimacombe, J. R. and Goddard, J. M. (1993). Leg lengthening in children – a retrospective review of anaesthetic management in 61 children including 14 with achondroplasia. *Paediatric Anaesthesia*, **3**, 89–93.

BCSH (British Committee for Standards in Haematology) (1992). Guidelines for the use of fresh frozen plasma. *Transfusion Medicine*, **2**, 57–63.

Campling, E. A., Devlin, H. B. and Lunn, J. N. (1989). The Report of the National Confidential Enquiry into Perioperative Deaths.

Casey, W. F. and Drake-Lee, A. B. (1982). Nitrous Oxide and middle-ear pressure. *Anaesthesia*, **37**, 896–900.

Cohen, M. M., Cameron, C. B. and Duncan, P. G. (1990). Paediatric anaesthesia morbidity and mortality in the perioperative period. *Anaesthesia and Analgesia*, **70**, 160–7.

Corssen, G., Gutierrez, J., Reves, J. G. and Huber, F. C. (1972). Ketamine in the anaesthetic management of the asthmatic patient. *Anesthesia and Analgesia*, **51**, 588.

Craft, T. M., Chambers, P. H., Ward, M. E. and Goat, V. A. (1990). Two cases of barotrauma associated with transtracheal jet ventilation. *British Journal of Anaesthesia*, **64**, 524–7.

Crean, P. M., Laird, C. R. D., Keilly, S. R. and Black, G. W. (1991). The influence of atropine premedication in the induction of anaesthesia with isoflurane in children. *Paediatric Anaesthesia*, **1**, 37–9.

Cropp, G. J. A. and Myers, D. N. (1972). Physiological evidence of hypermetabolism in osteogenesis imperfecta. *Pediatrics*, **49**, 375–91.

Dalens, B. and Chrysostome, I. (1991). Intervertebral epidural anesthesia in paediatric surgery: success rate and adverse effects in 650 consecutive procedure. *Paediatric Anaesthesia*, **1**, 107–17.

Delphin, E., Jackson, D. and Rothstein, P. (1987). Use of succinyl choline during elective paediatric anesthesia should be revaluated. *Anesthesia and Analgesia*, **66**, 1190.

Di Sito, M., Patel, R. I., Soliman, I. E. and Hanallah, R. S. (1988). Changes in oxygen saturation following general anaesthesia in children with upper respiratory signs and symptoms undergoing oto-laryngological procedures. *Anesthesiology*, **68**, 276.

Dralle, D., Muller, H., Zierski, J. and Klug, N. (1985). Intrathecal baclofen, for spasticity. *Lancet*, **II**, 1003.

Dubois, M. C., Gouyet, L., Murat, I. and Saint-Maurice, C. (1992). Lactated Ringer with 1% Dextrose: an appropriate solution for peri-operative fluid therapy in children. *Paediatric Anaesthesia*, **2**, 99–104.

Gillick v. *West Norfolk and Wisbech AHA*, 1986, A.C. 112.

Gillespie, J. A. and Norton, N. S. (1992). Patient controlled analgesia for children: a review. *Paediatric Anaesthesia*, **2**, 51–9.

Goldstein-Dresner, M. C., Davis, P. J., Kretchman, E., Siewers, R. D., Certo, N. and Cook, D. R. (1991). Double-blind comparison of oral transmucosal fentanyl citrate with oral Meperidine, Diazepam and Atropine as pre-anaesthetic medication in children with congenital heart disease. *Anesthesiology*, **74**, 28–33.

Goresty, G. V. and Maltby, J. R. (1990). Fasting guidelines for elective surgical patients. *Canadian Journal of Anaesthesia*, **37**, pp. 493–5.

Goudsouzian, N. G. (1991). Neuromuscular blocking agents in children. *Paediatric Anaesthesia*, **1**, 75–88.

Gourlay, G. K., Kowalski, S. R., Plummer, J. L., Cherry, D. A., Szekely, S. M., Mather, L. E., Owen, H. and Cousins, N. J. (1990). The efficacy of transdermal fentanyl in the treatment of post-operative pain: a double blind comparison of Fentanyl and placebo systems. *Pain*, **40**, 21–8.

Green, S. A. (1991). Post-operative management during leg lengthening. *Orthopaedic Clinics of North America*, **22**(4), 723–34.

Hackl, W., Maurity, W., Schemper, M., Winkler, M., Sporn, P. and Steinbereithner, K. (1990). Prediction of malignant hypothermia susceptibility: a statistical evaluation of clinical signs. *British Journal of Anaesthesia*, **64**, 425–9.

Hall, R. M. O., Hemming, R. D., Brown, T. C. K. and Cole, W. G. (1992). Anaesthesia for children with osteogenesis imperfecta – a review covering 30 years and 266 anaesthetics. *Paediatric Anaesthesia*, **2**, 115–22.

Hathaway, W. E. and Solomons, C. C. (1970). Abnormalities of platelet function in Osteogenesis Imperfecta. *Clinical Research*, **18**, 209.

Hertzka, R. E., Gauntlett, I. S., Fisher, D. M. and Spellman, N. J. (1989). Fentanyl-induced ventilatory depression: effects of age. *Anesthesiology*, **70**, 218–18.

Hongnat, J. M., Murat, I. and Saint-Maurice, C. (1991). Evaluation of current paediatric guidelines for fluid therapy using two different dextrose hydrating solutions. *Paediatric Anaesthesia*, **1**, 95–100.

Irwin, M., Gillespie, J. A. and Norton, N. S. (1992). Evaluation of a disposable patient-controlled analgesia device in children. *British Journal of Anaesthesia*, **68**, 411–13.

Kobel, M., Creighton, R. E. and Steward, D. J. (1982). Anaesthetic considerations in Down's Syndrome. Experience with 100 patients and a review of the literature. *Canadian Anesthesia Society Journal*, **29**, 593–9.

Korolenko, A. O. and Klimenko, V. A. (1990). Correction of autonomic nervous system hyperreactivity during surgery in children with cerebral spastic paralysis. *Anesteziologica 1 Reanimatologiia*, **3**, 68–70 (English Abstract).

Leary, N. P. and Ellis, F. R. (1990). Masseteric spasm as a normal response to suxamethonium. *British Journal of Anaesthesia*, **64**, 448–92.

Lee, S. S., Hershey, D. S., Drummond, M. D., Zanoth, R. M., Ecker, M. L. and Nubarak, S. J. (1991). Complications of posterior arthodesis of the cervical spine patients who have Down Syndrome. *Journal of Bone and Joint Surgery*, **73A**, 1547–54.

Lynn, A. M., Fischer, T., Brandford, H. G. and Pendergrass, T. W. (1986). Systemic responses to tourniquet release in children. *Anesthesia and Analgesia*, **65**, 865–72.

Lynn, A. M. and Slattery, J. T. (1987). Morphine Pharmacokinetics in early infancy. *Anesthesiology*, **66**, 136–9.

Marat, I., Delleur, N. N., Esteve, C., Eyn, J. F., Raynaud, P., Saint-Maurice, C. (1987). Continuous extradural anaesthesia in children – clinical and haemodynamic implications. *British Journal of Anaesthesia*, **69**, 1441–50.

Mason, D. G. (1990). The laryngeal mask airway in children. *Anaesthesia*, **45**, 760–3.

Maunuksela, E-L. and Korpela, R. (1986). Double-blind evaluation of a lignocaine-prilocaine cream (EMLA) in children. The effect on the pain associated with venous cannulation. *British Journal of Anaesthesia*, **58**, 1242–5.

McGrath, P. J. (1990). Paediatric pain: a good start. *Pain*, **41**, 253–4.

McNicol, L. R. (1985). Sciatic nerve block for children. Sciatic nerve block by the anterior approach for post-operative pain relief. *Anaesthesia*, **40**, 410—14.

McNicol, L. R. (1986) Lower limb blocks for children: Lateral cutaneous and femoral nerve blocks for post-operative pain relief in paediatric practice. *Anaesthesia*, **41**, 27–31.

Meakin, G., Shaw, E. A., Baker, R. D. and Morris, P. (1988). Comparison of atrcurium-induced neuromuscular blockade in neonates, infants and children. *British Journal of Anaesthesia*, **60**, 171–5.

Meakin, G. (1988). Underdosage with succinyl choline may lead to incorrect diagnosis of masseter spasm in children. *Anesthesiology*, **69**, 1025–6.

Meretoja, O. A. (1989). Is vecuronium a long-acting neuromuscular blocking agent in neonates and infants? *British Journal of Anaesthesia*, **62**, 184–7.

Moore, R. A., McNicholas, K. W. and Warren, S. P. (1987). Atlanto-axial subluxation with symptomatic spinal cord compression in a child with Down's Syndrome. *Anesthesia and Analgesia*, **66**, 89–90.

Morrison, J., Abrams, R., Villasenor, A., Hencmann, D. and Fonseca, N. (1992). Safety and effectiveness of intranasal Ketamine, Midazolam and Sufentanil for sedation during urgent paediatric dental procedures. Abstract presented at the Association of Paediatric Anaesthetists Meeting 1992.

MP concerned by surgery on babies (1987). *The Times*, London 5/8/87.

MPs attack 'paralysing' pain tests on babies (1987). *Today*, London 5/8/87.

NAWCH 'National Association for the Welfare of the Child in Hospital' Charter (n.d.). NAWCH Ltd, Argyle House, 29/31 Euston Road, London NW1.

Pace, N. A. (1991). Legal and ethical considerations of informed consent in children: implications for anaesthetists. *Paediatric Anaesthesia*, **1**, 89–94.

Purcell-Jones, G., Dormon, F. and Sumner, E. (1988). Paediatric anaesthetists perception of neonatal and infant pain. *Pain*, **33**, 181–7.

Rose, E., Simon, D. and Naberer, J. P. (1990). Premedication with intranasal midazolam in paediatric anaesthesia. *Annales Francaises de Anesthesie et de Reanimination*, **9**, 326–30.

Salch, M. and Burton, M. (1991). Leg lengthening: Patient selection and management in Achondroplasma. *Orthopaedic Clinics of North America*, **22**(4), 589–99.

Sandhar, B. K., Goresby, G. V., Maltby, J. R. and Shaffer, E. A. (1989). Effects of oral liquids and ranitidine on gastric fluid volume and pH in children undergoing out-patient surgery. *Anesthesiology*, **71**, 327–30.

Shapiro, L., Jedeikin, R., Shaler, D. and Hoffman, S. (1984). Epidural morphine analgesia in children. *Anesthesiology*, **61**, 210.

Sneyd, J. R. (1992). Excitatory events associated with propofol anaesthesia: a review. *Journal Royal Society of Medicine*, **85**, 288–91.

Splinter, W. N., Stewart, J. A. and Muir, J. G. (1989). The effect of pre-operative apple juice on gastric contents, thirst and hunger in children. *Canadian Journal of Anesthesia*, **36**, 55–8.

Stevens, J. E. (1992). Pain after Surgery. *Journal of Bone and Joint Surgery*, **72–2**, 321.

Steward, D. J. (1989). Psychological preparation and premedication. In G. A. Gregory (ed.), *Paediatric Anaesthesia*, Vol. 1. Churchill Livingstone, New York, pp. 523–7.

Steward, D. J. (1992). Hyperglycaemia, something else to worry about. *Paediatric Anaesthesia*, **2**, 81–3.

Sury, M. R. J., Johnstone, G. and Bingham, R. M. (1992). Anaesthesia for magnetic resonance imaging of children. *Paediatric Anaesthesia*, **2**, 61–8.

Tait, A. R. and Knight, P. R. (1987). The effects of general anaesthesia on upper respiratory tract infections in children. *Anesthesiology*, **67**, 930.

Tait, A. R., DuBoulay, P. M. and Knight, P. R. (1988). Alterations in the course of and histopathologic response to influenza virus injections produced by enfluran, halothane and diethyl ether anaesthesia in ferrets. *Anesthesia and Analgesia*, **67**, 671.

Taylor, E. A. S., Mowbury, M. J. and McLellan, I. (1991). Central venous access in children via the external jugular vein. *Anaesthesia*, **46**, 265–6.

Terrence, C. F. and Fromm, G. H. (1981). Complications of baclofen withdrawal. *Archives of Neurology*, **38,** 588–9.

Tiret, L., Nicoche, T., Hatton, F., Desmonts, J. M. and Youre, H. G. (1988). Complications related to anaesthesia in infants and children. *British Journal of Anaesthesia*, **61,** 263–9.

Underwood, S. M., Rowlson, C. J. and Savage, T. M. (1991). Intramuscular injections through indwelling cannulae. *European Journal of Anesthesiol*, **8,** 465–8.

Walbergh, E. J., Wills, R. J. and Eckhert, J. (1990). Plasma concentrations of midazolam in children following intranasal administration. *Anesthesiology*, **74,** 233–5.

Warde, D. L. (1992). What is the appropriate anaesthetic technique for Duchenne muscular dystrophy patients? Presented at Association of Paediatric Anaesthetists meeting, London, 1992.

Wark, H. J. (1983). Postoperative jaundice in children. The influence of Halothane. *Anaesthesia*, **38,** 237.

Watt, I. (1991). Magnetic Resonance Imaging in Orthopaedics. *Journal of Bone and Joint Surgery*, **73B,** 539–50.

Westrin, P. (1991). Induction dose of propofol in infants 1–6 months of age and in children 10–16 years of age. *Anesthesiology*, **74,** 455–8.

Whitburne, R. H. and Sumner, E. (1986). Halothane hepatitis in an 11-month old child. *Anaesthesia*, **41,** 611.

Wilhoit, R. D., Brown, R. E. and Bauman, L. A. (1989). Possible malignant hyperthermia in a 7-week old child. *Anesthesia and Analgesia*, **68,** 688–91.

Williams, O. A., Mills, R. and Goddard, J. M. (1992). Pulmonary collapse during anaesthesia in children with respiratory tract symptoms. *British Journal of Anaesthesia*, 411–13.

Willis, R. B. and Rorabeck, C. H. (1990). Treatment of compartment syndrome in children. *Orthopaedic Clinics of North America*, **21**(2), 401–12.

Chapter 8

Paediatric spinal surgery

John Stevens

Introduction

Surgery for correction of scoliosis is orthopaedic surgery and anaesthesia at its most heroic, combining an extensive incision and massive bone destruction with prolonged surgery in a group of patients amongst whom coexisting disease, often severe, is common.

Table 8.1 Paediatric scoliosis surgery in Oxford

From October 1989–November 1992	
Idiopathic	29
Congenital	18
Acquired	19
Cerebral Palsy	8
Rett's Syndrome	2
Neurofibromatosis	4
Muscular Dystrophies	4
Prader-Willi	1
Total 66 patients 11 aged 7–11, 55 aged 12–16	

Scoliosis may be congenital, acquired or in up to 70 per cent of cases idiopathic. The motive behind surgery in idiopathic scoliosis is primarily cosmetic, both to prevent further unsightly deformity, and to correct, as far as possible, the existing curvature. It is surprising how late many patients present and the curve is frequently too rigid to allow much correction. Long-term follow-up of untreated cases presenting in adolescence demonstrated no excess mortality and only a slightly increased incidence of hypertension, compared with population norms (Pehrsson, 1992). Presentation in infants or juveniles was, however, associated with premature death from respiratory and cardiac causes. There is some evidence that surgery improves respiratory function long-term (Gagnon *et al.*, 1989), but may cause deterioration in the short term (Baydur *et al.*, 1990; Kinneur *et al.*, 1992). The indications for and timing of surgery are dictated by the degree and rate of change of curvature thus regular monitoring of patients with scoliosis is required. The curvature tends to accelerate at times of rapid growth regardless of the aetiology thus surgery is mostly commonly considered in adolescence.

The indications for and timing of surgery in the non-idiopathic group are more varied. In wheelchair bound patients such as those with muscular dystrophy or spina bifida, spinal fusion may facilitate a more erect and comfortable sitting position but does not appear to prevent or delay deterioration of respiratory function or prolong life (Miller *et al.*, 1991, 1992). In patients able to walk either unaided or with the help of orthoses, a straightened and stiffened spine improves the mechanics of motion. However, the prolonged rehabilitation required may lead to a worsening of associated problems such as contractures and compromise mobility in some groups unless vigorous physiotherapy is employed (Muller *et al.*, 1992).

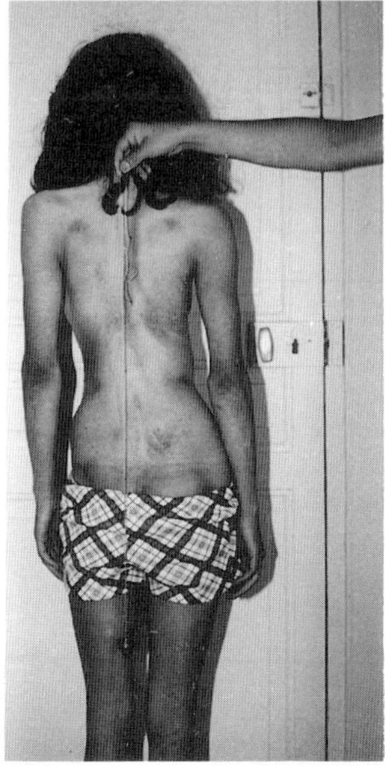

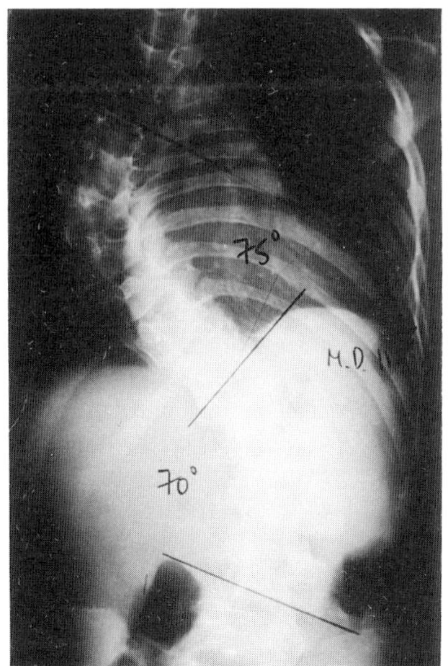

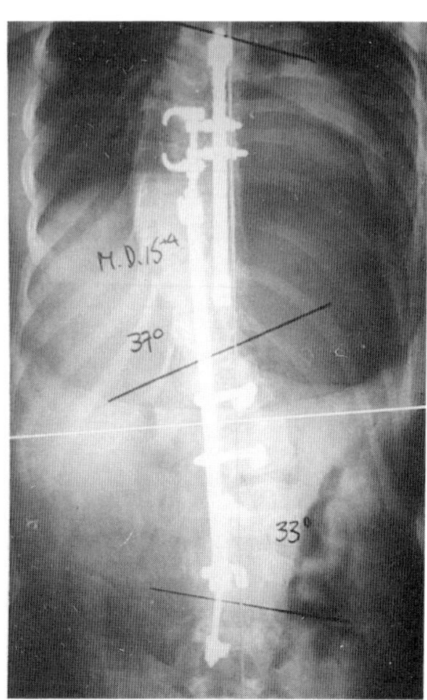

Fig 8.1 A 14 year-old girl with a double-curve idiopathic scoliosis (a). An upper angle of 75° and a lower angle of 70° (b) have corrected to 37° and 33° respectively after surgery (c).

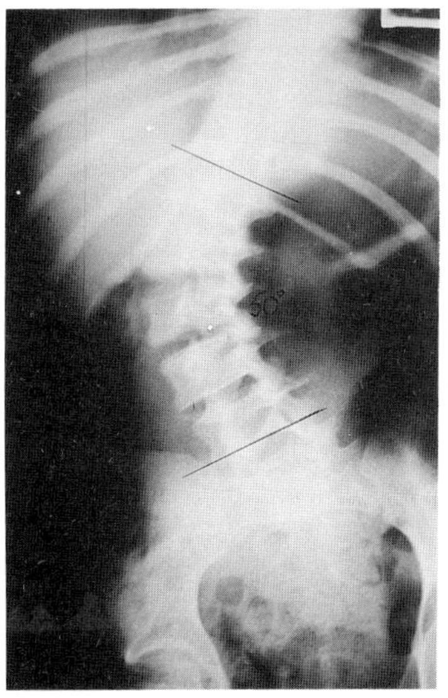

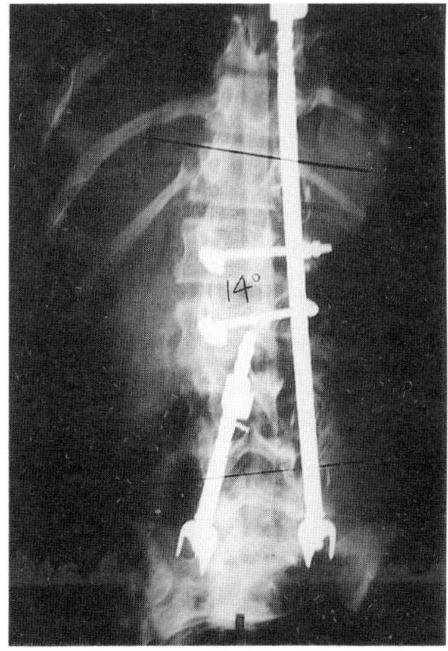

Fig 8.2 Acquired scoliosis in a boy with cerebral palsy. A 50° curve (a) has been corrected to 14° (b).

Preoperative assessment

The majority of patients will be fit young girls and routine investigations only will be required. Explanations of methods of pain management, the reasons for a wake-up test if planned, and the use of urinary catheters, CVP and arterial lines should be covered. Premedication is a matter for the individual and may or may not be deemed appropriate but for many of the patients this will be their first experience of hospital, thus some form of sedation is often helpful. Parental involvement should be encouraged, and a visit to the intensive care unit or high dependency unit, if admission is likely, suggested, to familiarize the patient with a new and challenging environment Respiratory function tests have been traditionally performed but rarely seem to provide unexpected information or are of great value in predicting intra or postoperative pulmonary problems (Gagnon *et al.*, 1989), and may be extremely difficult to perform in some children, often those in whom the most useful information is to be gained. The presence and function of ventricular shunts should be ascertained, particularly if these are venotriculo-atrial, as internal jugular cannulation may be contraindicated if both sides have been previously used for shunting.

Anaesthetic considerations

This form of surgery presents numerous problems for the anaesthetist, particularly in the following areas.

Temperature control

A large incision with considerable exposure and consequent loss of heat by evaporation is combined with the requirement for large volume, sometimes very rapid, blood and fluid administration.

Temperature monitoring is mandatory as should be efficient humidification of inspiratory gases. The use of electric or water heating blankets is compromised by the need to position the patient on some sort of support, and hot-air circulators, are more effective. The patient should be 'insulated' as far as possible, using sterile sheets of polythene through which the incision can be made, and the room temperature should be as warm as is practical, bearing in mind the physical nature of the surgery. Attention should be paid to warming fluids and it is important to keep the run of tubing from the heating system as short as possible.

Positioning

Patient positioning varies according to the surgeons preference. Numerous systems are available, and most are designed to attempt to reduce pressure on the abdomen and consequent epidural venous congestion. A bean-bag (Vac-Pac, Howmedica UK) which solidifies when a vacuum is applied, has the advantages that weight bearing is more evenly distributed in patients with considerable deformity than is possible with fixed systems like the Relton-Hall frame, and that the solid flat base is more stable. If a sand bag is placed under the abdomen before the bag is evacuated, and then removed, a well is created to relieve abdominal pressure. The greater the degree of curvature of the spine the more tortuous the course of the great vessels and the more likely compression against the vertebral bodies is to occur. A recent patient, in whom CVP measured at the Superior Vena Cava/atrial junction, in the supine position, measured 6 cms H_2O registered a pressure of 20–24 cms H_2O when turned prone. This could not be improved despite meticulous attention to position, and surgery was complicated by considerable venous oozing, particularly from the upper portion of the wound. Postoperatively periorbital and upper extremity oedema developed and subsided over 24–48 hours. Presumably compression or torsion had occurred at the SVC when the patient was turned prone.

Attention to pressure on the face must be paid. Many of these adolescent patients will be receiving orthodontic treatment and dental braces should be protected and padded to prevent trauma to the lips. Cases of retinal artery occlusion during surgery in the prone position have been recorded (West *et al.*, 1990; Wolfe *et al.*, 1992) as have cases of pancreatitis (Leichtner *et al.*, 1991), which could perhaps have been triggered by compression and venous or arterial occlusion particularly in the event of accidental or deliberate hypotension and massive transfusion. Postoperative ileus may also be prolonged and a naso-gastric tube should always be inserted. In the prone position, the epidural veins are several centimetres above the right atrium and air embolism is a further potential risk (Lany *et al.*, 1989; McCarthy *et al.*, 1990), particularly if the venous pressure falls too low. A venous pressure of 8–10 cms is probably ideal. Access to the endotracheal tube is limited, and a non-kinking reinforced tube relieves a further area of concern. Ventilatory difficulty may be encountered when the patient is turned and correct positioning of the tube in the trachea must be confirmed before surgery proceeds. Severe spinal deformity may also lead to bronchial torsion or compression and ventilatory problems (Colin *et al.*, 1988; Scuderi *et al.*, 1989), which may be exacerbated by surgical manipulation.

Haemorrhage

The extent of bony decortication inevitably leads to considerable haemorrhage, as does the harvesting

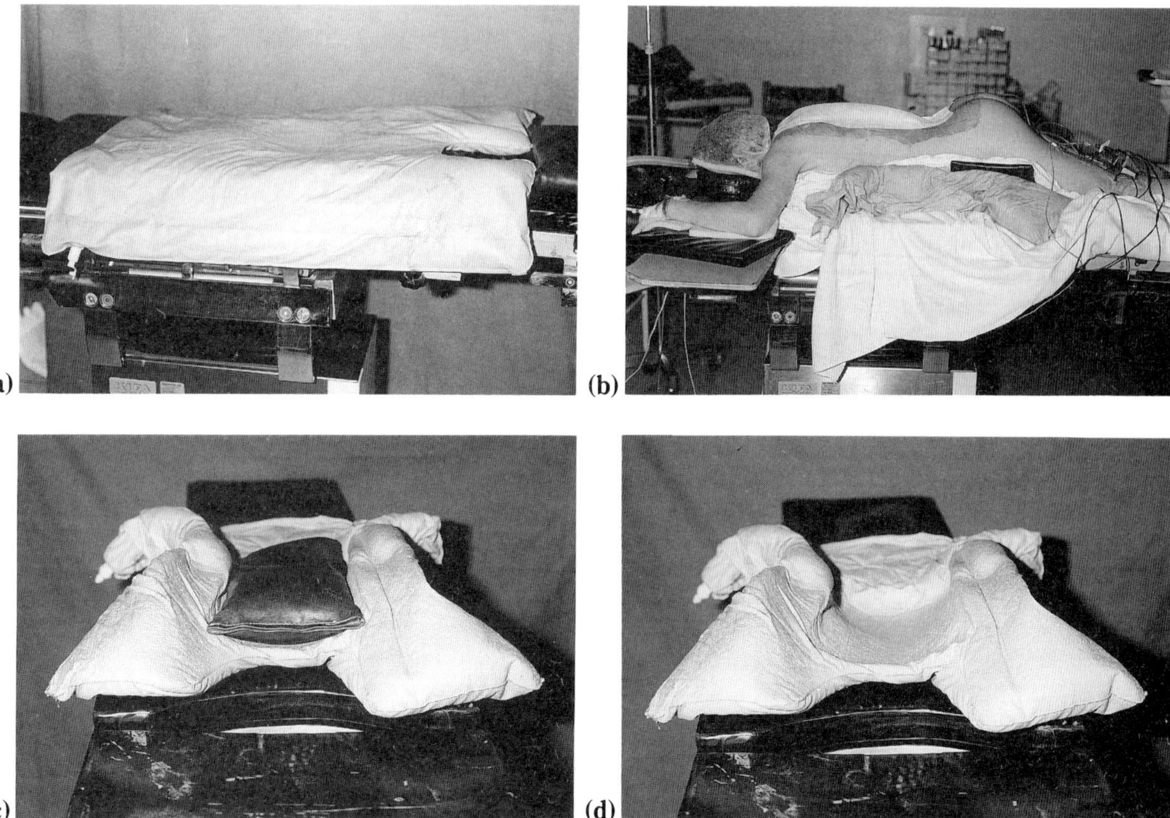

Fig 8.3 The Vac-Pac patient support (Howmedica UK). (a) Deflated. (b) in use. (c) and (d) to show the creation of a well for the abdomen by the use of a sand bag.

of bone grafts, and much attention has been paid to methods of reducing blood loss. Hypotensive anaesthesia has been advocated by many, but may increase the risk of spinal cord damage. Moderate hypotension, achieved by the use of paralysis and ventilation with a volatile agent, complimented by prevention of tachycardia with beta-blockade is a technique used by many anaesthetists. A study in Jehovah's Witnesses (Brodsky *et al.*, 1991) using hypotensive anaesthesia demonstrated that blood loss was more closely related to surgical time than to blood pressure control. This is not surprising as most of the bleeding from bone is venous and would not be greatly diminished by arterial hypotension. Administration of desmopressin does not decrease blood loss (Guay *et al.*, 1992), but the use of fibrin sealant at the sites of bone graft harvest and decortication reduces loss by more than 20 per cent (Tredwell and Scuvatzby, 1990). The use of allograft bone saves surgical time, decreases blood loss from the donor site, reduces postoperative pain and produces one less scar (Montgomery *et al.*, 1990). Transfusion may be associated with many complications (Landin and Nachemson, 1989) and much attention has been focused on alternatives to homologous blood. Preoperative bleeding and subsequent transfusion can reduce the amount of homologous blood required. McEuen *et al.* (1990) in 118 patients ranging from 30–45 kg body weight who donated an average of 800 mls of blood preoperatively, found that 63 per cent required no homologous blood and that the remainder had a much reduced need. They present a useful framework for managing blood donation. Preoperative donations can be enhanced by the administration of erythropoietin and iron supplements (Roye *et al.*, 1992). Auto-transfusion of salvaged blood at the time of surgery (Goodnough and Marcus, 1992) and in the postoperative period (Flynn *et al.*, 1991) can also improve outcome, is applicable to children, and is cost-effective (Elawad *et al.*, 1991), particularly if the risk of transmitted diseases is included in the equation, but may be associated with coagulopathies (Murray *et al.*, 1992). Central venous and arterial pressure monitoring are necessary to manage such massive losses effectively, as is urinary catheterization. Rib osteotomies, performed to correct the accompanying deformity of the chest wall will increase blood loss, and in patients with brittle bones, such as in osteogenesis imperfecta, the force of scoliosis surgery may lead to unrecognized distant fractures and occult blood loss (Sperry, 1989).

Anterior spinal fusion, which requires a thoracotomy, may also result in occult blood loss in the pleural cavity, and undue hypotension in these patients in the postoperative period, even if chest drains appear to be functioning correctly, should be viewed with suspicion and chest auscultation and *X*-ray performed to exclude a haemothorax.

Spinal cord function

Perhaps the most worrying aspect of scoliosis surgery is spinal cord damage, due either to direct surgical trauma or ischaemia from distraction (Naito *et al.*, 1992), and subsequent permanent disability. Much attention has therefore been paid to methods by which spinal cord dysfunction can be detected at an early stage before damage has become irreversible. The 'wake-up' test has been, for many years, the gold standard of such observations (Brustowicz and Hall, 1988), but may not be appropriate in retarded or deaf patients, may be distressing for the patient, is crude and sometimes difficult to perform, and may result in loss of tubes and vascular lines if not smoothly controlled. Despite apparent observation of voluntary movement of the lower limbs during wake-up, permanent dysfunction may occur and attention has been turned to electro-physiological monitoring, in the form of somato-sensory and motor evoked potentials. Somato-sensory evoked potentials (SSEP), recorded cortically, are prone to alteration by anaesthetic agents, hypotension, and hypo- or hyper-thermia (Perlik *et al.*, 1992), but when recorded at spinal level above the operative site are less variable as this involves fewer synapses, and electrodes inserted by the surgeon into the thoracic epidural space, or via an epidural needle at cervical level (Anderson *et al.*, 1990) have been utilized and shown to be of value. Motor evoked potentials can be produced by transcranial magnetic stimuli, a technique which is non-invasive, not unpleasant and can be used in the unanaesthetized patient pre- and post-operatively, but which is probably too sensitive to variations in anaesthesia and other physiological conditions for reliable intraoperative monitoring (Schmid *et al.*, 1992). A combination of motor (Owen *et al.*, 1991) and sensory potentials evoked or recorded at spinal level above the site of surgery seems to offer the best chance of detecting damage to motor and sensory pathways before it becomes irreversible (Mustam and Kendig, 1991). Such monitoring however, requires technical skill, close and constant observation and may distract the anaesthetist from other tasks, and should be the province of physiological measurement staff and the surgical team. The anaesthetists role should be to provide stable levels of anaesthesia and physiological conditions which facilitate meaningful interpretation by others, whilst bearing in mind the potential requirement for a wake-up test, should other monitoring prove equivocal (Loughnan and Hall, 1989).

Pain management

Scoliosis surgery is painful, but large doses of analgesic agents may compromise already suboptimal respiratory function in the postoperative period, and epidural local anaesthesia, although effective and practical, may prevent postoperative monitoring limb function. Epidural and intrathecal opiates are effective, require lower total doses of opiates and do not interfere with functional assessment (Loughnan *et al.*, 1991). Catheters are easily inserted by the surgeon at operation and are applicable to all patients. However, the risk of infection or of shearing of catheters on removal against irregular jagged bony surfaces are potential risks. Patient-controlled analgesia is also effective but may not be feasible in patients with muscle weakness, cerebral palsy or mental retardation. If postoperative ventilation and sedation is deemed necessary then continuous infusions of opiate are appropriate. Often the most pain emanates from the upper end of the incision where muscles of the shoulder girdle are stripped. Thoracotomy pain after an anterior approach can be controlled by cryosurgery, intrapleural local anaesthetic infusion, or by insertion of a catheter extrapleurally into the paravertebral space.

Ventilation

Preoperative respiratory dysfunction may indicate that postoperative ventilation may be required, but weaning may be difficult, particularly in advanced muscular dystrophy and other conditions with associated lung or muscle pathology and is worth avoiding if possible. Nasal CPAP may allow the maintenance

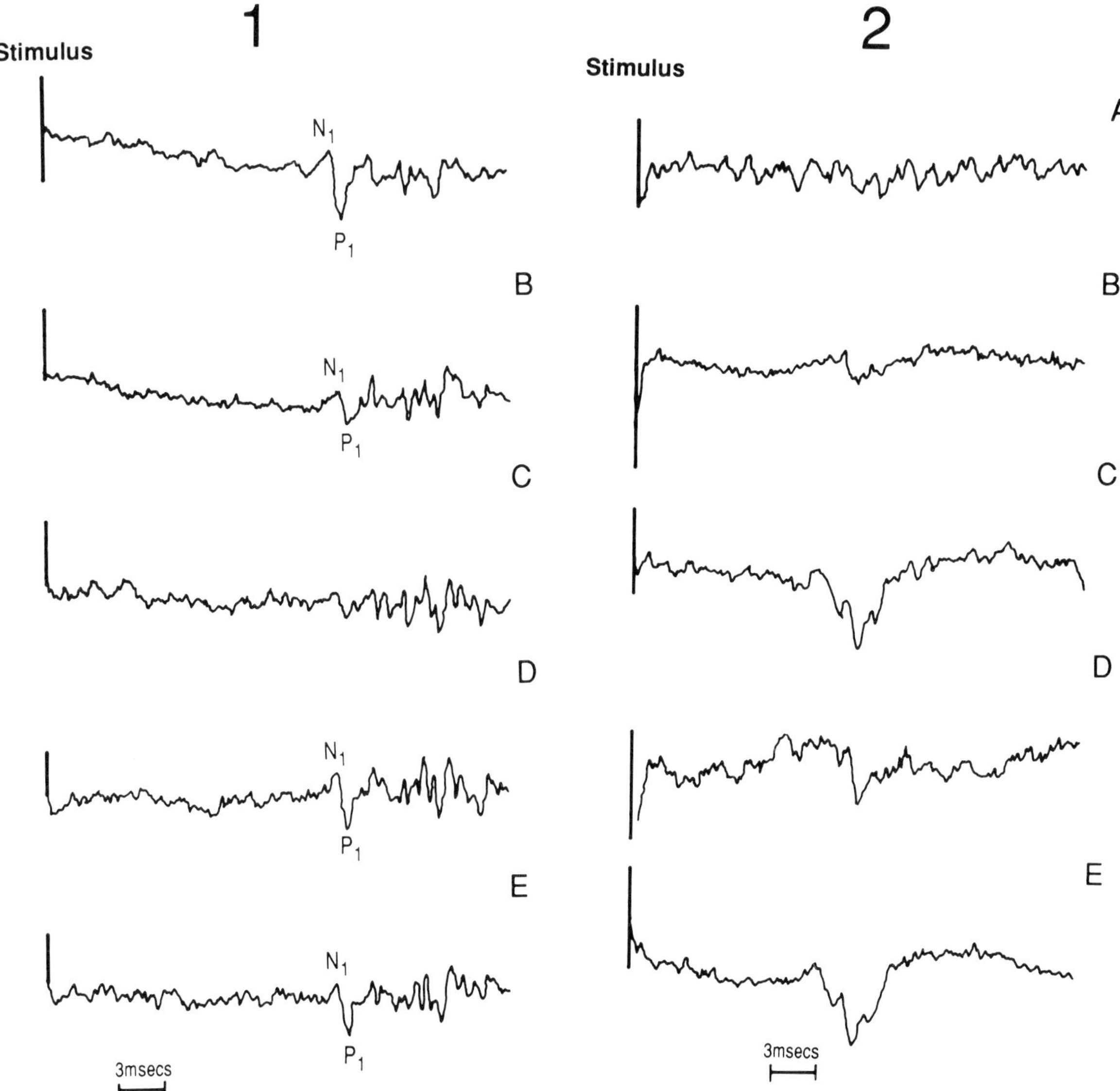

Fig 8.4 Somato sensory evoked potentials recorded by an epidural electrode inserted, at operation, above the site of surgery, with stimulating electrodes placed over the common peroneal nerve delivering a supra-maximal stimulus which is averaged over 512 stimuli. In Trace 1, during surgery in an adolescent female with idiopathic scoliosis, as distraction is produced with Harrington Rods, the amplitude of N and P, decreases in B and C and the latency increases. When the distraction was reduced recovery occurred in D and E. In Trace 2, from a young male with a crush fracture of L1 and L2 with numbness and paresis of the left leg before surgery, no potential can be recognised initially in A, but as the fracture is reduced surgically a potential appears in B, and increases in amplitude, with reduction of latency in C, D and E.

reasonable lung volumes, and renders coughing and physiotherapy more effective (personal data). Perhaps the most important factor in preventing respiratory complications is early correction before lung function has become too perilous. Such surgery should only be performed in units where intensive or high-dependency postoperative care is available and close monitoring of ventilatory function can be instituted. The elective nature of the surgery and the shortage of paediatric intensive care beds nationally inevitably leads to disappointments, and patients and parents, who will have spent many weeks or months building up to such a major event should be made aware of the likelihood of potential cancellation to avoid heart-rending disruptions in their programme.

References

Anderson, S. K., Loughnan, B. A. and Hetreed, M. A. (1990). A technique for monitoring evoked potentials during scoliosis and brachial plexus surgery. *Annals of Royal College of Surgeons*, **72**, 321–3.

Baydur, A., Swank, S. M., Stiles, C. M. and Sassoon, C. S. (1990). Respiratory mechanics in anaesthetised young patients with Kypho scoliosis. Immediate and delayed effects of corrective spinal surgery. *Chest*, **97**, 1157–64.

Brodsky, J. W., Dickson, J. H., Erwin, W. D. and Rossi, C. D. (1991). Hypotensive anaesthesia for scoliosis surgery in Jehovah's Witnesss. *Spine*, **16**, 304–6.

Brustowicz, R. M. and Hall, J. E. (1988). In defence of the wake-up test. *Anaesthesia and Analgesia*, **67**, 1019.

Colin, A. A., Allen, J. L., Berde, C. B., Griscom, N. T., Hall, J. E. and Young, L. V. (1988). Bronchial compression and ventilatory dysfunction in scoliosis. *American Journal of Diseases in Childhood*, **142**, 545–6.

Elawad, A., Benoni, G., Montgomery, F., Hyddnak, U., Persson, U. and Fredin, H. (1991). Cost-effectiveness of blood substitution in elective orthopaedic operations. *Acta Orthopaedica Scandinavica*, **62**, 435–9.

Flynn, J. C., Price, C. T. and Link, W. P. (1991). The third step of autologous blood transfusion in scoliosis surgery. Harvesting blood from the post-operative wound. *Spine*, **16**, S328–9.

Gagnon, S., Jodwin, A. and Martin, R. (1989). Pulmonary function test study after spinal fusion in young idiopathic scoliosis. *Spin*, **14**, 486–90.

Goodnough, L. T. and Marcus, R. E. (1992). Effect of autologous blood donation in patients undergoing elective spine surgery. *Spine*, **17**, 172–5.

Guay, J., Reinberz, C., Poitras, B., David, M., Mathews, S., Lottie, L., Rivard, G. E. (1992). A trial of desmopressin in reduced blood loss in patients undergoing spinal fusion for idiopathic scoliosis. *Anesthesia and Analgesia*, **75**, 405–10.

Kinneur, W. J. M., Kinnear, G. C., Watson, L., Webb, J. K. and Johnson, I. D. A. (1992). Pulmonary function after spinal surgery for idiopathic scoliosis. *Spine*, **17**, 708–13.

Landin, P. and Nachemson, A. (1989). Transfusion-related non-A non-B Hepatitis in elective spine deformity surgery in Gothenburg, Sweden. *Spine*, **14**, 1033–5.

Lany, S. A., Duncan, P. G. and Dupuis, P. R. (1989). Fatal air embolism in an adolescent with Duchenne muscular dystrophy during Harrington instrumentation. *Anesthesia and Analgesia*, **69**, 132–4.

Leichtner, A. M., Banta, J. V., Etienne, N., Schwartz, A. N., Renshaw, T. S., Solari, L. D., Ascione, J. and Hyams, J. S. (1991). Pancreatitis following scoliosis surgery in children and young adults. *Journal of Pediatric Orthopaedics*, **11**, 594–8.

Loughnan, B. A. and Hall, G. M. (1989). Spinal cord monitoring. *British Journal Anaesthesia*, **63**, 587–94.

Loughnan, B. A., Yan, K. W., Mensford, A. O. and Hall, G. M. (1991). Effects of epidural diamorphine on the somato-sensory evoked potential to posterior fibral nerve stimulation. *Anaesthesia*, **46**, 912–14.

MacEwen, G. D., Bennett, E. and Guille, J. T. (1990). Autologous blood transfusions in children and young adults with low body weight undergoing spinal surgery. *Journal of Pediatric Orthopaedics*, **10**, 750–3.

McCarthy, R. E., Lonstein, J. E., Mertz, J. D. and Kuslich, S. P. (1990). Air embolism in spinal surgery. *Journal of Spinal Disorders*, **3**, 1–5.

Miller, R. G., Chalmers, A. C., Dao, H., Filler-Katz, A., Holman, D. and Bost, F. (1991). The effects of spinal fusion on respiratory function in Duchenne Muscular Dystrophy. *Neurology*, **41**, 38–40.

Miller, F., Moseley, C. F. and Koreska, J. (1992). Spinal fusion in Duchenne Muscular Dystrophy. *Developmental Medicine and Child Neurology*, **34**, 775–86.

Montgomery, D. M., Aronson, D. D., Lee, C. L. and LaMont, R. L. (1990). Posterior spinal fusion: allographt versus autographt bone. *Journal of Spinal Disorders*, **3**, 370–5.

Muller, E. B., Nordwall, A. and VonWendt, L. (1992). Influence of surgical treatment in children with spina bifida on ambulation and motor skills. *Acta Paediatrica*, **81**, 173–6.

Murray, D. J., Gress, K. and Weistein, S. L. (1992). Coagulopathy after reinfusion of autologous scavenged red blood cells. *Anesth. Analgesia*, **75**, 125–9.

Mustam, W. D. and Kendig, R. J. (1991). Dissociation of neurogenic motor and somato-sensory evoked potentials. A case report. *Spine*, **16**, 851–3.

Naito, M., Owen, J. H., Bridwell, K. H. and Sugioka, T. (1992). Effects of dystraction on physiologic integrity of the spinal cord, spinal cord blood flow and clinical status. *Spine*, **17**, 1154–8.

Owen, J. H., Bridwell, K. H., Grubb, R., Jenny, A., Allen, B., Padberg, A. M. and Stimen, S. M. (1991). The clinical application of neurogenic motor-evoked potentials to monitor spinal cord function during surgery. *Spine*, **16**, S385–90.

Pehrsson, K., Larsson, S., Oden, A. and Nachemson, A. (1992). Long-term follow-up of patients with untreated scoliosis. *Spine*, **17**, 1091–6.

Perlik, S. J., Van Egeren, R. and Fisher, M. A. (1992). Somato-sensory evoked potential surgical monitoring. Observations during combined isoflurane-nitrous oxide anaesthesia. *Spine*, **17**, 273–6.

Roye, D. P., Pothstein, P., Richert, J. B., Verdico, L.

and Farcy, J. P. (1992). The use of pre-operative erythropoietin in scoliosis surgery. *Spine*, **17**, 5204–5.

Schmid, U. D., Boll, J., Liechti, S., Schmid, J., Hess, C. W. (1992). Influence of some anaestheic agents of muscle responses to transcranial magnetic cortex stimulation. *Neurosurgery*, **30**, 85–92.

Scuderi, G., Sanders, D. P., Brustowicz, R. M., Berle, C. B., Colin, A., Allen, J., Healy, G. B. and Hall, J. E. (1989). Post-operative Iordo-scoliosis causing extrinsic compression of the right main stem bronchus and respiratory insufficiency. *Spine*, **4**, 110–14.

Sperry, K. (1989). Fatal intraoperative haemorrhage during spinal fusion surgery for osteogenesis imperfecta. *American Journal of Forensic Medicine and Pathology*, **10**, 54–9.

Tredwell, S. J. and Scuvatzby, B. (1990). The use of fibrin sealant to reduce blood loss during Cotrel–Subousset instrumentation for idiopathic scoliosis. *Spine*, **15**, 913–15.

West, J., Askin, G., Clarke, M. and Vernin, S. A. (1990). Loss of vision in one eye after scoliosis surgery. *British Journal of Ophthalmology*, **74**, 243–4.

Wolfe, S. W., Lospinuso, M. F. and Barke, S. W. (1992). Unilateral blindness as a complication of patient positioning for spinal surgery. *Spine*, **17**, 600–5.

Chapter 9

Regional Anaesthesia

Introduction

Regional anaesthesia finds its best application in orthopaedic surgery, where most surgical procedures on the limbs can be carried out after suitable nerve block. Old people and others who fear general anaesthesia may prefer to have a local anaesthetic whilst, in the accident and emergency department, suturing of wounds and reduction of fractures can be performed even though the patient has recently had a meal.

In the past decade, three factors have brought about a reappraisal of regional anaesthesia. First, the suggestion by Scott (1984) of using a local block in combination with light general anaesthesia (which he called 'controllable sedation'), has had considerable impact. This method overcomes both the reluctance of some patients to stay awake during surgery and the surgeon's distrust of an incomplete block. A second factor, has been a general realization of the importance of postoperative pain relief and the ease with which regional anaesthesia can provide it. Finally, the increase in microvascular surgery for limb repair and grafting procedures (Chapter 3), and the growth in day surgery (Chapter 10), have increased the demand for regional anaesthesia.

The addition of a sequence of light general anaesthesia to regional anaesthesia frees the anaesthetist from the imperative of providing a perfect block every time. This means that blocks can be used much more often to minimize the requirement for general anaesthesia, give postoperative pain relief and gain practice. Thus, when there is a strong indication for local anaesthesia, the required block can be performed accurately and confidently. The regional block may form a small part of the anaesthetic sequence, as in an ankle block for subtalar fusion, or it may be the major part, e.g. when a brachial block is used with sedation for surgery of the arm. The beauty of the arrangement is its flexibility.

Many agents have been used for sedation but currently the most interesting are midazolam and propofol given as increments or an infusion in each case. Fanard *et al.* (1988) compared midazolam and propofol during orthopaedic surgery under epidural anaesthesia and found that there was a greater variation of dose required for midazolam but better sedation, whilst propofol gave a quicker recovery. Midazolam has the advantage of being a potent anticonvulsant so that any potential for seizures arising from the local anaesthetic agent is countered. If benzodiazepines are used they should be given in small aliquots until a suitable level of sedation is achieved: too large a dose produces a state of restlessness and confusion, which may render surgery impossible and can be treated only by proceeding to full general anaesthesia. An infusion of propofol may be used to produce any degree of sedation from drowsiness to general anaesthesia with a very short recovery time. Fanard *et al.* (1988) found than an infusion of only 1.74 mg/kg/hr provided adequate sedation with epidural anaesthesia.

In the elderly, the sedation produced by the local anaesthetic injected for the block should be assessed before giving additional sedation when usually only minuscule doses are required. It is in any case preferable to have the patient's cooperation whilst performing the block to report paraesthesia or anything untoward.

The two most important factors in successful regional anaesthesia are the relative obesity of the patient and the time available to perform the block. Patients who are obese are often poor subjects for local anaesthesia because anatomical landmarks may be difficult to define and it becomes impossible to position the needle precisely enough. Time is needed to perform the block and then to allow the block to become fully effective. All this will probably occupy half an hour, for, whilst the most accurate injection of lignocaine will produce rapid results, diffusion of the agent to the nerve trunk more usually takes 20 minutes or so to give a slowly progressive block. This time should be allowed for in planning the operating list.

The choice of regional technique must take into account whether a tourniquet is to be used, and analgesia should be provided for the ischaemic pain of the tourniquet. Tourniquets are applied as far proximally up the limb as possible to leave the operating field clear. Particularly with brachial blocks, it may sometimes be necessary to infiltrate subcutaneous lignocaine around the proximal border of the tourniquet cuff to abolish pain from the tourniquet itself.

The effectiveness of the block should be checked after a suitable interval and its distribution mapped out. If a block is incomplete, the missing element should be identified and blocked further peripherally with a small additional dose of local anaesthetic, so that the final result is perfect.

Pharmacokinetics of nerve blocks

Local anaesthetic bathing a nerve trunk will soak into the trunk from the periphery on an advancing front (Fig. 9.1). Transmission in fibres in the periphery of the trunk will be blocked first (Fig. 9.1B) and in those in the centre of the trunk last (Fig. 8.1A). Further, transmission in peripherally placed fibres will be blocked over a greater length of fibre than it will be for central fibres, so anaesthesia will appear earlier and last longer in territory supplied by peripherally placed fibres of a nerve trunk than in territory supplied by central fibres. If the pool of local anaesthetic is too small or the concentration too low, then fibres in the centre of the trunk will escape blockade; the thicker the nerve trunk, the more prominent these effects of distribution are likely to be.

In the nerve trunks supplying the limbs, the central fibres are the longest, supplying the extremity of the limb (Fig. 9.2), whilst shorter fibres are arranged more peripherally as their area of supply is more proximal. This explains why an incomplete block of the brachial plexus is likely to spare the fingers, and how the loss of motor power in the upper arm occurs before loss of sensation in the hand even though motor fibres are larger and more resistant to nerve block. Winnie *et al.* (1977) have expanded this argument, considering first a peripheral bundle of fibres in a trunk of the brachial plexus – 'a mantle bundle' – and, secondly, a central of 'core bundle' of fibres (Fig. 9.3). Within the mantle bundle, there are motor and sensory fibres: all the early branches of the brachial plexus from roots, trunks and upper cords are motor and therefore are arranged more peripherally within the mantle bundle than the sensory fibres. Thus, as local anaesthetic enters the nerve trunk, the first fibres to be blocked are motor to the

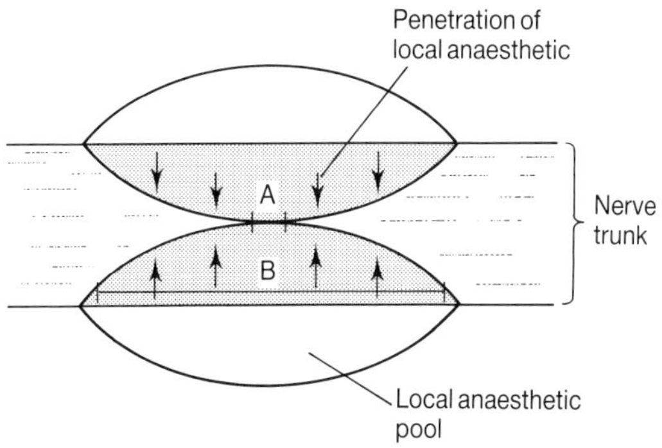

Fig 9.1 Pharmacokinetics of nerve block. A pool of local anaesthetic surrounding a nerve trunk will penetrate the trunk on an advancing front. Block of peripheral fibres B will occur first, followed by more central fibres A later. The length of nerve fibre blocked will be greater for peripheral fibres than for central fibres.

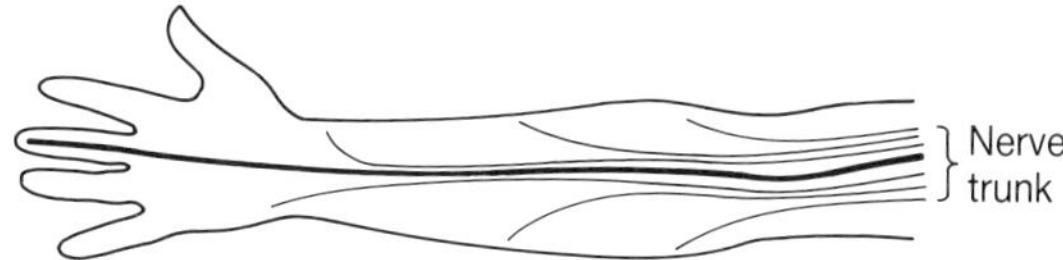

Fig 9.2 Arrangement of fibres in a nerve trunk. The central fibres are those supplying the most distal part of the limb.

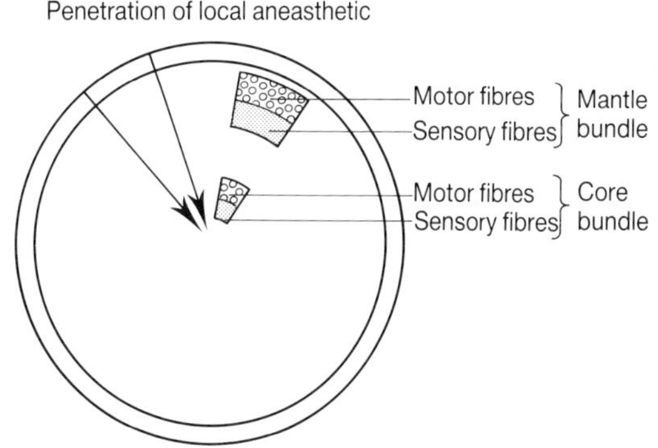

Fig 9.3 Arrangement of motor and sensory fibres in a cross-section of an upper limb nerve trunk of the brachial plexus. (Redrawn, with permission, from Winnie*et al.*(1977).)

upper arm, followed by sensory fibres to the upper arm. Within a core bundle the situation is similar: the peripheral fibres of the core bundle are motor, supplying the muscles of the forearm, and the deepest most central fibres run the longest course to provide sensation to the hand. Thus, as for the upper arm, motor power is lost before sensation, provided that the concentration of local anaesthetic remains great enough after dilution. At critical concentration of local anaesthetic, proximal motor power may be lost whilst distal motor power is presened. This simple model correctly predicts the pattern of loss of nerve function in the arm after brachial plexus block (Winnie *et al.*, 1977); it neglects, however, the effect of the vascular plexus within the nerve trunks which will tend to increase both the transport of local anaesthetic into the nerve trunk and that of its removal.

Techniques of regional anaesthesia

The remainder of this chapter is devoted to techniques of regional anaesthesia of particular value in orthopaedic surgery. More comprehensive descriptions of techniques are given in any text illustrated by Buckhoj and a useful guide to regional anaesthesia in children is that edited by Saint-Maurice and Shulte Steinberg.

Local infiltration

A muscle biopsy, generally taken from the quadriceps femoris, is required to establish a diagnosis of myopathy or dystrophy and occasionally to investigate the susceptibility of a patient to malignant hyperthermia (MH), General anaesthesia in these patients carries obvious risk from cardiomyopathy, poor respiratory function or in the case of MH, of inducing the disease. Yet surgeons are reluctant to use local infiltration for the procedure because it is often ineffective or the specimen is spoiled by the introduction of artefacts. Bupivacaine injected into muscle is directly toxic and causes rapid cellular degeneration (Newman and Radda, 1983) thus reducing the value of any specimen taken. An elegant solution to this problem is suggested by Gielen and Viering (1986), who used the inguinal paravascular technique of Winnie *et al.* (1973) to provide regional anaesthesia distant from the site of biopsy. They further noted that the amide local anaesthetics prilocaine and bupivacaine used in this way did not provoke hyperthermia crises in 22 patients subsequently considered to be susceptible to malignant hyperthermia.

Intravenous regional anaesthesia

Intravenous regional anaesthesia (IVRA) is an important area of local anaesthesia if only because of the very large number of such blocks administered each year: the clutch of broken arms produced by the first icy pavement of winter would probably be unmanageable without such a simple technique. IVRA is quick and reliable, producing dense anaesthesia of the arm. The technique involves inserting a needle into a distal vein, applying a tourniquet and exsanguinating the arm, before injecting 40 ml of local anaesthetic solution. Anaesthesia is of rapid onset and lasts as long as the tourniquet is inflated, but with no lasting analgesia after deflation. Because it is so simple, requiring only the ability to insert a needle into a vein, IVRA is often performed by junior staff, many of them non-anaesthetists with scant training. Nevertheless, close attention to detail and meticulous care of equipment are necessary if IVRA is to be used safely. In this respect, anaesthetists must set standards and educate orthopaedic and accident and emergency colleagues in the correct procedures. For all its simplicity, IVRA is not without risk; Grice *et al.* (1986) record that by 1986 the technique had been associated with at least 7 deaths, 2 cardiopulmonary arrests, 10 generalized seizures and many milder toxic symptoms. These mishaps have occurred through the escape of local anaesthetic into the systemic circulation either because of failure or early release of the tourniquet or through leakage of the solution beneath the tourniquet. A Health Notice (Hazard) issued by the Department of Health in 1982 drew attention to tourniquet failure and stressed the need to maintain the equipment, paying particular attention to hoses, connections and the accuracy of the pressure gauge. This notice also required the presence of someone (not necessarily an anaesthetist) whose sole duty was to supervise the tourniquet: the casualty officer should not both perform the block and carry out the procedure.

Leakage past the tourniquet has been reported by many workers and radio contrast studies show that this leakage commonly occurs through the venous system although other possibilities are; the interosseous circulation, which will bypass the tourniquet (Cotev and Robin, 1966) and the failure of a tourniquet to occlude calcified arteries (Jeyaseelan *et al.*, 1981). In the elderly with peripheral vascular disease or known Paget's disease, IVRA is best avoided.

After a near disaster, experimental work was carried out by El Hassan *et al.* (1984) to determine the factors that were associated with leakage of solution beneath the tourniquet. They found that in order to minimize the risk of leakage, the injection site should be distal, that is, in the hand rather than in the antecubital fossa; the injection should be performed slowly over 90 seconds to allow run-off of the solution; the volume of blood in the arm should be reduced as much as possible by exsanguination with an Esmarch bandage to create room for the volume of injectate and adequate pressure should be maintained in the tourniquet. These suggestions were confirmed in a later paper by Grice *et al.* (1986). However, thorough exsanguination of the arm may be difficult if it is painful, or undesirable if the lesion is neoplastic or contains glass.

It was also found that tourniquet width was important – the narrower the tourniquet, the higher the pressure required to prevent venous leakage beneath it since vessels beneath the tourniquet acted as collapsible 'spillover' resistors. Davis *et al.* (1984) found that narrow tourniquets (5–6 cm wide), such as those included in proprietary double cuffs for Bier's block, required a pressure 58 mmHg higher to occlude vessels than wide (12–14 cm) tourniquets. Grice *et al.* (1986) considered that a pressure of at least 300 mmHg was necessary for safe use of IVRA. However, such pressures are not without risk; Larsen and Hommelgaard (1987) reported a case of nerve damage produced by a tourniquet and argued that tourniquet pressure should be related to arterial pressure. In the view of Larsen and Hommelgaard, the tourniquet should be inflated to systolic pressure plus 100 mmHg, and the occlusion time should not be greater than 2 hours. Pfeiffer (1986) reported a case of renal failure caused by rhabdomyolysis in a 14 year old during IVRA when a pressure of 520 mmHg was used in the cuff. The leakage of myoglobin into the circulation occurred either because of ischaemic damage to burned tissue or, more likely, because of severe compression from the cuff.

IVRA is suitable only for operations on the forearm and hand which can be completed in the tourniquet time limit: for more proximal work the bulky tourniquet begins to intrude on the operative field. For fine work on the hand many surgeons are unhappy with the degree of exsanguination possible with an awake patient and full sensation in the arm. Mottling of the arm after induction of the block is caused by poor exsanguination and better results are obtained if the exsanguination is carried up and over the lower tourniquet when a double cuff is being used. In the leg a thigh tourniquet is required for adequate vascular occlusion but the dose of local anaesthetic required for that bulk of tissue is hopelessly toxic: if the tourniquet is applied to the lower leg then vascular occlusion is incomplete because the vessels of supply lie protected between the tibia and fibula. However, efforts continue to be made to adapt IVRA for use in the leg. Davis and Walford (1986) were able to measure plasma concentrations of bupivacaine leaking out from beneath a leg tourniquet even before surgery had begun and also noted that this loss of local anaesthetic tended to produce a patchy block.

Prilocaine is the agent of choice for IVRA, because of its low toxicity, should leakage into the circulation occur, although it is clear that other more toxic agents continue to be used. An editorial published nearly thirty years ago (JAMA, 1965) urged the abandoning of IVRA until a safer agent than lignocaine was available.

The timing and manner of deflation of the tourniquet are important in minimizing the escape of local anaesthetic agent into the circulation. If the tourniquet is released too soon, after a very quick procedure, the drug has not had time to bind to tissue, so the tourniquet should be left in place for 20 minutes; released briefly before reinflation and then released at intervals over several minutes. This procedure parcels out any unbound drug and reduces the plasma concentration which results (Tucker and Boas, 1971).

Whilst IVRA is a simple and successful technique, the potential toxicity of the volume of local anaesthetic agent injected must never be forgotten. Tourniquets must be serviced and checked regularly and resuscitation equipment and a second tourniquet should be immediately available.

Local anaesthesia of the arm

Introduction; brachial plexus blocks

The happy arrangement of the innervation of the upper limb within the confines of a single plexus has encouraged anaesthetists to develop many approaches to blockade of the brachial plexus. In essence, the attempts have been made to devise a technique as consistently successful as the supraclavicular approach without serious hazard of its own. This is clearly difficult because, within the area of the root of the neck and the thoracic inlet, many important structures are at risk. Nevertheless, in addition to axillary, supraclavicular and interscalene approaches, others have been described: a parascalene approach (Vongvises and Panijayanond, 1979), an infraclavicular approach (Raj *et al.*, 1973; Sims, 1977) and a longitudinal supraclavicular approach (Hempel *et al.*, 1981).

Each anatomical approach describes a way of entering the neurovascular fascial sheath which is drawn off from the fascia clothing the anterior and middle scalene muscles by the emerging brachial plexus. This sheath is funnel-shaped, growing smaller in diameter until it disappears at the level of the junction of upper and middle thirds of the upper arm (Fig. 9,4). The extent of any block depends upon the level at which the fascial funnel is entered and upon the volume of agent injected. In general, the interscalene and the axillary approaches demand a greater volume to secure the same block compared with the supraclavicular approach. Winnie (1975) has suggested that an approximate guide to the volume of solution required, in millilitres, may be calculated as equal to half the patient's height in inches.

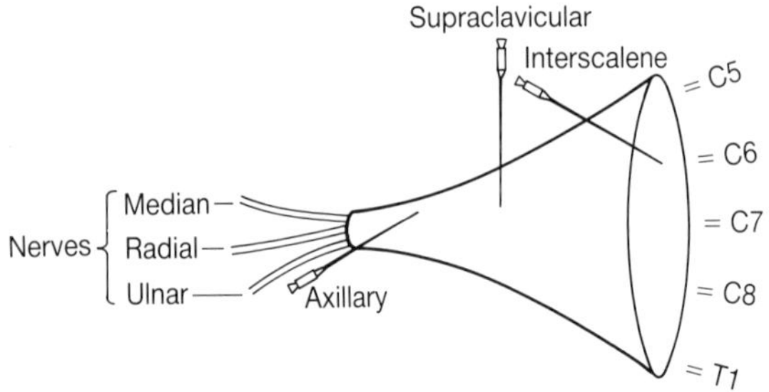

Fig 9.4 Schematic diagram of the fascia investing the brachial plexus; needle positions of the axillary, supraclavicular and interscalene approaches are indicated.

The axillary approach

The axillary approach is gaining in popularity because its freedom from complications makes it specially suitable for day surgery and outpatient use: successful blocks can be achieved in 90 per cent of patients (Selander, 1987). For longer term blocks the axillary approach is the easiest to use with a catheter technique.

The block is performed with the patient's arm abducted and externally rotated, with the hand positioned behind the head in the 'sunbathing' position. If the arm is abducted at more than a right angle, the axillary vessels will become difficult to palpate. After a skin bleb of local anaesthetic has been raised, the needle should be advanced medially along the line of the axillary artery as described by Winnie (1975) until the neurovascular sheath is entered with a 'pop' (Figs. 9.5; 9.6). When correctly positioned, the needle clearly transmits arterial pulsation. Accurate injection is often marked by distension of the neurovascular sheath as a visible linear prominence across the axilla, whilst the development of a circular mound is less promising. As the needle is withdrawn, 5 ml of local anaesthetic should be injected superficial to the sheath in order to block the intercostobrachial nerve which at this point overlies the neurovascular bundle (Fig. 9.7). If this nerve is not blocked, pain is likely to be felt from the medial aspect of an arm tourniquet.

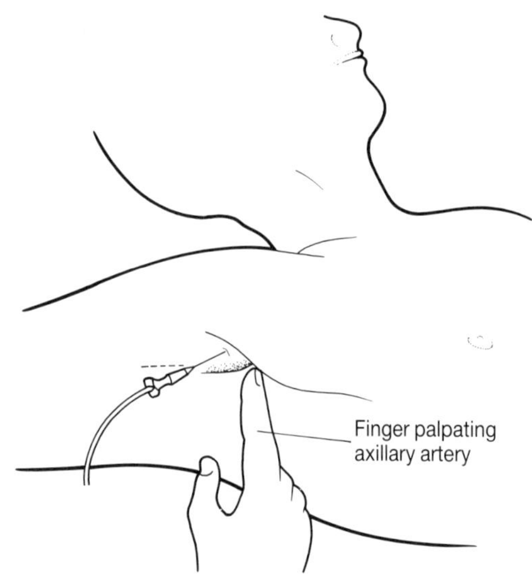

Fig 9.5 Axillary block; the axial approach. (Redrawn, with permission, from Winnie (1975).)

Common reasons for lack of success are failure to locate the artery especially in obese patients; use of too small a volume of solution and injecting too deeply. Bryce-Smith (1976) stressed how superficial the neurovascular bundle is in the axilla, where it lies subcutaneously. The volume of solution required was studied by Vester-Anderson *et al.* (1984) who found that 50 ml was superior to 40 ml of 1 per cent mepivacaine and that 60 ml gave no improvement.

Other manoeuvres will improve the likelihood of success. Using a tourniquet around the upper arm will reduce the peripheral streaming of solution noted by Ang *et al.* (1984) in radiological studies and will ensure that the solution encircles the artery to

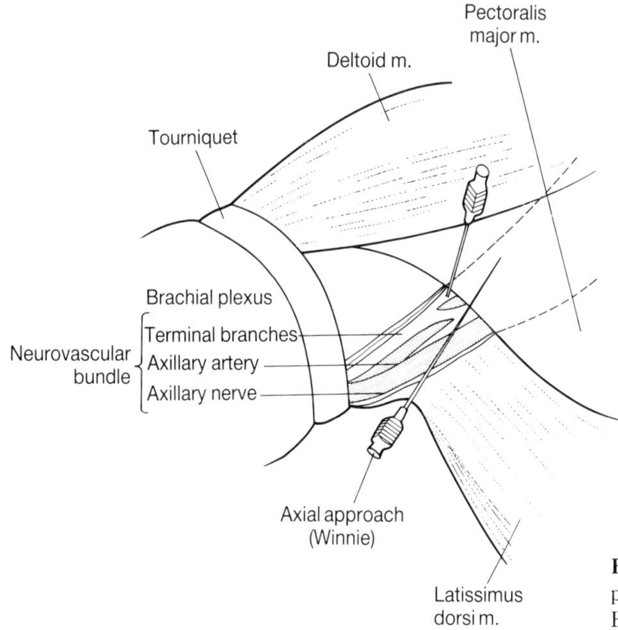

Fig 9.6 Axillary block: the axial approach contrasted with the perpendicular approach. (Redrawn, with permission, from Eriksson (1979).)

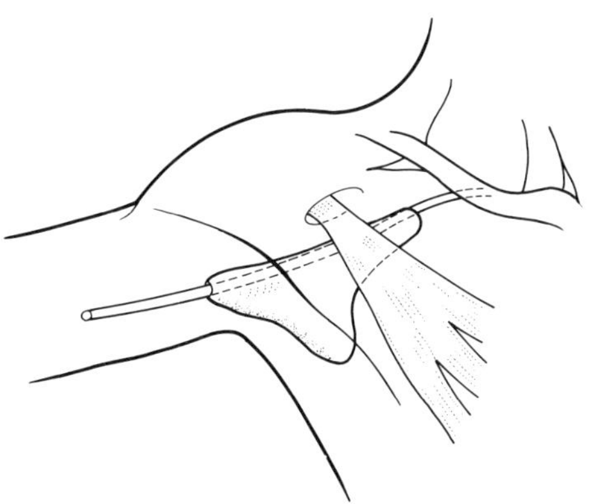

Fig 9.7 The morphology of the axillary sheath. The sheath is not a tubular structure investing the axillary vessels but has an extension inferiorly down the thoracic wall. (Redrawn, with permission, from Vester-Andersen*et al.*(1986).)

reach the radial nerve posteriorly. Proximal spread of solution can be encouraged by reducing the degree of abduction at the shoulder prior to injection. In full abduction the head of the humerus compresses the sheath posteriorly, reducing proximal spread and also restricting access to the posterior elements of the brachial plexus (Winnie, 1975).

This block depends upon the concept of a tightly fitting fascial sheath, which binds together the brachial plexus, axillary artery and vein, and serves to hold injected local anaesthetic solution in contact with the nerve trunks long enough for transmission block to occur. A tightly enclosing sheath is well represented in illustrated textbooks (Erikson, 1969; Winnie, 1983). However, there is an inconsistency between the concept of a tight fascial sheath and the large volumes of solution required to fill it and ensure a block. The answer seems to lie with further work by Vester-Anderson *et al.* (1986) who studied the morphology of the sheath by injecting gelatine into cadavers. After allowing time for the gelatine to set, the axilla was dissected. The sheath was found not to be tubular as supposed but to possess a tongue inferiorly, which extended down the lateral chest wall (Fig. 9.8) and, presumably, serves to permit the wide range of movement enjoyed at the shoulder. Thus an additional volume of solution is required to fill this space. Furthermore, it was noted that while the median and ulnar nerves were in direct contact with the injected gelatine at all cross-sections of the sheath, the musculocutaneous, radial and axillary nerves left the cast proximally and showed no direct contact in several cross-sections, thus explaining the observed difficulty in blocking these nerves by the axillary route.

Thompson and Rorie (1983) suggested that patchy axillary blocks may be caused by fibrous septa within the axillary sheath, which might loculate injected local anaesthetic and limit its spread to the plexus. These workers argued that it was necessary to make separate injections for each of the 3 major branches

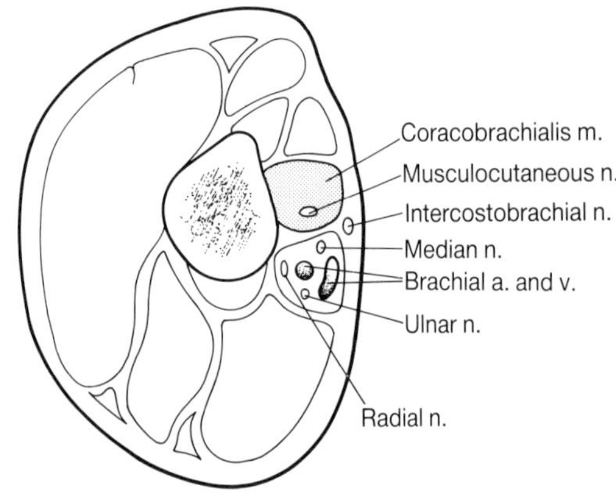

Fig 9.8 Cross-section of the upper arm, showing the position of the musculocutaneous nerve in the substance of the coracobrachialis muscle and the intercostobrachial nerve. (Redrawn, with permission, from Winnie (1975).)

of the plexus, despite common experience that a single injection will give a good block in most cases. In a further anatomical study, Partridge *et al.* (1987) found only incomplete feeble fibrous septa and no effective partitioning of the sheath. They also found that the sheath was not a single layer fibrous tube but was made up of numerous thin layers closely applied, which could easily be stripped by injection. When dye was injected, it spread without difficulty to radial, ulnar and median nerves in each case. While attempting to place needles in the axillary sheath, Partridge and colleagues noted that resistance was felt at a layer superficial to the sheath which could easily give rise to false positive injections and account for some of the failed blocks. These workers argued that a single injection is all that is required to produce a block and that multiple injections will only increase the likelihood of nerve damage.

The musculocutaneous nerve commonly escapes block because it leaves the neurovascular sheath very early at the level of the second part of the axillary artery. The musculocutaneous nerve supplies sensory innervation to the radial side of the forearm, so its block is essential for common surgery of the forearm (e.g. Colles' fracture). The nerve may be blocked whilst in the substance of coracobrachialis muscle by injecting 5 ml of solution into the fascial sheath of coracobrachialis (Fig. 9.7) immediately beneath pectoralis major muscle, and above the brachial artery. Alternatively, the musculocutaneous nerve may be blocked at the elbow where it lies superficially in the groove immediately lateral to the tendon of biceps muscle. The needle should be advanced subcutaneously in this groove 2.5 cm from the skin crease of the elbow joint and 5 ml of solution injected.

Catheter techniques

The duration of a block may be increased using a higher dose of local anaesthetic, by adding adrenaline to the solution or by using a catheter and topping-up the block. Long-term brachial blocks are important for the management of pain after major repair of the forearm and hand and also for preserving vasodilatation by sympathetic vasoconstrictor blockade. Avoidance of vasoconstriction is an essential element of postoperative management of replanted parts and free flaps.

The axillary approach is especially suitable for a catheter technique because no great angulation is required of the catheter to leave the needle and enter the perivascular space. Selander (1977) used a simple cannula inserted over a needle and taped in position to allow repeated injections for a prolonged block. Plancarte *et al.* (1987) introduced a 22-gauge epidural catheter through a 17-gauge Tuohy needle: the needle was rotated gently as it was inserted to ease its passage, and 6 ml of 1.5 per cent lignocaine was injected to distend the sheath before inserting the catheter. Repeated injections were given as necessary for up to 72 hours. Gaumann *et al.* (1987) used a very similar technique and attempted to thread the catheter as far proximally as possible in order to obtain the benefits of a proximal block without the risks of a supraclavicular approach. The mean distance of insertion was 12 cm from the skin and the block was maintained for up to 11 days. In 2 patients who had undergone replantation procedures, the catheter was reinserted after its initial removal had been followed by deterioration in limb blood flow. In both of these papers, the reported success rate (90 per cent and 99 per cent respectively) is higher than usual with axillary blocks, suggesting that using a catheter may be a good way of performing the block.

Continuous brachial plexus blockade has also been used to treat reflex sympathetic dystrophy and to provide analgesia for the treatment of adhesions of the elbow by continuous passive motion.

Because of the relatively slow metabolism of amide local anaesthetic agents, studies have been carried out to measure the plasma concentrations resulting from continuous brachial blocks. Tuominen *et al.* (1983) found that toxic levels were not reached with either supplementary dosage or with continuous infusion at the rate of 25 mg/hour of bupivacaine through an axillary catheter. Similar findings were reported with continuous infusion of bupivacaine through an interscalene catheter (Tuominen, 1986). Although 3 patients out of 40 were described as experiencing mild toxic symptoms, two in fact had common side-effects of interscalene block (hoarseness and Horner's syndrome); one patient suffered from dizziness which resolved when the infusion was stopped. Care should be used with any infusions of local anaesthetics in patients with multiple organ failure (Putensen, 1992) and plasma concentrations should be measured.

The supraclavicular approach

This approach to the brachial plexus utilizes the best landmarks which, even in the obese patient are seldom obscured, and it does not require the movement or manipulation of an injured arm. Because the trunks of the plexus are tightly grouped on the first rib a smaller volume of solution is required, which is an advantage in elderly patients. The resulting block gives anaesthesia for a tourniquet on the upper arm and also of the shoulder joint (although not the skin covering). The block may be used to provide anaesthesia for reduction of a dislocated shoulder when the classically dropped shoulder provides easier access to the brachial plexus. For surgery to the shoulder itself, it is necessary to inject local anaesthetic subcutaneously proximal to the shoulder to block branches of the supraclavicular nerves which supply the overlying skin. In obese patients the supraclavicular fossa often remains relatively free from fat so that the landmarks are still palpable and a brachial plexus block may be performed in preference to a difficult general anaesthetic.

When performing a supraclavicular block the modification of approach suggested by Winnie *et al.* (1975) should be used and any backwards (dorsal) angulation of the needle avoided. The patient should be positioned with his head turned away from the side of operation, and he should be asked to reach down towards his knee with the arm to be blocked, in order to drop the shoulder. The interscalene groove between the anterior and middle scalene muscles is found by palpating the posterior border of the sternomastoid muscle and then running the finger dorsally over the belly of the anterior scalene muscle until a groove is felt – usually overlaid by the external jugular vein. From this groove emerge the cervical nerve roots forming the brachial plexus, drawing out with them the fascial neurovascular sheath (Fig. 9.4). The finger should be allowed to drop downwards until the pulsations of the subclavian artery can be felt as it emerges also from the groove. With

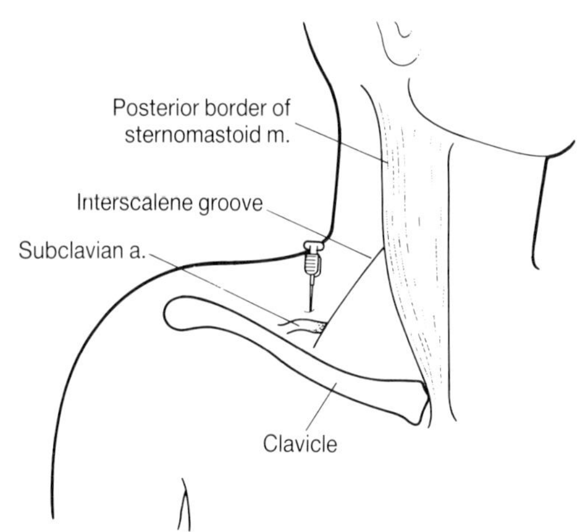

Fig 9.9 Supraclavicular approach to the brachial plexus. The needle should be inserted into the interscalene groove and advanced directly caudally. (Reproduced, with permission, from Winnie (1975).)

the finger remaining on the artery, a needle should be introduced behind (i.e. dorsal to) the finger, and thus the artery, and advanced directly caudally without angulation medially or dorsally so as to cross the neurovascular sheath in its vertical axis from above downwards (Fig. 9.9).

Beneath the needle is the first rib into which the scalene muscles are inserted. Although a click may be felt as the sheath is entered, this is less noticeable than when using the axillary approach and the end-point is paraesthesiae shooting down the arm to the hand or fingers. This usually occurs before the rib is contacted and is often at a surprisingly superficial plane. Paraesthesiae in the chest wall or shoulder should be ignored since they are probably caused by stimulation of peripheral nerves, especially the suprascapular nerve, and are a poor guide to the plexus itself. The needle should be short – no more than 4 cm – and of fine gauge, since the feel of the tissues is of little importance with this approach, and care should be taken not to aim the needle dorsally which might enter the bow of the first rib and the pleura. Upon injecting local anaesthetic, the paraesthesiae may become worse briefly before rapidly improving, and patients should be warned to prevent them moving and dislodging the needle.

This second sensation seems duller and longer-lasting than the initial electric shock and Winnie (1983) suggests that it is provoked by an increase in tissue pressure resulting from injection. If severe pain occurs, which might indicate intraneural injection, the needle should be withdrawn a little and injection recommenced. The volume of local anaesthetic required is 20–30 ml, depending on the size and the age of the patient. The development of shoulder-tip pain or a fit of coughing are associated with pleural irritation and, again, the needle should be withdrawn and landmarks checked. The patient should be observed postoperatively for development of a pneumothorax.

Accidental pneumothorax is the most serious complication of supraclavicular block and has a reported incidence of 0.6–6 per cent. However, if each patient is *X*-rayed postoperatively, the incidence rises to 25 per cent (De Jong, 1977). This means that supraclavicular block is unsuitable for day surgery, for patients with chronic respiratory disease and for patients who are to be ventilated, because of the risk of a tension pneumothorax. The clinical signs of a pneumothorax may be very slow in developing – taking 6 or 7 hours – as air leaks only slowly from a punctured lung. The patient complains of pleuritic pain and increasing difficulty in breathing. In the first instance a pneumothorax may be treated by aspiration, using a needle, three-way tap and 50 ml syringe; only if it reaccumulates is a chest drain necessary.

The interscalene approach

This approach was reported by Winnie (1970) as a logical development of the supraclavicular approach and avoids the possibility of pneumothorax by introducing the needle medial to the dome of the pleura. However, with this approach other structures are put at risk and the assembling brachial plexus is more spaced out so it is necessary for injected local anaesthetic to spread over a wide area to achieve a complete block (Fig. 9.4).

Technique of interscalene block

The patient should be positioned as for supraclavicular block and the cricoid cartilage palpated. This is the next prominent cartilage of the trachea beneath the thyroid cartilage and lies at the level of the sixth cervical vertebra. The interscalene groove is found at this level as described in the previous section, and at this point (i.e. where a line projected laterally from the cricoid cartilage crosses the interscalene groove) a needle should be inserted perpendicular to the skin in all planes through a bleb of local anaesthetic solution. The needle is thus angled slightly down, medially and slightly backwards. It should be advanced until paraesthesiae are elicited: if unsuccessful, the transverse process of the cervical vertebra is contacted and the needle should be withdrawn and reintroduced in a slightly more dorsal direction. Once paraesthesiae have been found, the desired volume of local anaesthetic should be injected. Paraesthesiae about the shoulder during interscalene block indicate successful anaesthesia in the arm in contrast to the supraclavicular approach (Roch *et al.*, 1992). Because the injection is being made at the level of C6 – that is, near the highest roots of the brachial plexus (C5-T1) – the lowest roots, which go on to form the ulnar nerve, are likely to escape blockade if an inadequate volume of solution is injected. With 20 ml of solution, the ulnar nerve is seldom blocked and must be blocked distally, whilst with 40 ml both the cervical and brachial plexuses will be blocked (Winnie, 1975). Blockade of the phrenic nerve (C4) and the recurrent laryngeal nerve on that side are to be expected so that the presence of a restrictive ventilatory defect or contralateral cord palsy are contraindications to interscalene block. Urmey and McDonald (1992) found a reduction in ventilatory function of approximately 25 per cent during interscalene block due to hemidaphragmatic palsy. Downward drainage of the local anaesthetic solution is encouraged if the block is performed with the patient sitting up, supported by a nurse. It is essential to aspirate before injection to ensure that the subarachnoid space has not been entered. After injection, further downward spread of solution may be encouraged by firm massage of the injection site. Despite these manoeuvres, the intercostobrachial nerve is rarely blocked and so pain from an arm tourniquet must be treated by subcutaneous infiltration as before.

The interscalene approach is the most proximal approach to the brachial plexus and provides excellent anaesthesia for the upper arm and shoulder, particularly if a large volume is used to include cervical blockade. Its freedom from late complications makes it suitable for day surgery of the shoulder, which is increasingly being performed. The surgery may be carried out in the 'beach chair' or sitting position which is a difficult requirement for general anaesthesia but ideal for interscalene plexus block. This approach is also suitable in the presence of infection or malignancy in the arm because it is remote from the path of lymphatic drainage.

Summary of brachial plexus blockade

Brachial plexus block is an extremely useful technique which may safely be used for any surgery of the arm – even amputation, if necessary. It is possible that, as has been found for the leg, continuous nerve blockade begun preoperatively may protect against phantom limb phenomena. The advantages of the approaches are compared in Table 9.1. The axillary approach is the most free from complications but the most restricted in application. It is suitable only for lesions of the forearm and hand but is useful for day cases and for patients with respiratory disease. The supraclavicular approach is technically the easiest but carries the worry of inducing a pneumothorax, although the likelihood is much diminished if the originally described backwards angulation of the needle is omitted and Winnie's approach adopted. The interscalene approach is suitable for day surgery and offers a more extensive block. However, although the risk of pneumothorax is remote, other complications occur; cardiorespiratory arrest after subarachnoid injection (Edde and Deutsh, 1977), phrenic nerve palsy, recurrent laryngeal nerve block, Horner's syndrome, arterial infusion (Tuominen *et al.*, 1991) and the development of transient carotid bruits (Siler *et al.*, 1973). Clearly, none of these blocks should be performed without a full appreciation of the risks and adequate resuscitation facilities.

The performance of all the blocks is improved by interposing a short length of flexible manometer tubing between the needle and the syringe so that any patient movement is neutralized and syringe changes can be accomplished without dislodging the needle (Winnie, 1969).

Peripheral blocks in the arm

Other blocks in the arm may be used to complete an incomplete brachial block or to allow distal surgery for which a tourniquet is not required: the techniques are described in standard texts of local anaesthesia. Wrist blocks and digital nerve blocks are very effective and are easily performed with only small volumes of local anaesthetic. The median nerve at the wrist and the ulnar nerve at the elbow are both subject to pressure neuritis at these sites and blocks here should be performed only when it is clear that no symptoms due to pressure are already present.

Local anaesthesia of the leg

The leg is innervated by 3 main nerve trunks arising in the lumbosacral plexus, so single-injection local anaesthesia of the leg can be achieved only with a subarachnoid or extradural technique. The cutaneous supply of the thigh is further complicated by contributions from the femoral branch of the genitofemoral nerve, the ilioinguinal nerve, the lateral cutaneous nerve of the thigh and the posterior cutaneous nerve of the thigh, all of which must be

Table 9.1 Comparison of the usual approaches of the brachial plexus

	Suitable for	Most likely failure	Complications	Contraindications
Axillary	Forearm	Musculocutaneous nerve	Intravascular injection Haematoma	Infection of the hand or arm
Supraclavicular	Arm Reduction of shoulder dislocations	Median nerve	Pneumothorax Stellate ganglion block	Respiratory disorders Day case surgery
Interscalene	Arm Shoulder	Ulnar nerve	Phrenic nerve block Subarachnoid injection Epidural injection Recurrent laryngeal nerve block	Respiratory disorders

blocked if an arterial tourniquet around the thigh is to be painless. Nevertheless, blocks of suitable peripheral nerves may usefully be combined with light general anaesthesia for surgery of the leg. Below the knee, innervation becomes simpler, involving only the terminal branches of the sciatic nerve and the saphenous branch of the femoral nerve. For surgery of the foot, nerve block at the ankle is simple to perform and, if no tourniquet is to be used, it is adequate for amputation of toes or debridement of wounds of the foot.

Femoral nerve block

Bryce-Smith (1976) proposed a refinement of the existing technique for femoral nerve block which improved the landmarks by giving an indication of the plane in which the femoral nerve lies. He suggested that the needle should be advanced lateral and cephalad to the femoral artery where it emerges from beneath the inguinal ligament so that the needle passes through this ligament. An indication of the depth of the femoral nerve is thus obtained from the loss of resistance as the needle leave the inguinal ligament. Paraesthesiae or involuntary movement of quadriceps femoris muscle may be obtained as the needle contacts the femoral nerve. Since the femoral nerve rapidly fans out into its terminal branches, the more proximal approach is likely to yield a more extensive block. The obturator nerve may be blocked in combination with the femoral nerve using the paravascular inguinal approach described by Winnie *et al.* (1973).

Paravascular technique of femoral nerve block

For this approach the needle should be directed proximally beneath the inguinal ligament immediately lateral to the femoral artery, which is marked on the skin by a finger on its lateral border (Fig. 9.10). The femoral nerve is located by obtaining paraesthesiae, and a volume of local anaesthetic should be injected while the marker finger applies pressure immediately distal to the needle to force the solution proximally towards the lumbar plexus. Finger compression should be continued after the needle is withdrawn. When volumes of local anaesthetic greater than 20 ml are injected and after paraesthesiae of the femoral nerve has been obtained, block of femoral, obturator and the lateral cutaneous nerve of the thigh should be obtained. Used alone, this technique provides analgesia of an extensive donor site for skin grafting procedures and, when combined with sciatic

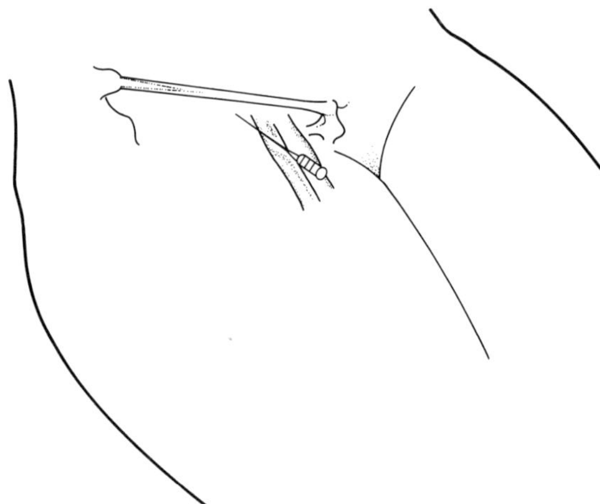

Fig 9.10 The inguinal paravascular technique of lumbar plexus anaesthesia (Reproduced, with permission from Winnie*et al.*(1973).)

nerve block, analgesia of the leg suitable for all but surgery of the proximal part of the thigh.

Sciatic nerve block

The sciatic nerve may be blocked using the elegant technique of Bryce-Smith (1966). The patient should be positioned on his side with the affected leg uppermost and slightly flexed at the hip. The sacral hiatus and greater trochanter should be identified and a 10 cm needle inserted at the mid-point of a line joining these two landmarks. This point overlies the sciatic nerve (Fig. 9.11). The needle is then advanced perpendicular to the skin and will penetrate the resistance offered by gluteus maximus muscle. Then, at a depth of about 5 cm, the nerve will be

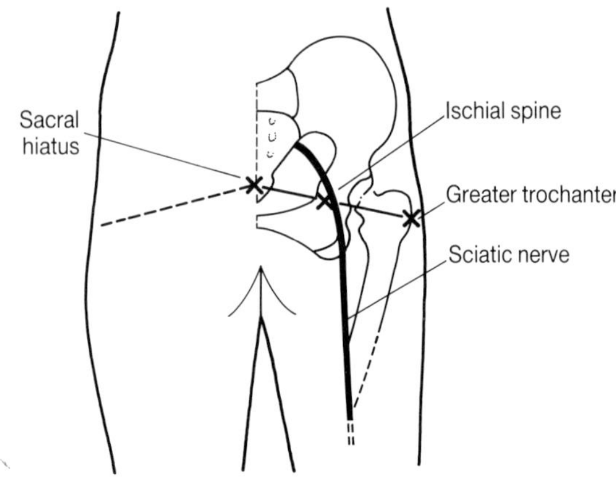

Fig 9.11 Landmarks for sciatic nerve block by a posterior approach (Reproduced with permission from Bryce-Smith (1976).)

encountered as a further, though lesser, resistance and the patient will experience paraesthesiae, often accompanied by involuntary muscle movement. At this point, 5 ml of 2 per cent lignocaine should be injected – the more concentrated solution is required because of the size of the sciatic nerve and therefore the distance over which diffusion of local anaesthetic agent must take place. Although methods are described for blocking the sciatic nerve by an anterior or lateral approach, in practice they are disappointing (Winnie, 1975; Bryce-Smith, 1976). Such techniques would clearly be very useful for patients who find it impossible to position themselves for the posterior approach because of pain in the limb or established traction apparatus. If high success rates are to be obtained using these techniques, the use of a nerve stimulator is advisable because the anatomical landmarks, by which the passage of the needle must be guided, are poor.

Nerve block at the ankle

The technique of nerve block at the ankle described by Bryce-Smith (1976) is simple to carry out and consistently successful, providing good analgesia of the foot. Whilst valuable as a technique for work in the accident and emergency department for the treatment of trauma of the foot, it is also an extremely useful block for the provision of pain relief after elective surgery of the foot and toes.

Intra-articular anaesthesia

Local anaesthesia of a joint may be produced by the injection of lignocaine or bupivacaine directly into the joint. Intra articular anaesthesia has been reported as a means of providing postoperative analgesia for day case arthroscopy (Allum and Ribbans, 1987); after Keller's arthroplasty (Porter and Davies, 1985) and even for management of osteoarthritic hip pain (Flanagan *et al.*, 1988). However, it is also possible to use intra-articular anaesthesia as sole anaesthetic for diagnostic arthroscopy and arthroscopic surgery of the knee. Intra-articular anaesthesia is particularly suitable for day cases and provides excellent postoperative analgesia with no loss in motor power such as that which follows femoral nerve block. Thus, the patient can climb onto the operating table and, at the end of the procedure, climb down and walk away.

The technique is very simple: the knee is flexed to 90° and the arthroscopy portals identified either side of the patella and infiltrated with lignocaine 1 per cent with adrenaline. In fact, only the skin and synovium are sensitive and movement of the needle in the intervening fat pad is barely noticeable. A needle is then advanced directly into the knee and the joint distended with 30 ml of bupivacaine 0.5 per cent with adrenaline. The patient should be asked to make bicycling movements with the leg for a minute or so in order to distribute the local anaesthetic throughout the knee and then left for 20–30 minutes for the block to become effective. There is obviously no analgesia for a tourniquet and the surgeon must be prepared to operate without one but, provided adrenaline containing local anaesthetic has been used, there is little need, for bleeding within the knee is minimal. For the surgeon, the only other noticeable difference from operating during general anaesthesia is that the knee is less relaxed and freedom of movement is limited. However, with the patient awake, the surgeon can demonstrate lesions in the patient's knee and discuss management options. Blood levels of the local anaesthetics injected are very low and there is a wide margin of safety (Eriksson *et al.*, 1986).

This technique is satisfactory for diagnostic arthroscopy, and minor arthroscopic surgery such as trimming of meniscal tears: it is less satisfactory in the presence of active synovitis when synovial hyperaemia may disperse the injected local anaesthetic.

Fairclough *et al.* (1990) compared intra-articular anaesthesia with femoral nerve block and general anaesthesia in 136 patients. They found the regional techniques gave rise to problems in 16 patients caused by restricted access due to poor relaxation, pain when a tourniquet was used (unsurprising) and bleeding into the joint. Femoral nerve block is likely to increase vascularity of the knee and Fairclough and colleagues used adrenaline free local anaesthetic for the intra articular block.

The use of a nerve stimulator

The performance of most regional blocks is made easier if a nerve stimulator is used. The purpose of the nerve stimulator is to locate mixed nerves by movement of muscles supplied by the motor component of the nerves in response to an applied electrical stimulus. The nerve stimulator (Fig. 9.12) should be capable of continuously variable output so

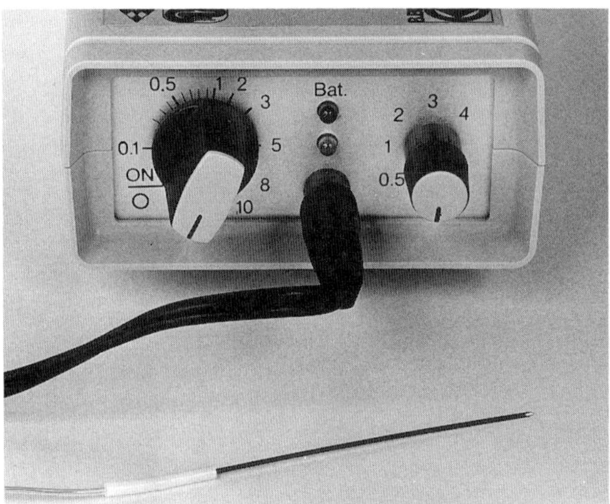

Fig 9.12 Nerve stimulator and insulated needle. The nerve stimulator has controls for stimulus size (left) and frequency (right) and indicator lights for battery condition and activity. The needle is insulated along the shaft leaving the tip bare.

that the smallest signal consistent with a response can be used to locate the nerve, and it should be capable of operating at 1–2 hertz so that the block can be performed speedily. Although originally specially prepared sheathed needles were used, Montgomery *et al.* (1973) demonstrated that it was not necessary to sheathe the shaft because the current density was so much greater at the tip than along the shaft: any needle of choice can be used.

To perform a block, the positive lead from the stimulator should be connected to a skin electrode up to 30 cm distant from the negative lead clipped to the hub of the needle, in order to create a depolarizing current at the axonal cell wall. After the needle has been introduced through the skin a high stimulus should be set, say 1ma, and the needle advanced with stimulation at 2 hertz: if no motor response is obtained, the stimulator is faulty and most likely needs a new battery. Once a response has been obtained, the stimulus should be reduced to 0.1–0.3 ma and the needle advanced to find the point of maximum response. At this point 2 ml of local anaesthetic should be injected: if the needle is positioned close to the nerve there will be almost immediate loss of muscle response (Raj, 1983) and the complete dose should be injected.

Complications of regional anaesthesia: nerve damage

In the series of regional blocks reported by Edmonds-Seal (1980) 2 patients had long-lasting neurological sequelae probably caused by direct damage to the nerve. In each patient the nerve damaged was the sciatic nerve which is particularly at risk: it is a large structure and many descriptions of sciatic nerve block urge transfixion of the nerve. Selander *et al.* (1977) investigated nerve damage from needles and published graphic photomicrographs of severed nerve fibres after transfixion with a long-bevelled cutting needle: they recommended that a 45° bevelled needle less frequently produces fascicular damage and should therefore be recommended for use in clinical anaesthesia.

More recently, Rice and McMahon (1992) examined the development of neurological lesions after transfixion injury of the rat sciatic nerve with both long and short-bevelled needles. In contrast to Selander and colleagues, who looked at nerve lesions immediately after impalement, Rice and McMahon studied the development of lesions and subsequent regeneration of nerve fibres over 28 days and came to a contrary conclusion. They found that when nerve fascicles are impaled, lesions occur less frequently, are less severe and (most important) are repaired more rapidly if they are caused by a long-bevelled needle. They further noted that damage was least if the bevel of the needle was aligned with the nerve fibres. Clearly more work is needed in this field, but for the present, the possibility of nerve injury must be borne in mind, disposable injection needles with a double-ground cutting bevel (i.e. to enter the skin easily) should be avoided and the bevel of the needle used should be aligned with the fibres of the nerve to be blocked. Whilst demonstrating that neurological injury is very rare, Wooley and Vandam (1959) advised that brachial blocks should not be used in patients such as musicians in whom a lasting minor neurological injury would be disabling.

Conclusion

Successful regional anaesthesia for operative surgery demands skill, practice and time: the techniques may be difficult but they are extremely rewarding and are often much appreciated by patients. It is important to explain to the surgeon what nerve blocks have been performed so that when he examines the patient postoperatively, he is not alarmed by loss of function and is aware that pain will not be a warning sign of developing complications. Fingers and toes should be left exposed and examined from time to time for colour and temperature.

References

Allum, R. L. and Ribbans, W. J. (1987). Day case arthroscopy and arthroscopic surgery of the knee. *Annals of the Royal College of Surgeons of England*, **69**, 225–6.

Ang, E. T., Lassale, B. and Goldfarb, G. (1984). Continuous axillary plexus block – a clinical and anatomical study. *Anesthesia and Analgesia*, **63**, 680–4.

Bryce-Smith, R. (1966). Local and regional analgesia. *Postgraduate Medical Journal*, **42**, 367.

Bryce-Smith, R. and Lee, J. A. (eds) (1976). *Practical Regional Anaesthesia*. Excerpta Medica and Elsevier, New York.

Cotev, S. and Robin, G. C. (1966). Experimental studies on intravenous regional analgesia using radioactive lignocaine. *British Journal of Anaesthesia*, **38**, 936–9.

Davis, A. H., Hall, I. D., Wilkey, A. D., Smith, J. E., Walford, A. J., Kale, V. R. (1984). Intravenous regional anaesthesia. The dangers of the congested arm and the value of occlusion pressure. *Anaesthesia*, **39**, 416–22.

Davis, J. A. H. and Walford, A. J. (1986). Intravenous regional anaesthesia for foot surgery. *Acta Anaesthesiologica Scandinavica*, **30**, 145–7.

De Jong, R. H. (1977). *Local Anaesthetics*. Thomas, Springfield, Ill.

Editorial (1965). Regional intravenous anesthesia. *Journal of the American Medical Association*, **193**, 300.

Edmonds-Seal, J., Paterson, G. M. C. and Loach, A. B. (1980). Local nerve blocks for postoperative analgesia. *Journal of the Royal Society of Medicine*, **73**, 111–15.

El Hassan, K. M., Hutton, P. and Black, A. M. S. (1984). Venous pressure and arm volume changes during simulated Bier's block. *Anaesthesia*, **39**, 229–36.

Eriksson, E. (1979). *Illustrated Handbook of Local Anaesthesia*, Lloyd Luke, London.

Eriksson, E., Haggmark, T., Saartok, T., Sebik, A. and Ortengren, B. (1986). Knee arthroscopy with local anaesthesia in ambulatory patients. *Orthopaedics*, **9**, 186–8.

Fanard, L., Van Steenberge, A., Demeire, X. and Van der Puyl, F. (1988). Comparison between propofol and midazolam as sedative agents for surgery under regional anaesthesia. *Anaesthesia*, **43** suppl., 87–9.

Fairclough, J. A., Graham, G. P., and Pemberton, D. (1990). Local or general anaesthesia in day case arthroscopy? *Annals of the Royal College of Surgeons of England*, **72**, 104–7.

Flanagan, J., Casale, F. F., Thomas, T. L. and Desai, K. B. (1988). Intra-articular injection for pain relief in patients awaiting hip replacement. *Annals of the Royal College of Surgeons of England*, **70**, 156–7.

Gaumann, D., Lennon, R. L. and Wedel, D. J. (1987). Axillary plexus block: proximal catheter technique for postoperative pain management. *Anesthesiology*, **67**, 3A, A242.

Gielen, M. J. M. and Viering, W. (1986). Three-in-one lumbar plexus block for muscle biopsy in malignant hyperthermia patients: amide local anaesthetic agents may be used safely. *Acta Anaesthesiologica Scandinavica*, **30**, 581–3.

Grice, S. C., Morrell, R. C., Balestrieri, F. J., Stump, D. A. and Howard, G. (1986). Intravenous regional anaesthesia evaluation and prevention of leakage under the tourniquet. *Anesthesiology*, **65**, 316–20.

Hempel, V., Van Finck, M. and Baumgartner, E. (1981). A longitudinal supraclavicular approach to the brachial plexus for the insertion of plastic cannulas. *Anesthesia and Analgesia*, **60**, 352.

Jeyaseelan, S., Stevenson, T. M. and Pfitzner, J. (1981). Tourniquet failure and arterial calcification: case report and theoretical dangers. *Anaesthesia*, **36**, 48–51.

Larsen, U. T. and Hommelgaard, P. (1987). Pneumatic tourniquet paralysis following intravenous regional analgesia. *Anaesthesia*, **42**, 526–9.

Montgomery, S. J., Raj, P. P., Nettles, D. and Jenkins, M. T. (1973). The use of the nerve stimulator with standard unsheathed needles in nerve blockade. *Anesthesia and Analgesia*, **52**, 827.

Newman, R. J. and Radda, S. K. (1983). The myotoxicity of bupivacaine, a 31P NMR investigation. *British Journal of Pharmacology*, **79**, 395–9.

Partridge, B. L., Katz, J. and Benirshke, K. (1987). Functional anatomy of the brachial plexus sheath: implications for anaesthesia. *Anesthesiology*, **66**, 743–7.

Pfeiffer, P. M. (1986). Acute rhabdomyolysis following surgery for burns – possible role of tourniquet ischaemia. *Anaesthesia*, **41**, 614–19.

Plancarte, A., Amascua, C., Marron, M., San Miguel, P. and Aldrete, J. A. (1987). Continuous brachial plexus block introducing catheters through a Tuohy needle in the axilla. *Anesthesiology*, **67**, 3A A287.

Porter, K. M. and Davies, J. (1985). The control of pain after Keller's procedure – a controlled double blind prospective trial with local anaesthetic and placebo. *Annals of the Royal College of Surgeons of England*, **67**, 293–4.

Putensen, C., Lingnau, W., Putesen-Himmer, G. and Herold, M. (1992). Plasma lignocaine concentrations associated with extradural analgesia in patients with and without multiple organ failure. *British Journal of Anaesthesia*, **69**, 513–17.

Raj, P. P., Montgomery, S. J., Nettles, D. and Jenkins,

M. T. (1973). Infraclavicular brachial plexus block – a new approach. *Anesthesia and Analgesia,* **52,** 897.

Raj, P. P. (1983). Mechanical aids. In Henderson, J. J. and Nimmo, W. S. (eds), *Practical Regional Anaesthesia.* Blackwell, Oxford.

Rice, A. S. C., McMahon, S. B. (1992). Peripheral nerve injury caused by injection needles used in regional anaesthesia: influence of bevel configuration, studied in a rat model. *British Journal of Anaesthesia,* **69,** 433–8.

Roch, J. J., Sharrock, N. E. and Neudachin, L. (1992). Interscalene brachial plexus block for shoulder surgery: a proximal paresthesia is effective. *Anesthesia and Analgesia,* **75**(3), 386–8.

Saint-Maurice, C. and Shulte Steinberg, O. (eds) (0000) *Regional Anaesthesia in Children.* Mediglobe, SA, Fribourg.

Scott, D. B. (1984). The use of local anaesthesia in the Accident and Emergency Department. Royal College of Surgeons Anniversary Forum: The Anaesthetist in the Accident and Emergency Department. Royal College of Surgeons, London.

Selander, D. (1977). Catheter techniques in axillary plexus block. *Acta Anaesthesiologica Scandinavica,* **21,** 324–9.

Selander, D., Dhuner, K. G. and Lundborg, G. (1977). Peripheral nerve injury due to injection needles used for regional anaesthesia. *Acta Anaesthesiologica Scandinavica,* **21,** 182–8.

Selander, D. (1987). Axillary plexus block: paresthetic or perivascular? *Anesthesiology,* **66,** 726–8.

Siler, J. N., Lief, P. F. and Davis, F. J. (1973). A new complication of interscalene brachial plexus block. *Anesthesiology,* **38,** 590.

Sims, J. K. (1977). A modification of landmarks for infraclavicular approach to brachial plexus block. *Anesthesia and Analgesia,* **56,** 554.

Thompson, G. E. and Rorie, D. K. (1983). Functional anatomy of the brachial plexus sheaths. *Anesthesiology,* **59,** 117–22.

Tucker, G. T. and Boas, R. A. (1971). Pharmacokinetic aspects of intravenous regional anesthesia. *Anesthesiology,* **34,** 538.

Tuominen, M. K., Rosenberg, P. H. and Kalso, E. (1983). Blood levels of bupivacaine after single dose and during continuous infusion in axillary plexus block. *Acta Anaesthesiologica Scandinavica,* **27,** 303–6.

Tuominen, M. K., Pitkanen, M. T. and Rosenberg, P. H. (1986). Continuous interscalene brachial plexus block with bupivacaine for postoperative pain relief. *Anesthesiology,* **65,** 3A A197.

Tuominen, M. K., Pere, P. and Rosenberg, P. H. (1991). Unintentional arterial catheterization and bupivacaine toxicity associated with continuous interscalene brachial plexus block. *Anesthesiology,* **75,** 356–8.

Urmey, W. F. and McDonald, M. (1992). Hemidiaphragmatic paresis during interscalene brachial plexus block: effects on pulmonary function and chest wall mechanics. *Anesthesia and Analgesia,* **74,** 352–7.

Vester-Anderson, T., Husum, B., Lindeborg, T., Borits, L., Gothgen, I. (1984). Perivascular axillary block IV: blockade following 40, 50, 60 ml of mepivacaine 1% with adrenaline. *Acta Anaesthesiologica Scandinavica,* **28,** 99–105.

Vester-Anderson, T., Broby-Johanson, U. and Bro-Rasmussen, F. (1986). Perivascular axillary block VI: the distribution of gelatine solution injected into the axillary neurovascular sheath of cadavers. *Acta Anaesthesiologica Scandinavica,* **30,** 18–22.

Vongvises, P. and Panijayanond, T. (1979). Parascalene technique of brachial plexus anesthesia. *Anesthesia and Analgesia,* **58,** 267.

Winnie, A. P. (1969). An 'immobile needle' for nerve blocks. *Anesthesiology,* **31,** 577.

Winnie, A. P. (1970). Interscalene brachial plexus blocks. *Anesthesia and Analgesia,* **49,** 455.

Winne, A. P., Ramamurthy, S. and Durrani, Z. (1973). The inguinal paravascular technic of lumbar plexus anesthesia: the three-in-one block. *Anesthesia and Analgesia,* **52,** 989–96.

Winne, A. P. (1975). Regional anaesthesia. *Surgical Clinics of North America,* **55,** 861–92.

Winnie, A. P., Tay, C. H., Patel, K. P., Ramamurthy, S. and Durrani, Z. (1975). Pharmacokinetics of local anaesthetics during plexus blocks. *Anesthesia and Analgesia,* **56,** 852.

Winnie, A. P. (1983). *Plexus Anaesthesia, Vol. 1: Perivascular Technics of Brachial Plexus Block.* Churchill Livingstone, Edinburgh.

Wooley, J. D. and Vandam, L. D. (1959). Neurological sequelae of brachial plexus nerve block. *Annals of Surgery,* **149,** 53–60.

Chapter 10

Day surgery

Introduction

'A surgical day case is a patient who is admitted for investigation or operation on a planned non-resident basis and occupies for a period a bed in a ward or unit set aside for the purpose' (Guidelines for Day Case Surgery, Royal College of Surgeons of England, 1985).

There is considerable financial and social pressure to extend the range and the amount of day case surgery because it is cheaper and faster than routine hospital admission. At present between 8 and 26 per cent of orthopaedic surgery is performed as day cases in the Oxford regional hospitals, with the smallest percentage at the teaching centre. National figures vary enormously due to confusion of day cases with outpatients or day-stay cases.

In general, orthopaedic surgeons have been slow to take up day surgery; there is a paucity of papers in the literature, and only a small number of cases is considered suitable (Table 10.1) although this is expanding. Patients over 65 years of age make up a large proportion of orthopaedic case load and rates of day surgery in this age group are generally low. The reluctance of surgeons arises from concern about the development of complications where the patient cannot be observed and the management of pain once the patient is home. Some of the problems are illustrated by Tibrewal and Foss (1991) who examined the difficulties associated with performing metatarsal osteotomy (Wilson's osteotomy) on day cases: of the 43 cases surveyed, none was re-admitted but difficulties arose in 13 patients over 55 years of age. These older patients felt it had been a struggle for their family for the first few days because they were very dependent, and 3 of the 13 had called their doctor for reassurance and a further supply of analgesics. Surgical results did not suffer and were similar to those obtained with full hospital admission, but this was bought at the expense of other agencies; general practitioners and carers.

Table 10.1 Orthopaedic operations suitable for day surgery (modified from Guidelines for Day-Case Surgery, RCS, 1992)

Manipulation of joints
Removal of pins, plates or screws
Change of plaster
Carpal tunnel release
Ganglionectomy and excision of synovial cysts and benign synoviomata
Removal of neuroma
Amputation of the fingers and lesser toes
Removal of foreign bodies
Scar revision and simple skin grafts
Excision of dupuytren's contracture
Relief of trigger finger
Diagnostic arthroscopy and arthroscopic surgery
Some radiological studies under anaesthesia
Chronic pain relief procedures and epidural injection

Day surgery is popular with patients because a firm date can be booked, without the likelihood of cancellation or postponement caused by other more urgent cases and because it interferes with work or domestic life much less. Day surgery is also patently less 'grave' than normal hospital admission.

Day surgery is particularly successful for children but it needs careful planning. Children should not be mixed with adult patients but rather the unit should be dedicated to children one day a week or fortnight. A play area should be set aside and easy chairs provided for parents. Children recover from anaesthesia very rapidly and it may be possible to have morning and afternoon operating lists.

In the face of a shortage of nurses and a dwindling number of inpatient beds, day surgery offers a means of using resources more efficiently and devoting inpatient operating sessions to major surgery only. There is, however, a growing fear that because minor cases can be dealt with much more speedily, general practitioners are offering minor surgery to patients more liberally so that although more work is being done, more work will need to be done! Difficulties also arise with teaching because common minor conditions are no longer available to students and junior medical staff on the wards.

Organization

The key to successful operation of a day surgery unit is thorough organization, from outpatient appointment to discharge from the day surgery unit. This will ensure that although contact with the patient is brief, management is as good as for in-patients because the use of protocols saves time. These protocols are drawn up for the unit and must be adhered to, but may be modified in the light of experience.

There are 2 ways in which day surgery fails; first, if preoperative selection is not rigorous, patients may be admitted who need extensive preoperative preparation and work is disrupted; and secondly, if junior anaesthetists or surgeons perform the operations, the complication rate rises and too many patients have to stay overnight.

At surgical outpatients, those patients whose operation falls within one of the suitable categories and who meet the other criteria for day surgery may be scheduled for the Day Surgery Unit (DSU). The patient should be ASA 1 or 2 and under 65–70 years of age, depending on what is proposed. This implies a different approach to the organization of surgical outpatient clinics. Time must be allowed for a complete medical and social history so that health risks and adverse social factors are not overlooked. If a procedure is intended under regional anaesthesia, then selection need not be quite so stringent. Time is saved if patients fill in a questionnaire about their previous medical history, living conditions and help at home, which should be checked by a nurse (a sample questionnaire is given in Guidelines for Day Surgery, Royal College of Surgeons, 1992). A date for operation can be discussed which fits in with school terms and holidays. If a patient is not considered suitable for day surgery, the reason should be explained to him and his doctor informed (Table 10.2).

Table 10.2 Patients who are unsuitable for day surgery

Those with severe systemic disease, insulin dependant diabetes mellitus, myocardial ischaemia
Those with coagulopathies or haemoglobinopathies
Obesity
Those who live more than half-an-hour away from the hospital
Social reasons; the patient lives alone; no escort can be found
Home circumstances inadequate, no lavatory nearby

Home circumstances are very important, since this is where the majority of postoperative care will take place. Patients must be questioned carefully about companions – will they be present throughout or simply look in – and about physical resources – how difficult will it be to make a cup of tea or go to the lavatory? If need be, the general practitioner or the district nurse should be consulted about the suitability of their patients for day surgery.

Patient information

A few days before admission patients should be sent details of the DSU and what is expected of them, together with confirmation of the admission date. If this letter is sent too soon, it is likely to be lost or disregarded. The information sent must contain a map showing the DSU and car parking facilities, and precise instructions for time of arrival with an escort, together with a list of what patients should bring with them. If patients are late arriving because the DSU is difficult to find, or no parking space is available, a full schedule of operating can become an impossible one. Patients should be instructed to have nothing to eat or drink that morning. This may be relaxed if regional anaesthesia is intended but to avoid confusion, it is helpful to keep separate lists for regional anaesthesia and general anaesthesia. A contact telephone number should be included so that any queries the patient may have can be answered. Finally, patients must be warned not to expect to drive or operate machinery in the 48 hours after general anaesthesia. It will be necessary to repeat this instruction after admission, and even so there is a suggestion that 30 per cent of patients disregard it.

Techniques of anaesthesia

The techniques of anaesthesia used in the DSU are simple and basic because the surgery is minor, taking 30 minutes or less. Nevertheless considerable skill and expertise in these techniques are necessary for the list to proceed smoothly and swiftly with no anaesthetic complications. It is a paradox of day surgery that the most minor cases demand the most senior staff.

At the beginnning of the morning, the anaesthetist should visit each patient and discuss anaesthesia with him or her whilst checking through their medical history. Any drugs the patient is taking should be identified and the time of the last dose verified. It is preferable that patients on regular medication should take it: the volume of water required to swallow tablets does not increase the risk of aspiration (Goodwin *et al.*, 1991). Premedication is usually unnecessary and, if given, may predjudice the patient's recovery after anaesthesia. If a patient is very apprehensive, a short-acting benzodiazepine can be given, such as midazolam 5 mg intramuscularly, and the operation scheduled for early in the day to allow ample time for recovery.

General anesthesia

Day surgery has been rendered a great deal easier by the development of ultra-short-acting intravenous anaesthetics and analgesics. The introduction of propofol, in particular, was the boost needed for day surgery to take off. In essence there are two techniques for general anaesthesia; a total intravenous technique (TIVA) based on propofol, and an inhalational technique (IT) based on isoflurane after propofol induction. All patients should be monitored; from before induction to recovery, with display of the electrocardiogram, blood pressure from a noninvasive device and haemoglobin saturation.

For TIVA, induction is accomplished with alfentanil 0.5 mg and a bolus of propofol 2.5 g/kg, and anaesthesia is maintained with either an infusion of propofol from a syringe driver or increments of propofol given manually at 9–15 mg/kg/hour (12 mg/kg/hr, Nightingale and Lewis, 1992, 10 mg/kg/hr, Gunawardene and White, 1988; 12–15 mg/kg/hr, Price *et al.*, 1988). The patients breathe oxygen-enriched air.

Alternatively, anaesthesia may be induced with alfentanil and propofol as above, and then followed with nitrous oxide, oxygen and isoflurane administered from either a laryngeal mask or a face mask and a Lack circuit. Little is saved by using a closed circle because the operating time is not much longer than that taken to fill the breathing system and denitrogenate the patient at high flows. When compared with TIVA, anaesthesia time is slightly increased by the time taken to reach surgical anaesthesia with the inhalational agent. For very minor operations, the opioid can be omitted from both sequences since it has been shown to confer little benefit in either the dose of propofol required or in quality of anaesthesia (Moffat *et al.*, 1989).

There is little to choose between the two techniques. The overall cost is similar and only subtle differences in quality of recovery over the first hour were found by Nightingale and Lewis (1992) on psychometric testing. This difference might have been accounted for by the slightly longer anaesthesia in the IT group and is of questionable clinical significance. Interestingly, although clinical recovery was complete by the time of discharge, none of the patients felt completely recovered 72 hours later. No patient was nauseated in hospital but 10 per cent of patients had been sick by 72 hours postoperatively. This is often prompted by the car journey home.

Alfentanil and propofol are known to cause very little nausea and vomiting (Gunawardene and White, 1988) and propofol may even have anti-emetic properties (McCollum *et al.*, 1988). In contrast both nitrous oxide (Alexander *et al.*, 1984) and isoflurane (Palazzo and Strunin, 1984) are associated with postoperative vomiting.

Intense pain during injection of propofol can be a problem, particularly if the patient is apprehensive or vasoconstricted and the injection vein is small. The pain can be reduced either by storing the propofol in a refrigerator and injecting it at 4° (McCrirrick and Hunter, 1990) or by adding lignocaine 0.1 mg/kg (Gehan *et al.*, 1991).

Each of these techniques can be accompanied by a suitable regional block, both to minimize drug dosage for general anaesthesia and to provide postoperative pain relief. With some of the more painful procedures, TIVA is difficult to manage without a regional block and IT may be easier.

Regional anaesthesia

A great deal of orthopaedic day surgery can be performed under regional anaesthesia and it is not difficult to construct regular local anaesthesia day surgery lists. Such lists can include all minor surgery of the arm and hand, many ganglions and other superficial lumps for biopsy, and diagnostic arthroscopies. Regional anaesthesia is particularly suitable for the elderly in order to avoid general anaesthesia. Techniques of peripheral nerve block are considered in Chapter 9.

Intrathecal anaesthesia

Intrathecal anaesthesia for day cases has not yet gained ground in the United Kingdom. Bridenbaugh (1983) reported 12 years experience of outpatient intrathecal anaesthesia in America whilst Atkinson and Lee (1985) blamed conservatism for lack of interest in Britain. Sarma and Bostrom (1990) reported their experience of intrathecal anaesthesia for day surgery in Sweden. Fifty-five of the 160 patients studied were undergoing orthopaedic procedures; arthroscopy, arthroscopic meniscectomy, hallux valgus correction, metatarsal osteotomy, achilles tendon repair and removal of intramedullary nails. Each patient received intrathecal bupivacaine 0.5 per cent heavy through either a 25 swg needle or a 26 swg needle, and intravenous fluids, vasopressors and sedatives as necessary: the blocks were performed before 1200 and all patients went home the same day. Despite not being instructed to lie flat for 24 hours only 15 patients (9.4 per cent) developed a postspinal headache. No patient required readmission for surgical complications but two patients needed a blood patch for a severe postspinal headache. The incidence of postspinal headache was 4 times as great with 25 swg needles as with 26 swg needles and decreased with age. The difference with age is confirmed elsewhere; Kortum *et al.* (1982) used a 22 swg needle and reported a 33 per cent incidence of headache in patients aged 20–29 but only a 6.2 per cent incidence in patients aged 60–69 years. Intrathecal anaesthesia clearly can be used for day surgery and 91 per cent of Sarma and Bostrom's cases were satisfied with the experience. Some of the surgery reported in this study is ambitious for day cases; removal of an intramedullary nail, for example, can take a long time if the nail is buried and difficult to find and is followed by severe postoperative pain. Nevertheless, if day surgery is to expand into more extensive surgery, then intrathecal anaesthesia may be a better alternative to deeper inhalational anaesthesia, and should not be overlooked.

Recovery and discharge

Recovery takes place in three stages; recovery of vital reflexes and conciousness, so that the patient may leave the recovery bay and does not need constant supervision; recovery from anaesthesia and surgery so that the patient is fit to go home; finally, complete recovery so that a patient may operate complex machinery. In addition to assessing recovery, anaesthetists must also consider postoperative analgesia and the need for anti-emetics.

Postoperative analgesia will depend upon residual analgesia from intravenous opioids given during the course of anaesthesia, any local blocks which have been performed and the use of NSAIDs. It is best to avoid potent opioids if possible because the drowsiness, respiratory depression and nausea make it unlikely that the patient will be fit to go home. Diclofenac 100 mg given as a suppository at the end of surgery can be supplemented if need be by an oral preparation. Pain after orthopaedic surgery is more amenable to NSAIDs than is pain after abdominal surgery where results have been disappointing. The place of prophylactic treatment with potent anti-emetics such as ondansetron is still being assessed but patients with a history of troublesome vomiting after general anaesthesia should receive an anti-emetic peri-operatively.

In the late afternoon the anaesthetist and surgeon should review the patients prior to discharge and make sure that recovery is clinically complete, that pain relief is adequate and the patient is not nauseated: if there is any doubt, overnight admission should be arranged. Before discharge patients should be given typewritten instructions about dressings and the care of their wound, whether stitches need removal and by whom, and whom to contact in an emergency, together with a supply of analgesics. They should be warned again not operate machinery or drive for 48 hours and not to make important decisions or sign documents for 24 hours. The hospital contact number should be repeated. A discharge letter to the general practitioner which gives details of what operation has been performed and what drugs have been given should be given to the patient to pass to his doctor or faxed directly to the surgery provided arrangements are made to guarantee confidentiality. More information about day surgery is available in the extensive review of day surgery published by White.

The design of the unit

Desirable features for a day surgery unit are sketched out in the Guidelines for day surgery (RCS, 1985). This report emphasizes that day surgery is minor or intermediate surgery performed on a day basis from a dedicated ward and requires similar surgical (and anaesthetic) facilities to inpatient surgery. The ward has minor modifications to enable it to act both as a receiving and discharge centre.

Units vary in size from 10–30 beds depending upon how may specialties use the unit and what type of surgery. At the Nuffield Orthopaedic Centre, the unit has 6 beds and two recovery bays serving one theatre to give a maximum day's operating of 8 cases, which should finish by early afternoon to allow time for recovery before discharge from 1600 onwards. A ground floor ward with easy external access is desirable with car parking nearby so that walking is reduced to a minimum. It is best if patients do not have to use a lift after anaesthesia since the vertical acceleration may provoke nausea. The ward itself should be light and airy (Fig. 10.1) with an adjacent waiting area for family and friends. The theatre should be close to the ward to avoid long delays between cases and, ideally, should interconnect with the main theatre block to reduce the isolation of staff. This arrangement also increases the flexibility of the theatre space which is accessible from the main hospital and can be used at the end of the day's operating for septic cases without contaminating the main theatres.

Conclusion

More day surgery is advocated by the Value for Money unit of the Department of Health ('Day surgery: making it happen', 1991) and the percentage of day cases performed will rise towards the 40–50 per cent of all cases expected, thus releasing resources for other improvements and increasing the number of patients treated.

The provision of purpose designed facilities for day surgery provides an enormous incentive for medical staff to explore what can be done as day cases and can easily be seen as a good investment with a good rate of return on capital. Day cases which are performed from inpatient wards and inserted into routine operating lists are relatively inefficient, allowing small financial savings, and interrupting operating lists. The anaesthetist must

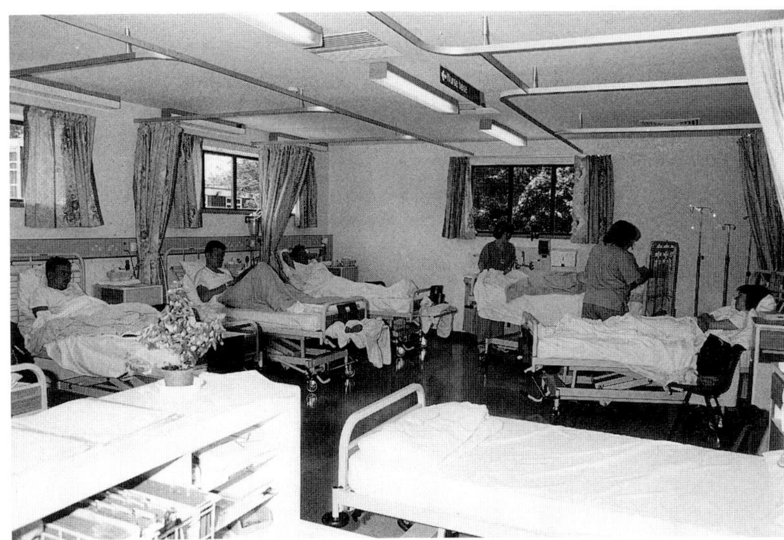

Fig 10.1 Day surgery ward. This is a ground floor ward with easy access and a light pleasant atmosphere.

absent himself from the list to see the patients pre-operatively and later to discharge them: it becomes difficult to give proper care to either group of patients.

Pitfalls in day case operating were highlighted by Bonney (1992), who reported 9 cases seen by him personally at the request of solicitors. Seven of the cases involved damage to nerves, one a non-union of an ulnar osteotomy and the last an operation performed on the wrong site. Particular failures which he identified included delegation of operations to in-experienced junior staff; the absence of any arrangement for the patient to be seen by any clinician before discharge; failure to provide patients with adequate instructions on going home and failing to make arrangements for patients to return and be seen and managed by the responsible clinician in the event of a postoperative emergency. All these cases concerned orthopaedic patients. Finally, enthusiasm should not outrun the wishes of patients: Senapati and Young (1989) found that whereas before operation 51 patients preferred the idea of day surgery to inpatient admission, only 14 still felt the same afterwards!

References

Atkinson, R. S. and Lee, J. A. (1985). Spinal anaesthesia for day case surgery? *Anaesthesia*, **40**, 1059–60.

Alexander, G. D., Skrupski, J. N. and Brown, E. M. (1984). The role of nitrous oxide in postoperative nausea and vomiting. *Anaesthesia and Analgesia*, **63**, 175.

Bonney, G. (1992). Pitfalls in 'day case' operating. *Journal of the Medical Defence Union*, **8**, 4–5.

Bridenbaugh, L. D. (1983). Regional anaesthesia for outpatient surgery – a summary of 12 years' experience. *Canadian Anaesthetists' Society Journal*, **30**, 548–52.

Day Surgery: Making it Happen (1991). Value for Money Unit, Department of Health and Social Security, HMSO, London.

Dundee, J. W., Nichol, R. M. and Moore, J. (1962). Studies of drugs given before anaesthesia III. A method for the study of their effects on postoperative vomiting and nausea. *British Journal of Anaesthesia*, **34**, 527–35.

Gehan, G., Karoubi, P., Quinet, F., Leroy, A., Rathat, C. and Pourriat, J. L. (1991). Optimal dose of lignocaine for preventing pain on injection of propofol. *British Journal of Anaesthesia*, **66**, 324–6.

Goodwin, A. P. L., Rowe, W. L., Ogg, T. W. and Samaan, A. (1991). Oral fluids prior to day surgery. *Anaesthesia*, **46**, 1066–8.

Gunawardene, R. D. and White, D. C. (1988). Propofol and emesis. *Anaesthesia*, **43**, suppl., 65–7.

Kortum, K., Nolte, H. and Kenkman, H. J. (1982). Sex difference related complication rates after spinal anaesthesia. *Regional Anaesthesia*, **5**, 1–6.

McCollum, J. S. C., Milligan, K. R. and Dundee, J. W. (1988). Antiemetic action of propofol. *Anaesthesia*, **43**, 239–40.

McCrirrick, A. and Hunter, S. (1990). Pain on injection of propofol: the effect of injectate temperature. *Anaesthesia*, **45**, 443–4.

Moffat, A. C., Murray, A. W. and Fitch, W. (1989). Opioid supplementation during propofol anaesthesia. *Anaesthesia*, **44**, 644–7.

Nightingale, J. J. and Lewis, I. H. (1992). Recovery from day-case anaesthesia: comparison of total iv anaesthesia using propofol with an inhalation technique. *British Journal of Anaesthesia*, **68**, 356–9.

NHS Management Executive. Value for Money Unit (1991). Day Surgery: Making It Happen. HMSO, London.

Palazzo, M. G. and Strunin, L. (1984). Anaesthesia and emesis I etiology. *Canadian Anaesthetists Society Journal*, **31**, 178–87.

Price, M. L., Walmsley, A., Swaine, C. and Ponte, J. (1988). Comparison of a total intravenous anaesthetic technique using a propofol infusion, with an inhalational technique using enflurance for day case surgery. *Anaesthesia*, **43**, 845.

Royal College of Surgeons (RCS) (1985). Commision on the Provision of Surgical Services: Guidelines for Day Case surgery. Revised 1992. Royal College of Surgery London.

Senapatic, A. and Young, A. E. (1989) Acceptability of day care surgery. *Journal of the Royal Society of Medicine*, **82** 735–6.

Tibrewal, S. B. and Foss, M. V. (1981) Is day surgery for Wilson's osteotomy safe? *Journal of Bone and Joint Surgery (BR)* **738** 340.

Sarma, V. S. and Bostrom, U. (1990), Intrathecal anaesthesia for day-care sugery. *Anaesthesia*, **45**, 769–71.

White, P. F. (ed.) (1993). *Outpatient Anaesthesia*. Churchill Livingstone, New York.

Part II

Acute Surgery

Chapter 11

Spinal injuries

Jennifer Goy

This chapter is intended as a guide for anaesthetists who are un-familiar with the management of patients with spinal cord injuries.

Incidence and aetiology

There are approximately 700 new cases of spinal cord injury recorded on the United Kingdom database each year (Gardner, *pers. comm.*). There appear to be an increasing number of traumatic cervical injuries reaching specialist centres, which may reflect compulsory wearing of seat belts, improved initial resuscitation techniques at the scene of the injury and a reduction in the initial mortality prior to transfer.

As a result, more patients with spinal cord injuries now present to non-specialist units for initial medical management and also for surgical fixation of an unstable spine, prior to referal and transfer to a specialist centre. Many aspects of the management of these patients may involve the anaesthetist.

Table 11.1 New patient admissions to the National Spinal Injuries Centre, Stoke Mandeville Hospital, 1991

Traumatic	134
Non-traumatic	55
Total	189
Tetraplegic – C8 and above	80
Paraplegic – T1 and below	105
Unspecified	4
	189

Table 11.2

Cause of spinal injury		Highest incidence
Traumatic		
Road traffic accidents	74	
Motor vehicle	56	24 male tetraplegics
Motor cycle	18	11 male paraplegics
Pedestrian	4	3 male tetraplegics
Sport	19	10 male tetraplegics
Domestic	18	9 male tetraplegics
Occupational	19	12 male tetraplegics
Non-traumatic	55	26 male paraplegics
e.g. surgery, vascular, tumour, transverse myelitis, infection		

Type of spinal cord injury

Spinal cord injuries may be complete or incomplete. Just over 50 per cent of patients have complete injuries, the remainder may show sparing of variable degrees of motor, sensory or autonomic function.

Patients with spinal cord injuries above T6 exhibit important differences in almost all aspects of their management and the greater the sensory and autonomic sparing which may occur, the fewer are the problems that may be experienced by the anaesthetist.

There are ‘recognized patterns’ of incomplete injuries most frequently found at the cervical levels.

Anterior cord syndrome

The anterior tracts of the cord are damaged by any interruption of the anterior spinal artery or one of its tributaries. This causes a complete motor loss below that level, loss of spinothalamic tracts; pain, temperature and touch, but sparing of the posterior columns; light touch, proprioception and position sense (typically flexion-rotation injuries).

Posterior cord syndrome

A fracture of the posterior part of a vertebra causes disruption to the posterior columns, causing loss of proprioception with ataxia, but leaving motor sparing together with pain, temperature and touch (typically hyperextension injuries).

Central cord syndrome

Central cord compression occurs with hyperextension injuries in patients with cervical spondylosis or stenosis. The central part of the cord is damaged causing a variable degree of arm weakness, with lesser involvement of the more peripheral tracts supplying the legs and bladder.

Brown–Sequard syndrome

Hemisection of the cord can be caused by a lateral fracture or a penetrating injury. This presents with motor loss on the same side and spinothalamic loss on the opposite side (pain, temperature and touch). Posterior columns, (proprioception) are little affected as some of the fibres cross.

Cauda equina lesions

Fracture dislocations below L1–2 usually exhibit variable neurological sparing because of the width of the canal at this level, and present as lower motor neurone lesions. Sensory or motor loss may occur and bladder function is frequently affected.

Sacral sparing

The periphery of the cord is supplied by radicular arteries, the largest entering between T9/L3. It is possible therefore that sensation from the lower sacral segments may be preserved in an otherwise complete lesion, as the radicular arteries supply a significant amount of blood to the lower cord.

Physiology

The anaesthetic management of patients with spinal cord injuries depends on an understanding of the physiological changes caused by the injury. Once these are appreciated, routine anaesthetic and intensive care management can logically be altered to suit the special needs of these patients.

Immediate physiological changes

At the time of the spinal cord injury an acute activation of the sympathetic nervous system and adrenal medulla occurs, lasting several minutes. It is accompanied by hypertension, reflex bradycardia, and bizarre dysrhythmias (Greenhoot *et al.*, 1972; Evans *et al.*, 1980). The physiological significance increases, the higher the spinal level.

Intense vasoconstriction may precipitate left ventricular failure and the development of subendocardial infarction (Eidelberg, 1973). This may lead to reduced myocardial function over the next few days. The hypertension generated by the sympathetic discharge may also disrupt the pulmonary capillary endothelium causing alveolar haemorrhage, which may lead to subsequent pulmonary oedema (Theodore and Robin, 1976).

Spinal shock

The spinal cord, below the level of the injury, becomes isolated from the control of the higher centres and initially there is substantial impairment of the function of the isolated spinal cord. There is loss of somatic and visceral sensation, generalized muscle flaccidity and loss of reflexes, with the occasional exception of sacral reflexes which may persist for a few days. Sacral parasympathetic activity is affected, manifested by large bowel and bladder atony. In injuries above T6 the sympathetic activity is markedly reduced, leaving unopposed vagal activity. Injuries at T6 and below have varying degrees of sympathetic impairment.

Table 11.3 indicates the physiological changes seen in injuries above T6. The lower levels of spinal cord injury will present with decreasingly modified changes, similar to those produced by spinal anaesthesia.

The above may be further modified by associated head, chest or abdominal injuries, frequently seen when these patients present after trauma.

Changes in established cord injuries

After a variable length of time, usually a few days to a few weeks depending on the level of the injury, the isolated spinal cord regains reflex activity. Inappropriate sympathetic activity is of most rel-

Table 11.3 Physiological changes following injury above T6

1. BP 80–90 mmHg systolic ← vasodilatation ← ↓ sympathetic tone
2. HR 50–60/min ← unopposed vagal activity
3. Respiration – ↓ vital capacity
   problems with secretions ← impaired cough
   ventilation/perfusion mismatch
4. Retention of urine
5. Paralytic ileus +/− gastric dilatation
6. Deep venous thrombosis and pulmonary emboli
   ← ↑ venodilation
   venous stasis
7. Poikilothermia ← vasodilation
   unable to shiver
8. Pressure sores ← ↓ blood supply
   ↓ sweating

Table 11.4 Autonomic dysreflexia

Arteriolar vasodilatation above the level

Arteriolar vasoconstriction below the level → ↑ BP

↓

	sinuatrial	X	vasomotor	1X	baroreceptors
↓ HR ←	node	←	centre	←	– aortic arch
		inhibitory stimuli		X	– carotid sinus

Peripheral capacitance vessels constrict → ↑ central venous pressure

↑ Cardiac output, ↑ Stroke volume, ↑ Systemic vascular resistance, ↑ Pulmonary arteriolar pressure

Cardiac arrhythmias

evance to the anaesthetist. Background autonomic inactivity leads to postural changes causing orthostatic hypotension and any fluid losses also cause a fall in blood pressure, whilst overactivity results in autonomic dysreflexias. These occur in most patients, but not all, with spinal cord injuries above T6. Table 11.4 shows the responses which may be caused by a cutaneous or visceral stimulus below the level of the spinal injury. The lower the injury is below T6, the more sympathetic outflow there will be above the injury, and the reflex will be increasingly under the control of higher centres (Frankel and Mathias, 1979; Mathias and Frankel, 1988). Dysreflexias are associated with an increase in circulating noradrenaline, not adrenaline, indicating they are directly due to increased sympathetic activity and not to the release of vasopressor from the adrenal medulla.

The awake patient may experience initial pallor followed by flushing and sweating of the face, nasal stuffiness also caused by vasodilatation, pupillary dilation, and a throbbing headache, the severity of which relates to the hypertensive response. In extreme circumstances this can lead to retinal, subarachnoid and intracerebral haemorrhage (Mathias and Frankel, 1983; Mathias *et al.*, 1988). Fits have also been reported (Kurmick, 1956; Frankel and Mathias, 1979).

Reflex hypertension associated with autonomic dysreflexia, and equally important to the anaesthetist, hypotension in response to fluid loss or repositioning is usually limited to injuries above T6. Below this level there is baroreflex control of the innervated circulation which includes the splanchnic bed (Mathias and Frankel, 1988), but caution must still be exercised. The resting blood pressure of patients with complete injuries begins to show a linear relationship with the level of the injury. The blood pressure progressively rises as the level falls from cervical down to lumbar levels (Frankel *et al.*, 1972). In time, vagal control may become more sensitive in tetraplegic patients (Mathias *et al.*, 1979).

During the initial period after injury, as reflex activity returns, the loss of the higher cortical inhibitory influences now leads to spasticity of the muscles. Muscular reflexes and spasms also develop, initially predominantly flexor and provoked by major stimuli, which cause radiation up and down the spinal cord leading to an extensive response. In time these can be provoked by minor cutaneous stimuli, e.g. insertion of a needle or straightening of a limb. Extensor reflexes may return later, associated with clonus and may be severely incapacitating for some patients.

General management – initial 6 months after injury

Treatment of spinal shock

The physiological changes associated with spinal shock are tabled in the previous section and are most appropriate to injuries above T6.

1. Low blood pressure, 80–90 mm Hg systolic

Once hypovolaemia has been corrected, attempts to increase the systolic blood pressure above 80–90 mm Hg with intravenous fluids may result in pulmonary oedema, to which these patients are susceptible. Fluid and blood replacement must be given conservatively. If good peripheral perfusion and a urine output of 0.5 ml/kg/hr are not achieved, a sympathomimetic may be started. Dopamine may be indicated if urine output is reduced. However, if the peripheral perfusion and blood pressure are poor, Dobutamine may be more appropriate. Monitoring central venous pressure is of limited value because of the disruption of central venous tone caused by the sympathetic paralysis. The central venous pressure may rise only slightly as the veins are filled until they become progressively so distended that the patient suddenly develops pulmonary oedema. However, it is sometimes a useful guide and offers a valuable route for drug therapy. Pulmonary wedge pressure measurement may be indicated in the more complex cases (Meyer *et al.*, 1971; Fraser and Edmonds-Seal, 1982), and occasionally cardiac output studies.

2. Low heart rate, below 50–60/minute

Unopposed vagal activity leads to a decreased heart rate. This does not usually increase in response to altered physiological states, e.g. hypovolaemia, but may develop into a profound bradycardia in the presence of hypoxia.

3. Respiration

Intubation and suction of the pharynx, endotracheal or tracheostomy tube may stimulate the vagus and precipitate a profound bradycardia, and even cardiac arrest, particularly in the presence of hypoxia. Atropine should always be available and pre-treatment with intravenous atropine is often indicated.

The muscles involved in respiration are the accessory muscles (C1,2,3,), the diaphragm, (C4,5,6,), the intercostals, (T1–11,), and the abdominal muscles, (T12-L1,). The diaphragm is the main muscle of inspiration, although the accessory muscles can be used for a limited period. The intercostals have inspiratory and expiratory functions, and the abdominal muscles are used in forced expiration and coughing.

Respiratory function should be monitored by vital capacity and blood gas measurements. Increased inspired oxygen may be necessary. Prophylactic chest physiotherapy must be started as soon as possible and atelectasis may necessitate bronchoscopy. A mini-tracheostomy can be useful to clear secretions. Intermittent positive pressure ventilation may be required.

Many patients with no previous history of atopy or asthma can develop bronchospasm, as a result of interruption of the sympathetic bronchodilator tone, which may require treatment. Asthmatics frequently develop severe bronchospasm. There should be a low threshold for treating patients with a high spinal cord injury, and a nebulized beta agonist and ipratropium are found to be useful.

4. Retention of urine

Immediately after an acute spinal cord injury there may be a decreased secretion of urine, which has a high specific gravity and low sodium content, differentiating it from acute tubular necrosis.

Urinary retention occurs after injury at any level, following loss of reflex detrusor contractions and persistent activity of the external urethral striated sphincter. At this stage in their management all patients need catheterization. Intermittent or suprapubic catheterization is preferable to reduce the incidence of associated infections, but is often impractical. Frequently an indwelling catheter is necessary initially, especially when hourly urine measurements are required. In males catheters should be strapped to the anterior abdominal wall to prevent angulation at the penile scrotal junction and consequent complications. Over distension of the bladder must be prevented, to avoid subsequent diminished bladder contractility.

5. Paralytic ileus and gastric dilatation

Most patients develop a paralytic ileus and oral fluids should not be given initially until bowel sounds return. A nasogastric tube should be passed if the stomach becomes distended and impairs respiration. An H_2 antagonist, antacids or sucralfate are usually given to reduce acidity. There is a significant incidence of gastrointestinal bleeding, due either to stress ulceration or exacerbation of a chronic ulcer, and most commonly presents in patients with cervical cord injuries. Early gastroscopy may be indicated. Suppositories can be given after 48 hours to stimulate the bowel (Silver and Williams, 1987).

6. Deep vein thrombosis and pulmonary emboli

Patients with spinal cord injuries have a very high risk of developing thromboembolic complications and in the absence of any other contraindicating injury anticoagulants should be started 24 to 36 hours post injury and continued for a minimum of 12 weeks (Silver and Williams, 1987; Silver and Williams, 1991).

7. Poikilothermia

The patient's temperature must be monitored throughout and resuscitation fluids should be warmed (Silver and Williams, 1987).

8. Pressure sores

Damage to vasomotor control of the skin blood flow and impaired sweating means the skin below the level of the spinal injury cannot respond to changes in temperature or accurately alter its blood flow. Patients must be turned every 2–4 hours to prevent the early development of pressure sores. All positions can be used to nurse patients, although tetraplegics may not tolerate being prone. The skin must be inspected for signs of pressure at each turn. The sacral skin is the most vulnerable.

9. Sepsis

It has been suggested that patients with spinal cord injuries are more susceptible to infection. However, it is rarely justifiable to use prophylactic antibiotic cover, and the advice of a microbiologist should be sought.

10. Development of contractures

Physiotherapy should be started as soon as possible after admission to give passive movements to all affected limbs.

Intensive care management

Patients who have spinal cord injuries without other associated trauma may be managed in a high dependency area, for initial assessment and stabilization. However, a significant number of these patients do present with other complicating injuries, which necessitate intensive care management. These patients can present a significant challenge.

The commonest cause for admission to the Intensive Care Unit at Stoke Mandeville Hospital is respiratory insufficiency (Bunsell, *pers. comm.*), usually neurological in origin and often complicated by aspiration of vomit whilst unconscious, an immersion incident in a diving accident, or associated chest trauma, e.g. fractured ribs, a pneumothorax or a haemothorax. Head injury and the consequent confusion make stabilization of the cord difficult, and sedation may affect respiratory function. The diagnosis of an acute abdomen is frequently made late; fever, shoulder tip pain, and after a few days, increased spasms may be the first indications. A plain *X*-ray of the abdomen may show air under the diaphragm, but appropriate positioning of the patient to demonstrate this may be difficult. Abdominal ultrasound can be useful. Fractures of long bones make nursing care difficult.

Patients also need to be transferred to the Intensive care unit to treat the secondary complications of the spinal cord injury previously referred to in relation to spinal shock. Reference has already been made to their outline management in that section.

Preparation for inter-hospital transfer

Most patients with spinal cord injuries will initially be admitted to non-specialist hospitals. Transfer to a specialist centre should be arranged as soon as the patient is resuscitated and stable, to minimize the onset of complications and to offer the patient and the family the psychological support required at this time. Transfer by helicopter should be considered, particularly if the distance is greater than 100 miles or road conditions are unpredictable. Alternatively, slow ambulance transfer may be used. Many patients have associated injuries and the possibility of these must be considered before transfer. Abrupt deterioration may occur with any level of recent spinal cord injury, particularly high thoracic and cervical injuries. Patients should be accompanied by an experienced doctor skilled in resuscitation, who is able to intubate, without moving the neck in tetraplegic patients. The patient should be nursed in a neutral position with the spine appropriately supported, following the advice of the specialist centre accepting the patient.

Clinical assessment is the most important guide to the fitness of the patient for transfer, and it is not possible to give absolute management guidelines. The following should be considered:

1. Respiratory System

1. Blood gases
   - consider the clinical trends since admission;
   - Increase inspired oxygen if indicated.
2. Vital capacity. Deterioration may indicate an ascending lesion or a tiring diaphragm. Absolute values are not as important.
3. Humidification is essential if the patient is intubated or has a tracheostomy.

4. Hypoxia causes vagal bradycardia, so patients should be pre-oxygenated and given intravenous atropine before suction of any secretions.
5. Restrict intravenous fluids to prevent pulmonary oedema.
6. Chest *X*-ray to exclude other injuries, especially in patients with thoracic and cervical fractures.
   - *Pneumothorax* – may be difficult to diagnose if the *X*-ray has been taken with the patient supine.
   - *Haemothorax* – not uncommonly misdiagnosed as it may present as a uniform opacity in one hemithorax if the patient is supine.
   - *Paravertebral haematoma* may be mistaken for a ruptured aorta. If there is significant doubt appropriate investigations must be carried out prior to transfer.
7. Chest physiotherapy is frequently of benefit. Nebulized terbutaline may be indicated prior to transfer of patients with high lesions, who are prone to bronchospasm.

2. Gastrointestinal tract

Patients should not have oral fluids and a nasogastric tube should be passed, and allowed to drain freely. Even in the presence of bowel sounds a pelvic colonic ileus may be present due to the loss of pelvic parasympathetic reflexes. A Ryles tube may not be necessary, if flatus has been passed.

3. Bladder

An indwelling catheter attached to a closed continuous drainage system is necessary, preferably a suprapubic.

4. Associated fractures

Spinal fractures below the level of the injury are frequently missed, and similarly pelvic and long bone fractures should be excluded. These may influence the estimated fluid losses. If the patient has a spinal and a long bone fracture, an intra-abdominal injury should be suspected and peritoneal lavage may be advisable prior to transfer.

Surgical fixation of the spine

Anaesthesia for early exploration of the cord and fixation of the spine in a potentially unstable patient, who may have other associated injuries, poses many problems for the anaesthetist. The dangers to the patient should never be underestimated.

More patients with spinal cord injury now have surgical exploration and stabilization of the spine in the admitting hospital, prior to transfer to a specialist unit. Penetrating wounds may need to be explored. Progressive ascent of the neurological signs may necessitate surgical decompression, and early restoration of cord alignment to improve or preserve neurological function may require surgical reduction of fracture dislocations. When surgery necessitates dissection of intact ligaments, stabilization is usually indicated. New internal fixation devices are being developed, especially for use in the thoracolumbar region. Earlier mobilization of these patients is possible, thus decreasing the period of prolonged recumbency and its associated problems.

Thorough preoperative assessment by both the surgeon and the anaesthetist is essential, to determine the presence of other possible associated life threatening injuries, before spinal surgery is commenced.

The management of patients with an acute spinal injury has already been discussed: the preoperative assessment and general principles of anaesthesia are outlined in the next section.

Anaesthesia

Preoperative assessment

First few days/weeks following injury – spinal shock

The preceeding sections on spinal shock and its management are summarized in Table 11.5 below, to enable the anaesthetist to make a logical preoperative assessment.

Established spinal cord injury

These patients are frequently extremely anxious about anaesthesia and the preoperative visit by the anaesthetist should include a full discussion of any previous anaesthetic experiences, including any problems that may have occurred in non-specialist hospitals. They are often well informed about the possible alternative methods of anaesthetic management, and in view of the frequency of the surgery they may need over the years, many patients appreciate an opportunity to express a choice, should this be appropriate. The preoperative assessment of these patients is summarized in Table 11.6.

Table 11.5 Preoperative assessment during the first few days/weeks following injury

1. Date of injury – if more than 3 days ago, avoid Suxamethonium
2. Level of injury – T5 and above, T6 and below
3. Complete/incomplete – record preoperative neurological signs
4. Is the spinal fracture stable?
5. Check for other injuries – chest, head, abdomen
6. Respiration
   Tidal volume
   CXR – ?pneumothorax, ?haemothorax, ?ruptured aorta
   Blood gases if clinically indicated
   PH chest problems, e.g. asthma
7. Blood pressure – ? hypovolaemia, check
   urine output >0.5 ml/kg/hr
   peripheral perfusion
8. Heart rate – <60/minute, prescribe atropine 0.6 mg i.m. preoperatively
   ECG – ? myocardial damage
9. Paralytic ileus/gastric distension
   Rx nasogastric tube
      metoclopramide 10 mg i.m.
      H_2 antagonist i.m.
      antacid immediately preoperatively
10. Indwelling urinary catheter – if not already *in situ*
11. Is the patient anticoagulated?
12. Medications, full blood count, urea and electrolytes
13. Allergies

Table 11.6 Preoperative assessment for patients with an established spinal cord injury

1. Date of injury – if more than 6 months ago, Suxamethonium may be used
2. Level of injury – T5 and above, T6 and below
3. Complete/incomplete, both motor and sensory components
4. History of other relevant injuries associated with the initial trauma
5. Respiratory system
   Recent chest infection – proceed with caution. It may be better to postpone surgery in a patient with a high injury
   PH chest diseases prior to injury. These may have been modified by the injury, e.g. bronchiectasis, asthma
   PH tracheostomy
   CXR
6. Blood pressure
   A baseline is useful and blood pressure is linearly related to the level of the injury
   Chronic injuries may have hypertension associated with renal problems
   Injuries above T6 may be prone to postural hypotension
7. Heart rate – important in injuries above T6, <60/minute consider i.m. atropine preoperatively.
8. Is the patient anticoagulated?
9. Is the patient prone to autonomic dysreflexia?
10. What degree of spasticity and spasms does the patient experience?
11. Medications
12. Allergies
13. Full blood count. Patients with chronic infection, e.g. pressure sores, have a low Hb which is tolerated poorly under general anaesthesia. These patients may respond better if they are transfused several days preoperatively
14. Urea and electrolytes – renal function may be impaired
15. Liver function tests – low proteins with chronic sepsis
16. Patients with cervical and high thoracic injuries should have their necks examined for mobility and possible difficult intubations

Premedication

Premedication is the personal preference of the anaesthetist and, where appropriate, the patient may be encouraged to express a choice. All patients with injuries above the mid-thoracic level may be more sensitive to standard premedication doses and those with cervical and thoracic injuries have an increased risk of acid aspiration, particularly in the recovery period; attention to preoperative fasting is important. A suggested regime:

metoclopramide 10 mg orally 2 hours preoperatively
H_2 antagonist orally 2 hours preoperatively

antacid immediately before theatre, if a difficult intubation is anticipated.

Injuries above T6

If postoperative pain is anticipated an opiate premedication may be useful to assess the patient's tolerance to opiates. A cervical patient may be given 50 mg Pethidine i.m., or if the patient is prone to spasms, preoperative Diazepam 10 mg may be useful. Depending on the nature of the surgery Atropine 0.6 mg i.m. one hour preoperatively may be indicated.

Injuries T6 and below

The personal preferences of the anaesthetist and the patient will influence the choice for these patients.

Choice of anaesthetic technique

At the time of the preoperative visit the possible ways of anaesthetic management should be discussed with the patient. The following factors may influence the final decision:

1. The nature of the surgery.
2. The level of injury in relation to the proposed surgery.
3. Complete/Incomplete – pain sensation may be absent in some types of incomplete injury.
4. Prone to autonomic dysreflexia?
5. Prone to spasms?

The choices currently available are:

1. No anaesthetic.
2. Topical local anaesthetic, e.g. local anaesthetic gel for cystoscopy.
3. Local anaesthetic infiltration.
4. Regional block.
5. Sedation with anxiolytic, e.g. Midazolam. (Diazepam may be more useful if the patient is prone to spasms.)
6. Propofol infusion – it may be necessary to give i.v. fluids to counteract a fall of blood pressure.
7. General anaesthesia.

Anaesthetic room management

In our unit patients are transferred to theatre on wide trolleys lying on pillows, on a canvas, with the exception of patients with new injuries for spinal fixation, who are transferred on their beds. All patients remain lying on pillows whilst in the operating theatre. Full monitoring should be attached in the anaesthetic room. Continuous, non-invasive blood pressure measurement from a finger is valuable to follow acute changes. An i.v. infusion should be started. The arm of a patient with an established spinal cord injury must be held firmly as, even in the absence of sensation, a marked spasm of the whole arm may be induced when the needle enters the skin. Cervical patients, especially C4–5, may have poor veins and contractures may make access difficult.

The following should be considered prior to induction for patients with injuries T5 and above:

1. Heart rate <60 /min give Atropine i.v. → HR 60–70 /min.
2. Blood pressure <100 mm systolic – give an initial 250 ml crystalloid to help counteract the fall in blood pressure caused by the induction agent.
3. Increase inspired oxygen prior to induction.

It is our practice to leave the traction attached to patients with new cervical injuries, and for a doctor trained in the management of spinal injuries or an orthopaedic surgeon to take responsibility for the position of the head, to avoid extension of the neck, and to apply cricoid pressure if a rapid sequence induction is indicated. Many cervical patients, with either acute or established injuries, can present as unexpectedly difficult intubations, so any necessary equipment should be assembled. A full range of endotracheal tubes and intubating aids should be available. Fibreoptic intubation may be indicated, but should be reserved for use by an experienced anaesthetist. Occasionally awake intubation may be necessary (Wood and Lawler, 1992).

Unless contraindicated, suxamethonium is used during the first 3 days after injury for ease of orotrachael intubation. If a non-depolarizing relaxant is indicated, the airway should be assessed again after the induction agent has been given.

Induction

Cervical and higher thoracic spinal patients are very sensitive to induction agents and these should be titrated cautiously, to minimize both the subsequent fall in blood pressure and the respiratory depression. Thiopentone and Propofol are both used routinely. An induction agent which does not cause involuntary movements is preferred for a patient with a new spinal cord injury. In patients with an established spinal cord injury there is an alteration in cerebral autoregulation, and they can tolerate lower cerebral perfusion pressures while maintaining cerebral blood flow (Eidelman, 1973).

Suxamethonium

The use of suxamethonium in a patient with a new spinal cord injury is associated with hyperkalaemia which may lead to cardiac arrest (Smith and Grenvik, 1970; Stone *et al.*, 1970; Mathias *et al.*, 1979). After reviewing the literature neither the onset nor the duration of the hypersensitivity has been well defined in man. In skeletal muscle where the nerve terminal approaches the muscle, there are discrete motor endplates with receptor sites for the depolarizing action of acetylcholine. After denervation the entire muscle membrane becomes receptive due to the development of receptor sites in extrajunctional areas, and the depolarization dose of acetylcholine is reduced by a factor of 10–4. In normal muscle ionic efflux of $K+$ and influx of $Na+$ ions take place at these endplate receptor sites. After a spinal cord injury suxamethonium will lead to a massive efflux of $K+$ from the increased number of receptor sites. It appears that a full paralysing dose of a non-depolarizer is needed to attenuate this response (Gronert and Theye, 1975).

Work in baboons, which have a similar response to man, showed that half peak increases occurred 8.4 days after denervation injury (mean increase 2.78 mEq/1) and peak increases at 14 days (mean increase of 5.5 mEq/1). However, an increase in potassium was noted as early as 4 days after injury (John *et al.*, 1976). As denervated muscle atrophies and fibrous tissue replaces the muscle fibres, the $K+$ content in the muscle decreases. Our current knowledge would suggest suxamethonium should be avoided from the fourth day after injury. Hyperkalaemia may also follow suxamethonium given to patients with major trauma and it is possible that extra caution should be observed regarding its use in these patients. It is our practice to recommence using suxamethonium 6 months after injury.

Laryngeal masks are becoming increasingly useful in short cases and those presenting with difficult intubations, but care must be taken not to increase intragastric pressure because of the poor cough reflex to protect against regurgitation in the recovery period. Endotracheal tubes are indicated in most patients requiring general anaesthesia, to enable the airway to be secured and protected against gastric contents, especially when the patient is to be ventilated.

Operating theatre management

When the patient is transferred into the operating theatre full monitoring equipment must be attached before the patient is positioned for surgery, to check for hypotension and bradycardias which not uncommonly occur at this time in injuries above T6, in response to the induction agents. They can usually be corrected with intravenous Atropine and more fluid. The transfer of a patient with a new spinal cord injury from a bed to the operating table must be jointly supervised by the anaesthetist and the surgeon. When the patient is stable, meticulous attention to positioning is essential, using sheepskins, to avoid pressure on the skin. As mentioned before, the altered control of the blood supply to the skin puts these patients at increased risk of pressure damage, even after short periods of time, and especially in the presence of dysreflexia.

Most patients with high injuries are more stable if IPPV is used. Spontaneous respiration may lead to hypercapnoea, and the altered V/Q ratios decrease the uptake of the volatile agents. Non-depolarizing relaxants are very rarely indicated above T6; atracurium is occasionally useful to settle a patient on the ventilator. The possible incomplete reversal of a non-depolarizing agent at the end of the case may cause respiratory problems postoperatively. The inspired gases should be humidified to prevent the formation of viscid secretions. Low inspiratory pressures should be used and a low pressure ventilator disconnect alarm is needed. It is also necessary to check that the urethral catheter, suprapubic catheter or condom is able to drain freely, as bladder distension during the case may cause an autonomic dysreflexia.

These patients are prone to hypothermia. They are poikilothermic and their temperature should be monitored throughout. The following may be helpful:

1. Warm theatre.
2. Blood warmer for i.v. fluids.
3. Irrigation fluids should be kept in a warming cabinet and the amount of fluid required must be anticipated in advance.
4. It is not possible to lie spinal patients on standard warming mattresses because of the pressure on their skin. When possible a dry heated mattress may be placed on top of the patient on a sheepskin.

Peri-operatively blood loss must be estimated continuously and replaced by the appropriate fluids.

Patients with high injuries, particularly above T6, tolerate fluid loss poorly, as they are unable to compensate by vasoconstricting. After spinal surgery the surgeon and the assistants should be present at the end of the case until the patient is safely transferred back to bed. Repositioning may cause hypotension due to pooling of blood, particularly in the presence of hypovolaemia, and haemorrhage can occur or become apparent when the patient is moved. After turning, full monitoring should immediately be reapplied and the patient observed in theatre until stable, before being transferred to the recovery area. Peri-operatively thoracolumbar dissections and fixations may have large blood losses which are poorly tolerated unless they are rapidly replaced.

Autonomic dysreflexia

An autonomic dysreflexia may be caused by any visceral distension and the most effective treatment of a dysreflexia is to remove the cause. Cardiac arrhythmias appear to be more frequent in the presence of hypercapnoea. Control is more difficult to achieve with vasoactive drugs in an anaesthetised patient because the causative stimuli are not sustained in the theatre, as they may be on the ward, and marked swings in blood pressure may result. An enhanced response occurs to pressor agents and to hypotensive drugs, which should both be titrated cautiously. Rapid lowering of blood pressure can sometimes be achieved by head-up tilt, which causes venous pooling.

Autonomic dysreflexia is particularly common during bladder surgery. Attention must be paid to the capacity of the bladder and to the volume of irrigation fluid needed to distend it. In a normocapnic patient reduction of the bladder distension and a temporary increase in the depth of the anaesthesia usually control the dysreflexia. Good control may be achieved with spinal anaesthesia by interrupting the afferent reflex arc (Alderson, 1990).

If general anaesthesia is used for genito-urinary surgery, male patients may need to be ventilated initially on a high concentration of a volatile agent to prevent an erection occurring during the initial instrumentation. Intravenous fluids and the surgical stimulus usually counteract hypotension secondary to the vasodilation caused by the volatile agent.

Postoperative management

Recovery area

It is often easier to recover these patients supine. Full monitoring should be attached and the following observed for:

1. Respiratory depression.
2. Reduced ability to cough and protect the airway if the patient vomits.
3. Reduced ability to compensate for any postoperative blood loss.
4. Hypothermia – may need a warming blanket.
5. Autonomic dysreflexia in injuries above T6, often caused by blocked urine drainage, particularly after bladder surgery when irrigation is *in situ*.

Later postoperative problems

1. *Postoperative vomiting.* To minimize the risk of postoperative vomiting oral fluids may be restricted for longer postoperatively. Therefore, intravenous fluids should be left *in situ* until the patient is drinking.
2. *Pulmonary oedema.* Care must be taken with postoperative fluids, particularly in patients with injuries above T6, to avoid pulmonary oedema.
3. *Atelectasis.* Viscid secretions may occur if inspired anaesthetic gases have not been humidified.
4. *Adequate pain relief.* There is reluctance to prescribe adequate opiate analgesia to these patients because of the increased risk of respiratory depression. In the absence of hypovolaemia they tolerate reduced doses of opiates well and the use of opiates in the preoperative period may indicate appropriate doses. Patient controlled analgesia (PCA) systems offer significant benefit. Some can be modified to be operated by the mouth for patients with poor hand control and a built-in respiratory monitor with feedback is an advantage to patients most at risk. It is our policy to nurse all patients using a PCA, who have injuries above T6, in a spinal high dependency area.
5. *Sepsis.* Spinal patients appear to be more prone to postoperative septic complications.

Long-term considerations

1. Bladder

Urinary sepsis was originally one of the highest causes of mortality and many patients died of renal failure secondary to chronic infections, renal stones and outflow problems. During initial rehabilitation, estimations of residual urine and videourodynamics may indicate bladder outlet obstruction or vesicoureteric reflux. Cystoscopy, litholapaxy and sphincterotomy are frequently required, and bladder distension during surgery may precipitate significant autonomic dysreflexia in patients with injuries above T6. Extracorporeal shock wave lithotripsy and percutaneous nephrolithotomy for removal of renal stones have markedly reduced the number of open kidney operations, with a subsequent reduction of morbidity.

Two further recent advances are artificial urethral sphincters for the management of neuropathic incontinence due to sphincter paralysis, and anterior sacral nerve root stimulators involving the insertion of a radio-linked implant to enable complete emptying of the bladder in a patient with an intact sacral parasympathetic nerve supply. Identification of S2, 3, 4 nerve roots depends on stimulating the individual motor roots and measuring the bladder contractions produced. It is preferable to avoid the use of Atropine, because of its muscarinic effect on the bladder, and also the use of longer acting non-depolarizing muscle relaxants. The posterior roots are similarly identified by direct stimulation. This operation is frequently carried out in patients with high spinal cord injuries and posterior root stimulation may cause autonomic dysreflexia, which ceases when stimulation stops. If the patient is prone to severe dysreflexia the posterior roots may be cut during surgery; this also has the effect of increasing bladder capacity.

Patients with spinal cord injury have a 20 times increased incidence of bladder cancer. Many of these tumours are squamous carcinomas. They present late, usually ten to twenty years after injury (El Masri and Fellows, 1981).

2. Post-traumatic syringomyelia

With the increasing use of nuclear magnetic resonance imaging post-traumatic cavitation is a more frequent finding. It may present as an extension of the neurological level and is treated by drainage, either into the subarachnoid space, the pleural cavity or the peritoneal cavity. When a syrinx is incised at T1–4 level the relief of pressure within the cord may cause direct stimulation of the cardiac nerves leading to a transient arrhythmia. When a syringopleural shunt is inserted care must be taken to minimize the risk of a pneumothorax in a patient who may already have a reduced respiratory reserve, and a post-operative chest *X*-ray in recovery is advisable.

3. Spasms

Some patients progressively develop reflex spasms which may become extremely incapacitating. These may prevent surgery in patients with complete spinal cord injuries from being performed without general anaesthesia, which abolishes the spasms.

Diazepam is commonly used to alleviate spasms. Many patients are managed with oral Baclofen which acts at a spinal level. It does not cause problems for the anaesthetist. Intrathecal Baclofen has been shown to reduce side-effects and to be more efficacious. For long-term management it may be given via a catheter into the cerebrospinal fluid from a reservoir pump, which is implanted subcutaneously on the anterior chest wall. The surgery does not present any special problems, but patients must be observed for Baclofen overdosage in the late post-operative period.

4. Pain

More than half the patients with spinal cord injuries experience chronic pain. This may be junctional pain, in the band between normal and abnormal sensation or deafferentation pain, occurring in areas where there is no normal sensation. It may also be related to muscle spasms. Neurosurgical opinion and intervention at a relatively earlier stage in the patient's management is now often appropriate, and newer techniques and operations are evolving, with varying degrees of success. Dorsal root entry zone (DREZ) radio-frequency lesions induced at the immediate point of entry of the dorsal root into the spinal cord are now an established procedure. Peri-operatively direct stimulation of the high thoracic nerves may cause dysreflexia. It is infrequently used in patients with cervical lesions because of the risk of increasing the neurological level.

5. Spinal deformities

Complete high spinal cord injuries occurring before vertebral growth has finished may cause a spinal deformity as the child grows, leading to the added problem of scoliosis.

6. Pathological fractures

Osteoporosis occurs in the bones of the paralysed limbs and pathological fractures can occur following minimal trauma. These are frequently managed conservatively but may require internal fixation.

7. Hand surgery for improvement of hand function in patients with cervical lesions

The emphasis of rehabilitation for all spinal patients is to use existing functions to their maximum potential. Restoration of active elbow extension and a functional hand grip by muscle and tendon transfers may be of great benefit.

8. Domicillary ventilation

Most patients who need ventilation soon after injury are weaned successfully. In the long-term some patients with very high tetraplegia are able to breath during the day, but may need ventilation overnight; others will require continuous ventilation. Pressure limited ventilators are usually preferred, e.g. East Radcliffe ventilator, which can easily be taught to the patient's family and carers. An uncuffed silver tracheostomy tube enables the patient to speak. Both simple humidification and suctioning are needed. Oxygen is infrequently required.

9. Obstetrics

Amenorrhoea is common in the initial 3 to 9 months after injury, following which female fertility is not affected by spinal cord injury at any level. During pregnancy, urinary tract infections, anaemia, deep vein thrombosis and increased osteoporosis are more common in these patients. They may have premature labours and are usually admitted to the spinal unit between 36 and 37 weeks awaiting transfer to the obstetric unit. Labour is frequently rapid and unattended births have occurred.

The first stage of labour involves nerves from T10-L1 levels and the second stage S2–4, so patients with an injury above T10 should not experience pain, but may experience a poorly characterized abdominal discomfort. Patients with an injury above T6 may experience autonomic dysreflexia with uterine contractions, and may also have muscle spasms which are either localized to the segments of sensory input or more generalized involving increased tone and spasms of the abdominal and leg muscles. It is our practice to control these dysreflexias with epidural Bupivicaine, commencing with 10 ml, 0.25–0.5 per cent given 1–2 hourly, as clinically indicated. Care must be taken to avoid an overdistended bladder. The patients should have full monitoring, which may include direct arterial pressure if the blood pressure swings are extreme. Non-invasive continuous finger arterial pressure may be adequate. When the level of the injury is above T5, all voluntary use of the abdominal muscles will be absent (Hughes *et al.*, 1991). Vaginal delivery is usual, but forceps may be required.

References

Alderson, J. D. (1990). Chronic care of spinal cord injury. In J. D. Alderson and E. Frost (eds), *Spinal Cord Injuries. Anaesthetic and Associated Care.* Butterworth, London, pp. 108.

Bunsell, R. P. (Personal communication).

Eidelberg, E. E. (1973). Cardiovascular response to experimental cord compression. *Journal of Neurosurgery*, **38**, 326–31.

Eidelman, B. H. (1973). Cerebral blood flow in normal and abnormal man. Unpublished DPhil Thesis. University of Oxford.

El Masri, W. S. and Fellows, G. J. (1981). Bladder cancer after spinal cord injury. *Paraplegia*, **19**, 265–70.

Evans, D. E., Kobrine, A. I. and Rizzoli, H. V. (1980). Cardiac arrhythmias accompanying acute compression of the spinal cord. *Journal of Neurosurgery*, **52**, 52–9.

Frankel, H. L., Michaelis, S., Golding, R. and Beral, V. (1972). The blood pressure in paraplegia I. *Paraplegia*, **10**, 193–8.

Frankel, H. L. and Mathias, C. J. (1979). Cardiovascular aspects of autonomic dysreflexia since Guttman and Witteridge (1947). *Paraplegia*, **17**, 46–51.

Fraser, A. and Edmonds-Seal, J. (1982). Spinal cord injuries – Review Article. *Anaesthesia*, **37**, 1084–98.

Gardner, B. K. (Personal communication).

Greenhoot, J. H., Shiel, F. O. M. and Mauck, H. P. (1972). Experimental spinal cord injury: electrocardiographic abnormalities and fuchsinophilic myocardial degeneration. *Archives of Neurology*, **26**, 524–9.

Gronert, G. A. and Theye, R. A. (1975). Pathophysiology of hyperkalaemia induced by succinylcholine. *Anesthesiology*, **43**, 89–99.

Hughes, S. J., Short, D. J., Usherwood, M. McD. and Tebbutt, H. (1991). Management of the pregnant woman with spinal cord injuries. *British Journal of Obstetrics and Gynaecology*, **98**, 513–18.

John, D. A., Tobey, R. E., Homer, L. D. and Rice, C. L. (1976). Onset of succinylcholine-induced hyperkalaemia following denervation. *Anesthesiology*, **45**, 294–9.

Kurnick, N. B. (1956). Autonomic hyperreflexia and its control in patients with spinal cord lesions. *Annals of Internal Medicine*, **44**, 678–86.

Mathias, C. J., Christensen, N. J., Corbett, J. L., Frankel, H. L. and Spalding, J. M. K. (1976). Plasma catecholamines during paroxysmal neurogenic hypertension in quadriplegic man. *Circulation Research*, **39**, 204–8.

Mathias, C. J., Christensen, N. J., Frankel, H. L. and Spalding, J. M. K. (1979). Cardiovascular control in recently injured tetraplegics. *Quarterly Journal of Medicine*, **190**, 273–87.

Mathias, C. J. and Frankel, H. L. (1988). Cardiovascular control in spinal man. *Annual Review of Physiology*, **50**, 577–92.

Mathias, C. J. and Frankel, H. L. (1983). Autonomic failure in tetraplegia. In Bannister, R. (ed.), *Autonomic Failure. A Textbook of Clinical Disorders of the Autonomic Nervous System*. (ed.) Bannister, R. Oxford University Press, pp. 453–88.

Meyer, G. A., Berman, I. R., Doty, D. B., Moseley, R. V. and Gutierrez, V. S. (1971). Haemodynamic response to acute quadriplegia with or without chest trauma. *Journal of Neurosurgery*, **34**, 168–77.

Silver, J. R. and Williams, S. J. (1987). Initial management of spinal injury. In J. Hadfield and M. Hobsley (eds), *Current Surgical Practice*, Vol. 4. Edward Arnold, London, pp. 62–79.

Silver, J. R. and Williams, S. J. (1991). Acute management of spinal injuries. In M. Swash and J. Oxbury (eds), *Clinical Neurology*, Vol. I. Churchill Livingstone, London, pp. 710–35.

Smith, B. R. and Grenvik, A. (1970). Cardiac arrest following succinylcholine in patients with central nervous system injuries. *Anesthesiology*, **33**, 558–60.

Stone, W. A., Beach, T. P. and Hamelberg, W. (1970). Succinylcholine – danger in the spinal cord injured patient. *Anesthesiology*, **32**, 168–9.

Theodore, J. and Robin, E. D. (1976). Speculations on neurogenic pulmonary oedema. *American Review of Respiratory Diseases*, **113**, 405–11.

Tobey, R. E. (1970). Paraplegia, succinylcholine and cardiac arrest. *Anesthesiology*, **32**, 359–64.

Wood, P. R. and Lawler, P. G. P. (1992). Managing the airway in cervical spine injury. *Anaesthesia*, **47**, 792–7.

Chapter 12

Anaesthesia for the accident service

Peter McKenzie

Fractures and associated problems

The most common fractures presenting to the accident service and requiring surgical treatments are those of the femoral neck. Femoral neck fractures and their management are discussed in detail later in this chapter.

Blood loss

Many fractures are associated with concealed blood loss. A tibial fracture loses about 500 ml of blood and a femoral fracture approximately 1 litre. Pelvic fractures can be associated with 2 litres loss or more, together with losses from the associated soft tissue injuries. These losses can be life-threatening. Spinal fractures cause considerable retroperitoneal bleeding.

Vascular

Many major fractures can lead to compromised circulation, either, for example to the skin by direct tension from a bony fragment, or by direct vascular pressure or disruption. These problems may lead to the need for very urgent reduction and/or exploration to preserve tissue viability.

Compartment syndrome

This complication can be potentially fatal with rhabdomyolysis, disseminated intravascular coagulation and renal failure. Less severe complications include Volkmann's ischaemic contracture. Compartment syndrome is grossly underdiagnosed and may occur, for example, in 10 per cent of tibial fractures. Pressure studies of suspect compartments may be used (Bulstrode *et al.*, 1989). Pulse oximetry may be of value in early detection of deterioration of circulation (David, 1991). Early treatment by fasciotomy can lead to a dramatic return of normal circulation.

Hypoxaemia after fractures

Clinically unsuspected hypoxaemia often occurs after fractures, particularly those of long bones (Tachakra and Sevitt, 1975). The rapid development of hypoxaemia would be consistent with some form of embolization. This might include fat globules and subsequent fibrin formation (Saldeen, 1970). Tissue thromboplastic products also reach the pulmonary circulation (Modig, 1977).

The degree of hypoxaemia can be very severe and occur in young, previously fit, people. It is remarkable that severe desaturation is often not noticed even by experienced clinicians. A high index of suspicion is thus required! While most patients do not go on to develop 'fat embolism' syndrome, routine measurement of oxygen saturation on air on admission, with blood gas analysis where significant desaturation is present, can enable appropriate management to be instigated. Postoperatively, particular care should be paid to ensuring safe levels of oxygen saturation.

Manipulation of the fracture under anaesthesia can also cause falls in saturation and vigilance is required.

Children requiring general anaesthesia following a fracture

Like most adults, children requiring general anaesthesia following a fracture should be treated as if having a 'full stomach'.

General anaesthesia may however, be avoided in some children by alternatives such as the use of entonox (50 per cent nitrous oxide in oxygen) self-administered during the reduction of closed fractures (Wattenmaker *et al.*, 1990).

Intravenous regional analgesia has proved a very successful method for the reduction of upper limb fractures and dislocations in children as young as 3 years of age (Olney *et al.*, 1988; Barnes *et al.*, 1991).

Children may present for the application of hip spicas. This will involve much manipulation of the child's position; in particular, being turned from the supine to the prone position and back again. An elegant way to overcome the problem of sedation/anaesthesia for this procedure without instrumentation of the airway, is the use of incremental doses of intravenous ketamine, *always* preceded by an effective antisialogogue, either intramuscular atropine or intravenous glycopyrrolate. The initial dose of ketamine may be 2–3 mg kg^{-1} with smaller incremental doses as required. If intravenous access is not possible, intramuscular ketamine (10 mg kg^{-1}) is an alternative. Ketamine may also prove useful for multiple general anaesthetics for change of dressings, with propofol also a useful alternative.

Anaesthesia for repair of fractured neck of femur

Patients having repair of fractured neck of femur are one of the highest risk groups commonly presented for anaesthesia. Most patients are elderly and there may be many intercurrent and associated medical problems. Great demands are placed on health care resources, and postoperative morbidity and mortality may be high. There is now clear evidence that anaesthesia may influence outcome, although interpretation of the evidence is open to a variety of points of view. Repair of the fracture is first aimed at pain relief and early mobilization, and thus few patients should be rejected for anaesthesia and surgery. This section will discuss preoperative assessment and preparation for anaesthesia and surgery of the patient with hip fracture and will describe the types of anaesthesia available and their advantages and disadvantages both immediate and in the long-term.

Incidence of fractured neck of femur

The incidence of fractured neck of femur is rising at an almost alarming rate and substantially faster than can be explained by the increasing proportion of elderly people in the population. The annual incidence in 1964 was 3 per 1000 in women over 75 years of age. By 1983 the comparable figure was 8 per 1000 rising to 16 per 1000 by 1981 (Knowelden *et al.*, 1964; Wallace, 1983). Boyce has reported that the incidence in Oxford, after compensating for the increase in elderly in the population, had doubled over a period of 30 years (Boyce, 1985). This type of fracture may comprise one sixth or more of all fractures (Keith, 1973). The incidence rises sharply with age and is twice as common in females as males.

The elderly patient: general considerations

The physiological and pathological consequences of ageing must be taken into account when assessing patients for anaesthesia and surgery.

Cardiovascular system

Arterial blood pressure tends to rise with age and there is debate as to what constitutes normal blood pressure in the elderly. Quite a proportion of elderly patients may be on treatment for hypertension and, for example, diuretic therapy may lead to relative dehydration and hypokalaemia. As a general rule all antihypertensive therapy should be continued in the peri-operative period. In elective surgery uncontrolled hypertension is a contraindication to anaesthesia, but in patients with fractured neck of femur, there is seldom time to stabilize uncontrolled hypertension. However, excessively high blood pressure should be treated as a matter of urgency. It is very important that preoperative electrocardiography is carried out in all patients presenting for repair of fractured neck of femur. Ischaemic heart disease is common and may be asymptomatic. A history of recent myocardial infarction greatly increases the risks of peri-operative reinfarction and associated mortality and this risk is greatest in the first 3 months after infarction. This may be one of the few major (but not absolute) contraindications to surgical treatment in the patient with fractured neck of femur.

Other conditions of particular importance are undiagnosed conduction defects such as heart block which will require a temporary cardiac pacing wire to be inserted before anaesthesia. Patients who are receiving beta-blockade for angina or hypertension must continue it throughout the peri-operative period.

Congestive cardiac failure is also fairly common and all medication should also be continued. If cardiac failure is uncontrolled then aggressive management should be instituted to improve the patient's condition within 12–24 hours.

Deep venous thrombosis occurs in a very high proportion of patients with hip fracture and this topic will be discussed subsequently.

Respiratory system

Arterial pO_2 tends to fall with age although data are scant as to whether this process continues above the age of about 60 years. It is the author's experience that it does not.

Chronic obstructive airways disease is fairly frequent in the elderly and if the condition is significant, then preoperative and postoperative physiotherapy may be of advantage. The very rare patient who has sufficiently severe pulmonary disease to render them in the category of 'Pink Puffer' or 'Blue Bloater' will present a very high risk for anaesthesia and general anaesthesia is strongly contraindicated. However for the patient with less severe disease with copious sputum, general anaesthesia and tracheal intubation will allow an opportunity for tracheobronchial toilet which may be of considerable benefit. Patients with a FEV_1 of less than 1 litre or a FEV_1 less than 50 per cent of vital capacity may be expected to produce postoperative problems if general anaesthesia is employed. An acute chest infection will not improve if the patient is immobile and is not, in the author's opinion, any contraindication to surgery; indeed it is an indication to proceed. General anaesthesia will again allow bronchial suctioning.

Central nervous system

The development of confusional states after admission to hospital with fractured neck of femur is a relatively common occurrence and the contribution of anaesthesia is controversial. This topic will be discussed later. Many patients who are admitted with fractured neck of femur are suffering from senile dementia. The benefits of early mobilization and pain relief from the operation are particularly noticeable in this type of patient. The aetiology of postoperative confusional states is multifactorial and postoperative hypoxaemia is a contributory factor. An unfamiliar environment may be sufficient to cause this condition in many elderly patients.

Metabolic disease

Severe uncontrolled diabetes should be adequately controlled before operation. The maturity onset diabetic will tend to be on either diet restriction or oral hypoglycaemic agents. It is relatively rare for an elderly patient to be receiving insulin. In the diabetic patient receiving diet alone, monitoring of blood sugar peri-operatively is required and occasionally hyperglycaemia may develop requiring intervention with insulin therapy.

In the patient on oral hypoglycaemic therapy the main problem is undiagnosed hypoglycaemia. Of particular concern are patients on chlorpropamide, as this drug has an extremely long duration of action up to 60 hours.

Medication

Many elderly patients are taking a variety of medication. Two of the most common categories of medication are discussed and their relevance to anaesthesia and surgery mentioned.

Digoxin

The risk of digitalis toxicity is a possibility particularly in the elderly but it is rarely possible to obtain serum digoxin levels before surgery. Suspicion of digoxin toxicity might be raised by the presence of vomiting or ventricular arrhythmias. The coexistence of hypokalaemia is an important contributory risk factor. In general, digoxin should be continued throughout the peri-operative period.

Diuretic therapy

Hypokalaemia may lead to cardiac arrhythmias and difficulty in reversal of muscle relaxants. Anaesthesia and surgery should be probably postponed if serum potassium is less than 3.0 mmol $litre^{-1}$ Very occasionally, 'potassium–sparing' diuretics such as triamterine cause hyperkalaemia and hyperkalaemia can also occur in patients receiving potassium supplementation with conventional diuretic therapy.

Specific problems in the preoperative period

'Dehydration'

Patients with fractures of the femoral neck are frequently dehydrated and hypovolaemic to a greater extent than is appreciated by many junior surgical colleagues. Careful consideration of the common pattern of events will reveal that this is not such a surprising finding:

1. elderly patients frequently do not have adequate oral fluid intake and it has been demonstrated that their thirst mechanism is depressed;
2. many patients are on concurrent long-term diuretic therapy;
3. patients often lie after the injury for some time before help arrives and during this time do not receive any fluids;
4. there is blood loss and oedema formation at the site of injury;
5. patients are fasted for a variable period of time before surgery and if surgery has to be postponed may have to suffer a second or even third period of fasting in the days that follow.

The above factors must be assessed for each individual patient and appropriate fluid replacement instituted. It is the author's view that every patient with fractured neck of femur should receive intravenous fluids as soon as they are admitted to hospital. Despite the widespread fear of fluid overload, in the author's experience this is rare and on the contrary, insufficient fluid replacement is extremely common. The presence of hypovolaemia is particularly hazardous if the use of spinal or epidural anaesthesia is contemplated.

Arterial hypoxaemia

While it is known that arterial pO_2 decreases with advancing age (Davis and Spence, 1972), it has been found that patients with fractured neck of femur have arterial pO_2 values which seem to be lower than would be predicted on the basis of age alone. Further deterioration occurs after general anaesthesia (Wishart *et al.*, 1977; McKenzie *et al.*, 1980). It is probably unnecessary to administer oxygen routinely to the majority of patients with fractured neck of femur in the preoperative period, but blood gas estimation is useful particularly where there is concurrent cardiorespiratory disease.

The reason for the preoperative arterial hypoxaemia is not known, but clinically unsuspected hypoxaemia occurs after long bone fractures and is thought to be due to subclinical fat embolus (Tachakra and Sevitt, 1975). Another possible explanation for the preoperative hypoxaemia could be the supine position (Ward *et al.*, 1966) or prolonged recumbency (Cardus, 1967).

Preoperative investigations

Full blood count is obviously essential as, in addition to the unknown losses occurring at the fracture site, undiagnosed anaemia is relatively common in the elderly patient. However dehydration will confuse the interpretation of haematocrit results.

Urea, creatinine and electrolyte determinations are helpful in assessing the degree of dehydration, and in determining whether renal function is adequate. The diagnosis of hypokalaemia or more rarely hyperkalaemia is extremely important in its relevance to anaesthesia. Preoperative electrocardiograph and chest X-ray are necessary both as a baseline and for diagnosis of a multiplicity of preexisting conditions.

Availability of cross-matched blood is a wise precaution in all such patients.

Preparation of patients for surgery

It is the view of the author that the ideal time for surgery is between 12–24 hours after admission to hospital. All patients should have adequate fluid replacement prior to surgery. On occasion measurement of central venous pressure may be of help in the patient with cardiac disease, in order to avoid fluid overload.

When is it justifiable to postpone operating?

Inevitably this is a matter of opinion and one has to balance the benefits of delay against the risks, for example, of hypostatic pneumonia or further increases in the risk of deep vein thrombosis. In the author's experience, clearly justifiable reasons for postponement of surgery and anaesthesia are: uncorrected hypovolaemia, severe hypokalaemia, severe anaemia, severe uncontrolled congestive cardiac failure, rapid uncontrolled atrial fibrillation, diabetic ketoacidosis, and any situation where the patient would not obviously benefit from the procedure. The latter may include patients who are moribund and who are expected to succumb in the very near future. For them an operative procedure would only add to their suffering.

Other workers believe in optimizing the patient's condition before proceeding with surgery, which may result in a delay of several days.

If a previously ambulant patient suffers a fall and is admitted rapidly to hospital, it may well be appropriate to operate as soon as convenient, after routine investigations have been performed.

Premedication

In the opinion of the author, specific premedication in the elderly patient with fractured neck of femur is unnecessary but analgesia should, of course, be given if required. Appropriate analgesia for the elderly may include any of the usual opiate analgesic drugs but care should be taken with dosage, particularly in the very elderly or in those with hepatic or renal impairment. Non-steroidal anti-inflammatory analgesics may be very effective but should not be used if there is any renal impairment. Nerve blocks of femoral and lateral cutaneous nerve of thigh may be very effective.

Surgical technique

Surgical procedures fall into 2 types: internal fixation (by screws or screw or pin and plate) or primary prosthesis of the femoral head. Patients having primary hip prosthesis (in common with patients having total hip replacement) may exhibit sudden arterial hypotension during reaming of the femoral shaft or during insertion of the prosthesis and/or cement. A sudden decrease may also occur in arterial pO_2 at this time (Modig *et al.*, 1975). There are anecdotal reports of fatalities on the operating table shortly after insertion of prosthesis and/or cement. There are several hypotheses for these circulatory and respiratory changes. Air embolism has been demonstrated (Michel, 1980) It has also been shown that thromboplastins are released into the circulation causing microaggregates to embolise to the lungs; fat embolism and acrylic monomers from the cement may also be involved (Modig *et al.*, 1975).

In view of the above it is obvious that the anaesthetist must take particular care in the patient having primary hip prosthesis and must ensure that the patient is not hypovolaemic or hypotensive and receives added inspired oxygen no matter what technique of anaesthesia is employed. The cautious use of a short-acting vasopressor drug (e.g. methoxamine) if acute hypotension is encountered may be helpful.

Anaesthetic technique

There is now clear evidence that anaesthetic techniques have effects on outcome after repair of fractured neck of femur. However the nature of the effects which have been seen is complex and controversial. Anaesthetic techniques available can be subdivided into general anaesthesia or some form of regional anaesthetic technique.

General anaesthesia

There is a wide variety of agents available for general anaesthesia and it is not the purpose of this text to discuss all the possibilities for a patient with fractured neck of femur. Some drugs may prove beneficial in the elderly unfit patient and it is proposed to mention a few of these drugs and their possible benefits.

Etomidate has excellent cardiovascular stability and rapid hepatic metabolism. These advantages may be particularly beneficial in the elderly patient. Problems include pain on injection, superficial thrombophlebitis in the arm, and myoclonic twitching movements. Pain on injection may be mitigated by mixing with some lignocaine, but does not seem to be a major problem in the elderly. Likewise, thrombophlebitis, in the experience of the author, is mainly a problem in the young patient and not in the elderly. Myoclonic movements are of no serious importance.

Etomidate is the author's first choice as an induction agent in the majority of patients having general anaesthesia for repair of fractured neck of femur. The older muscle relaxants have a greatly increased duration of action in the elderly compared with younger patients and are contra-indicated.

Atracurium and vecuronium are thus the non-depolarizing relaxants of choice. Atracurium need not necessarily be reversed and this may offer a small advantage over vecuronium but either drug is eminently satisfactory.

In anaesthetic practice in the United Kingdom most anaesthetists will choose a technique involving intravenous induction of anaesthesia followed by tracheal intubation and then maintenance of anaesthesia with either spontaneous respiration with nitrous oxide, oxygen and volatile anaesthetic agent or controlled ventilation using a volatile anaesthetic agent and opiate supplementation with or without muscle relaxant as required. Controversy exists as to which of these two major types of anaesthesia is preferable. This topic will be discussed later under the section on effects of anaesthetic techniques on outcome. In general terms cardiovascular stability is aimed for, with fentanyl prior to induction, along with avoidance of hypoxia and hypocarbia at any stage and assurance of lack of residual muscle relaxation at the end of the procedure. If possible, centrally acting anticholinergics such as atropine should not be used.

A technique using spontaneous ventilation via a laryngeal mask airway might be used in suitable patients. Propofol would appear to be the induction agent of choice in this circumstance, but it should be given very slowly and cautiously after preoxygenation in this type of patient to avoid undue falls in arterial blood pressure and oxygen saturation. Experience with this technique in the patient with hip fracture is limited, and it is suggested that the patient must not be at risk of regurgitation and not have significant respiratory problems.

Regional anaesthesia

Although various combinations of nerve blocks have been employed, by far the most common regional anaesthetic technique for repair of fractured neck of femur is spinal (subarachnoid) block. Epidural block is occasionally employed but because of the osteoarthritic changes frequently present in these elderly patients epidural anaesthesia may be technically difficult, and onset is much slower. The discussion will therefore be restricted mainly to spinal anaesthesia.

Spinal subarachnoid block

In the patient with fractured hip this necessitates turning the patient into the lateral position and inserting a spinal needle at the L3, 4 or L4, 5 interspace. Positioning of the patient with a fractured hip may be unpleasant and uncomfortable for the patient. Careful handling will minimize the discomfort, and lifting the patient off the bed to turn them into the lateral position rather than rolling them may be less painful. A most useful adjunct to this is the administration of intravenous ketamine in analgesic dosage, i.e. 20–30 mg.

Many different local anaesthetic agents have been used but at present in the United Kingdom, choice is restricted to bupivacaine either in a plain or 'heavy' solution.

Some workers advocate the use of a unilateral block using very low doses of 'heavy' anaesthetic agent in repair of fractured neck of femur (McLaren *et al.*, 1978). This has the advantage of minimizing cardiovascular effects consequent upon the sympathetic block produced by the spinal anaesthesia. However it does mean that the patient may be uncomfortable lying on some types of orthopaedic table as the uninjured leg may not be anaesthetized. Many patients fall asleep as the block takes effect as this is the first time they have been pain free since the injury. If additional sedation is thought necessary a low dose propofol infusion may be utilized. If a satisfactory block is not obtained then recourse should be made to full general anaesthesia without delay. Attempts to cover an inadequate block with sedation and/or analgesia are almost invariably unsatisfactory.

Cardiovascular effects of spinal anaesthesia

In the elderly, profound falls in blood pressure may occur. Intravenous fluids are routinely given to patients receiving spinal anaesthesia in an attempt to compensate for the expansion in the capacity of the circulatory system. On occasions when the fall is profound vasopressor drugs are used and indeed in some countries (for example USA) the use of vasopressors is almost routine. The drugs most commonly used are methoxamine which has mainly alpha-agonist properties, or ephedrine which has both alpha and beta-agonist properties. In patients with ischaemic heart disease, methoxamine is the drug of choice as it does not cause tachycardia or have an inotropic effect and thus should not adversely affect the oxygen supply/demand ratio of the myocardium. In addition to its alpha-agonist activities it has a small degree of beta-blockade. Bradycardias are sometimes associated with its use, mainly as a reflex response to the rise in arterial pressure and from the beta-blockade. Thus if the heart rate is relatively slow prior to administration, it is wise to consider the prophylactic use of glycopyrrolate or, if the effect required is urgent, atropine.

Effects of anaesthetic technique

Controversy over the choice of anaesthetic technique for the patient with fractured neck of femur was fuelled by publication of the paper by McLaren *et al.* (1978), demonstrating in a study of 55 patients randomly allocated to receive spinal or general anaesthesia, that the mortality in the first 4 weeks after surgery was 4 per cent in the spinal anaesthetic group compared with 31 per cent in the general anaesthetic group. The authors did not attempted to elucidate the cause of the difference in mortality but suggested a difference in the incidence of thromboembolism as a possible reason. The mortality in the general anaesthetic group was 25 per cent at 2 weeks and 31 per cent at 4 weeks – figures which are high in comparison with most other studies which have been published. None the less, this is a striking and statistically significant difference.

The present author and colleagues also examined comparative outcome after spinal subarachnoid anaesthesia compared with general anaesthesia (McKenzie *et al.*, 1984). Methodology differed from McLaren and colleagues in that patients having general anaesthesia were intubated but breathed spontaneously. Spinal anaesthesia was unilateral in the study by McLaren, and all patients were sedated by nitrous oxide and althesin infusion. In the study by the present author, blocks were bilateral and minimal or no sedation was employed.

Figure 12.1 shows cumulative mortality over the first 2 months following surgery (McKenzie, 1984). There is significantly lower mortality in the spinal anaesthetic group by 2 weeks after surgery. In addition, there is a marked clustering of deaths in the general anaesthetic group between the fifth and fifteenth days after operation. However by the end of 2 months after surgery, survival was virtually

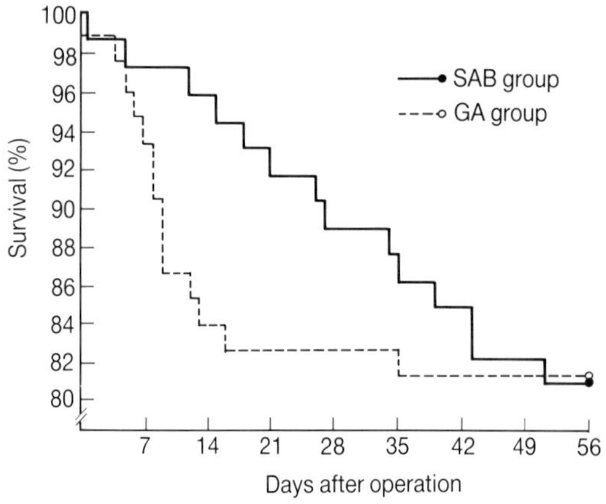

Fig 12.1 Cumulative total mortality in each group in first 56 days after operation. Individual deaths occurred on the following days after operation: *General anaesthesia* (GA) group (n = 75; 14 deaths) – 0, 4, 5, 6, 7, 8, 8, 9, 9, 9, 12, 13, 16, 35; *subarachnoid blockade* (SAB) group (n = 73; 14 deaths) – 1, 5, 12, 15, 18, 21, 26, 27, 34, 35, 36, 43, 43, 51.

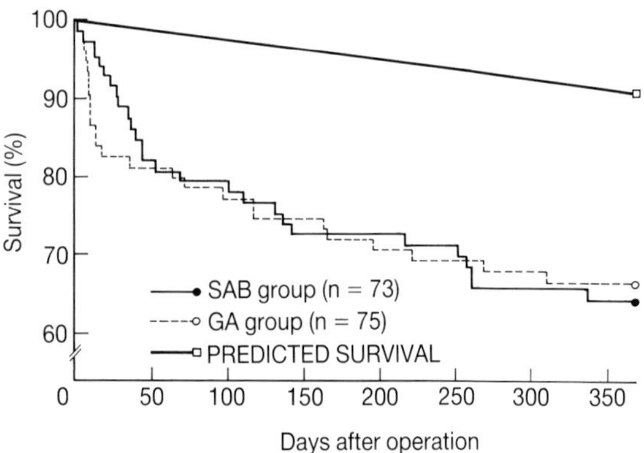

Fig 12.2

identical in both groups and remained identical up to 1 year (Fig 12.2). Predicted survival in a Scottish population matched for age and sex is also shown at the top of the figure. The pattern of mortality in the general anaesthetic group closely resembles in distribution that which might be expected from deaths caused by pulmonary embolism. Causes of death which had been certified were recorded, but were not supplemented by autopsy findings and are probably of dubious value. Interestingly, there were a greater number of deaths ascribed to thromboembolic complications in the general anaesthetic group. Respiratory complications were, perhaps surprisingly, the main cause of death recorded in the group who had spinal anaesthesia.

Other larger studies have now confirmed that there is no long-term difference in mortality after spinal or general anaesthesia (Valentin *et al.*, 1986; Davis *et al.*, 1987).

Spreadbury (1980), found a significant difference in early postoperative mortality between patients receiving conventional general anaesthesia and anaesthesia with intravenous ketamine. Mortality in the first 14 days following general anaesthesia was 20 per cent compared with 3.3 per cent in the ketamine group. However, when followed up for a longer period (duration not stated), the mortality became identical at 30 per cent. Both McLaren and Spreadbury used controlled ventilation with opiates and muscle relaxation. Spreadbury condemns this technique as being fundamentally unsafe in the patient with fractured neck of femur.

However, a randomized study in Oxford of spontaneous or controlled ventilation for hip fracture surgery has shown no difference between the techniques in mortality up to 6 months after surgery (Coleman *et al.*, 1988). Indeed, mortality was low in comparison to many other studies being 5.2 per cent at 4 weeks and 15.1 per cent at 6 months. No change was made to routine patient management other than the study protocol. This included intubation utilizing suxamethonium and, in the controlled ventilation group, atracurium only if indicated clinically, and in a small dose. Added oxygen was given after anaesthesia to all patients absolutely continuously for a minimum of 6 hours.

Other effects of anaesthetic technique

Deep venous thrombosis

The incidence of deep venous thrombosis (DVT) in patients after surgery for repair of fractured femoral neck, when detected by the most accurate method (venography) is probably the highest of any surgical procedure. There is evidence to support the hypothesis that the difference in early mortality after spinal or general anaesthesia may be due to a difference in incidence of thrombo-embolic events. Thorburn (1980) was the first to show that regional anaesthesia (spinal) was associated with a reduced incidence of DVT as detected by venography. In a study of patients having hip replacement the incidence of DVT after general anaesthesia was 53 per cent, but only 29 per cent after spinal anaesthesia. Modig (1983) then demonstrated a similar finding with epidural block in hip replacement; 77 per cent of patients had DVT after general compared to 40 per cent after epidural anaesthesia.

The same pattern has been demonstrated in patients after repair of fractured neck of femur. When detected by venography the incidence of DVT was 76 per cent after general anaesthesia and 40 per cent after spinal anaesthesia (McKenzie *et al.*, 1985).

It is probable that general anaesthesia itself contributes to the development of DVT, while spinal and epidural blocks are protective, but only if they affect the lower limbs. Thoracic epidural blocks for abdominal surgery have no demonstrable effect (Hendolin *et al.*, 1982; Mellbring *et al.*, 1983). General anaesthesia causes a considerable reduction in lower limb venous return on induction (Clark and Cotton, 1968): an effect which occurs even when controlled ventilation is not used. Blood viscosity changes may also be involved and this is discussed later.

Postoperative changes in coagulation including increases in clotting factors, increased blood viscosity, increase in platelet numbers and stickiness, fibrinolytic 'shut-down' and depressed levels of the heparin co-factor, antithrombin III, all further contribute to the development or further propagation of clot. With most surgical procedures clots are thought to start 'on the table' but some patients with hip fracture may already have DVT by the time they reach surgery.

Spinal and epidural anaesthesia may increase blood flow to the lower limbs. Arterial inflow and venous outflow velocities are increased after epidural block (Modig *et al.*, 1983) and it is likely that this also occurs with spinal anaesthesia. In a study of a subgroup of patients from the present author's series on DVT, blood viscosity changes were examined along with its main determinants: haematocrit, fibrinogen levels and red cell deformability (Drummond *et al.*, 1980). Measured blood viscosity was found to fall very significantly after spinal anaesthesia and to remain unchanged after general anaesthesia. This effect was thought to be mainly a result of haemodilution consequent upon vasodilatation and the increased fluid requirements necessitated by this in the spinal anaesthesia group. However, when the effects of haematocrit change were eliminated by the use of a Nomogram to correct results to a standard haematocrit of 0.45, there still existed a significant difference in viscosity, both during and after surgery between the 2 groups. No changes were evident in fibrinogen levels but there was an increase in red cell deformability in the spinal anaesthetic group and a decrease in deformability in the general anaesthesia group. *In vitro* testing with halothane (used in the clinical study) revealed a dose dependant stiffening of red cells. The mechanisms are unknown. Changes in blood viscosity in fractured neck of femur are known to affect the incidence of DVT when viscosity is lowered by a defibrinating agent, arvin, derived from snake venom (Lowe *et al.*, 1978).

The importance of the viscosity changes is difficult to estimate as their effects are not only on DVT but also on micro-circulatory perfusion of vital organs.

Other possible mechanisms for the effects of anaesthesia on DVT have been suggested. Modig *et al.* (1983) has shown that after epidural block there was less suppression of fibrinolysis, release of plasminogen activator and decreased clotting factor activation. Lignocaine itself as an infusion has been shown to reduce DVT after hip replacement (Cooke *et al.*, 1977).

Postoperative oxygenation

After operation, patients who have had spinal anaesthesia show no change in blood gases (McKenzie *et al.*, 1980). However, in the first hour after general anaesthesia there is evidence of a dramatic and sometimes alarming fall in pO_2 if patients are allowed to breathe room air (Fig. 12.3). The minimum mean pO_2 is reached between about 5 and 7 minutes after discontinuation of anaesthetic gases. Some patients in the study (McKenzie, 1984) achieved extremely low pO_2 levels and the study was discontinued after 10 patients and all subsequent patients in that hospital having hip fracture surgery received supplemental oxygen! It is therefore vitally important to ensure that added oxygen is given, particularly including the time of transfer from the operating theatre to the recovery area, which is probably the time when patients would otherwise be most at risk of unrecognized hypoxaemia. The study showed no patient to have hypercarbia; none of the patients had obstruction or apnoea and none were thought to be cyanosed at any time in good daylight.

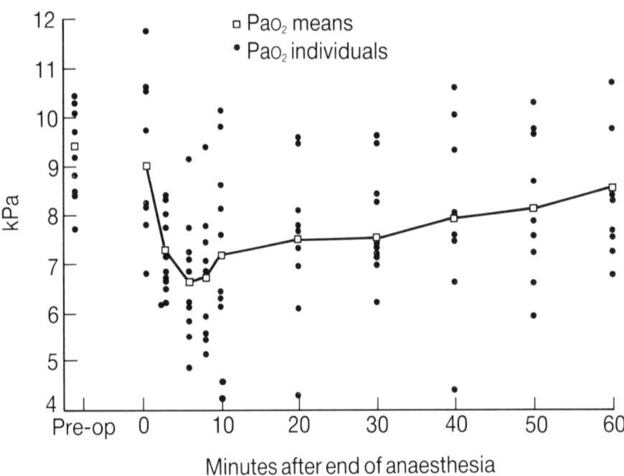

Fig 12.3

Confusional states

Following on from the above paragraph, hypoxaemia in the early postoperative period has been shown to be associated with confusional states after hip fracture surgery (Berggren *et al.*, 1987). The aetiology of confusional states is multi-factorial but there has been a clinical impression that elderly patients are less confused after spinal anaesthesia than after general anaesthesia. However, controlled studies have refuted this (Riis *et al.*, 1983; Bigler *et al.*, 1985; Berggren *et al.*, 1987). Berggren found anticholinergics and a history of depression to be the main risk factors and confused patients had more complications and their length of hospital stay was increased by nearly 4 times.

Perhaps the routine administration of oxygen has removed a real increase in confusional states associated with general anaesthesia which may have existed in the past.

Choice of technique

In experienced hands and with meticulous technique there should be no difference in outcome associated with spinal or general anaesthesia for the average patient. Spinal anaesthesia can be uniquely useful for some patients and even life saving by avoidance of general anaesthesia, for example, in the patient with severe respiratory disease. However there are disadvantages including technical difficulty in the elderly; the use of a 22 g needle is helpful and spinal headache is very rare in this type of patient. Spinal anaesthesia takes time and has a limited duration, may fail partially or completely, may be stressful and painful for the patient, and can cause profound falls in arterial pressure if the patient is more 'dry' than one suspects. There are also the usual contra-indications of sepsis and coagulation problems.

General anaesthesia has its large quota of potential problems which are inappropriate to discuss here but is (usually!) controllable, reliable, quick and of almost unlimited duration. It is for the above reasons that the present author favours general anaesthesia as his preferred method for the majority of patients with hip fracture. However, it is most important that trainees in anaesthesia should learn the skills of spinal anaesthesia in this type of patient for the situations where it is uniquely useful.

Repair of bracheal plexus injury

This procedure may take place relatively soon after the injury or many weeks later. It may take many hours and the duration may be unpredictable. Surgeons may wish to use a nerve stimulator. A technique where intubation and controlled ventilation are initially established with a medium acting non-depolarizing muscle relaxant and continued using opioids, volatile agent and mild hyperventilation is satisfactory (avoiding suxamethonium; vide infra). Care must be taken to humidify inspired gases, warm intravenous fluids and to monitor and maintain body temperature, which may necessitate active and passive warming blankets.

The use of suxamethonium after nerve or tissue trauma can lead to potentially lethal rises in serum potassium. This response can occur as little as 5 days after injury and persist for up to 6 months. It can be seen after apparently minor upper motor neurone lesions and also after immobilization, for instance in patients in the intensive care unit.

References

Barnes, C. L., Blasier, R. D. and Dodge, B. M. (1991). Intravenous regional anesthesia: a safe and cost-effective outpatient anesthetic for upper extremity fracture treatment in children. *Journal of Pediatric Orthopedics*, **11**, 717–20.

Berggren, D., Gustafson, Y., Eriksson, B., Bucht, G., Hansson, L. I., Reiz, S. and Winblad, B. (1987). Post-operative confusion after anaesthesia in elderly patients with femoral neck fractures. *Anesthesia and Analgesia*, **66**, 497–504.

Bigler, D., Adelhoj, B., Petring, O. U. and Pederson, N. O. (1985). Mental function and morbidity after acute hip surgery during spinal and general anaesthesia. *Anaesthesia*, **40**, 672–6.

Bulstrode, C. J. K., Ecker, J. and Laws, G. (1989). In S. Westaby (ed.), *Trauma. Pathogenesis and Treatment*. Heinemann, Oxford.

Boyce, W. J. and Vessey, M. P. (1985). Rising incidence of fracture of the proximal femur. *Lancet*, **i**, 150–1.

Cardus, D. (1967). O_2 alveolar-arterial tension difference after 10 days recumbency in man. *Journal of Appled Physiology*, **23**, 934–7.

Clark, C. and Cotton, L. T. (1968). Blood-flow in deep veins of leg. Recording technique and evaluation of methods to increase flow during operation. *British Journal of Surgery*, **55**, 211–14.

Coleman, S. A., Boyce, W. J., Cosh, P. H. and McKenzie, P. J. (1988). Outcome after general anaesthesia for repair of fractured neck of femur: a randomised trial of spontaneous versus controlled ventilation. *British Journal of Anaesthesia*, **60**, 43–7.

Cooke, E. D., Lloyd, M. J., Bowcock, S. A. and Pilcher, M. F. (1977). Intravenous lignocaine in prevention of deep venous thrombosis after elective hip surgery. *Lancet*, **ii**, 797–9.

David, H. G. (1991). Pulse oximetry in closed limb fractures. *Annals of the Royal College of Surgeons of England*, **73**, 283–4.

Davis, A. G. and Spence, A. A. (1972). Postoperative hypoxemia and age. *Anesthesiology*, **37**, 663–4.

Davis, F. M., Woolner, D. F., Frampton, C., Wilkinson, A., Grant, A., Harrison, R. T., Roberts, M. T. S. and Thadaka, R. (1987). Prospective, multi-centre trial of mortality following general or spinal anaesthesia for hip fracture in the elderly. *British Journal of Anaesthesia*, **59**, 1080–8.

Drummond, A. R., Drummond, M. M., McKenzie, P. J., Lowe, G. D. O., Smith, G., Forbes, C. D. and Wishart, H. Y. (1980). The effects of general and spinal anaesthesia on red cell deformability and blood viscosity in patients undergoing surgery for fractured neck of femur. In J. F. Stolz and P. Drouin (eds), *Haemorheology and Diseases*. Doin Editeurs, Paris, pp. 445–51.

Hendolin, H., Tuppurainen, T. and Lahtinen, J. (1982). Thoracic epidural analgesia and deep venous thrombosis in cholecystectomised patients. *Acta Chirurgica Scandinavica*, **148**, 405–9.

Keith, S. (1973). The hospital in-patient enquiry. 1970. *Health Trends*, **5**, 13–14.

Knowelden, J., Buhr, A. J. and Dunbar, O. (1964). Incidence of fractures in persons over 35 years of age. A report to the M.R.C. working party on fractures in the elderly. *British Journal of Preventive and Social Medicine*, **18**, 130–41.

Lowe, G. D. O., Meek, D. R., Campbell, A. F., Forbes, C. D. and Prentice, C. R. M. (1978). Subcutaneous ancrod in prevention of deep-vein thrombosis after operation for fractured neck of femur. *Lancet*, **ii**, 698–700.

McKenzie, P. J. (1984). Anaesthesia for repair of fractured neck of femur. A comparison of spinal and general anaesthesia. MD Thesis, University of Glasgow.

McKenzie, P. J., Wishart, H. Y., Dewar, K. M. S., Gray, I. and Smith, G. (1980). Comparison of the effects of spinal anaesthesia and general anaesthesia on post-operative oxygenation and perioperative mortality. *British Journal of Anaesthesia*, **52**, 49–54.

McKenzie, P. J., Wishart, H. Y., Gray, I. and Smith, G. (1985). Effects of anaesthetic technique on deep vein thrombosis. A comparison of subarachnoid and general anaesthesia. *British Journal of Anaesthesia*, **57**, 853–7.

McKenzie, P. J., Wishart, H. Y. and Smith, G. (1984). Long-term outcome after repair of fractured neck of femur. Comparison of subarachnoid and general anaesthesia. *British Journal of Anaesthesia*, **56**, 581–5.

McLaren, A. D., Stockwell, M. C. and Reid, V. T. (1978). Anaesthetic techniques for surgical correction of fractured neck of femur. *Anaesthesia*, **33**, 10–14.

Mellbring, G., Dahlgren, S., Reiz, S. and Sunnegardh, O. (1983). Thromboembolic complications after major abdominal surgery: effect of thoracic epidural analgesia. *Acta Chirurgica Scandinavica*, **149**, 263–8.

Michel, R. (1980). Air embolism in hip surgery. *Anaesthesia*, **35**, 858–62.

Modig, J. (1977). Posttraumatic pulmonary microembolism. *Annals of Clinical Research*, **9**, 164–72.

Modig, J., Borg, T., Karlstrom, G., Maripuu, E. and Sahlstedt, B. (1983). Thromboembolism after total hip replacement: role of epidural and general anesthesia. *Anesthesia and Analgesia*, **62**, 174–80.

Modig, J., Busch, C., Olerud, S., Saldeen, T. and Waernbaum, G. (1975). Arterial hypotension and hypoxaemia during total hip replacement: the importance of thromboplastic products, fat embolism and acrylic monomers. *Acta Anaesthesiologica Scandinavica*, **19**, 28–43.

Olney, B. W., Lugg, P. C., Turner, P. L., Eyres, R. L. and Cole, W. G. (1988). Outpatient treatment of upper extremity injuries in childhood using intravenous regional analgesia. *Journal of Pediatric Orthopedics*, **8**, 576–9.

Riis, J., Lomholt, B., Haxholdt, O., Kehlet, H., Valentin, N., Danielsen, U. and Dyrberg, V. (1983). Immediate and long-term mental recovery from general versus epidural anaesthesia in elderly patients. *Acta Anaesthesiologica Scandinavica*, **27**, 44–9.

Saldeen, T. (1970). Fat embolism and signs of intravascular coagulation in a posttraumatic autopsy material. *Journal of Trauma*, **10**, 273–86.

Spreadbury, T. H. (1980). Anaesthetic techniques for surgical correction of fractured neck of femur. A comparative study of ketamine and relaxant anaesthesia in elderly women. *Anaesthesia*, **35**, 208–14.

Tachakra, S. S. and Sevitt, S. (1975). Hypoxaemia after fractures. *Journal of Bone and Joint Surgery*, **57**, 197–203.

Thorburn, J., Louden, J. R. and Vallence, R. (1980). Spinal and general anaesthesia in total hip replacement: frequency of deep vein thrombosis. *British Journal of Anaesthesia*, **52**, 1117–21.

Valentin, N., Lomholt, B., Jensen, J. S., Hejgard, N. and Kreiner, S. (1986). Spinal or general anaesthesia for surgery of the fractured hip? *British Journal of Anaesthesia*, **58**, 284–91.

Wallace, W. A. (1983). The increasing incidence of fractures of the proximal femur: an orthopaedic epidemic. *Lancet*, **i**, 1413–14.

Ward, R. J., Tolas, A. G., Benveniste, R. J., Hansen, J. M. and Bonica, J. J. (1966). Effect of posture on normal arterial blood gas tensions in the aged. *Geriatrics*, **21**, 139–43.

Wattenmaker, I., Kasser, J. R. and McGravey, A. (1990). Self-administered nitrous oxide for fracture reduction in children in an emergency room situation. *Journal of Orthopedics and Trauma*, **4**, 35–8.

Wishart, H. Y., Williams, T. I. R. and Smith, G. (1977). A comparison of the effect of three anaesthetic techniques on postoperative arterial oxygenation in the elderly. *British Journal of Anaesthesia*, **49**, 1259–63.

Index